Previews

Our world today is filled with illness: mental, emotional, physical, environmental, and political. Sometimes things can seem hopeless, and we ourselves helpless to bring about any positive change. Yet there are subtle laws of healing, success, and harmony that have been discovered and used for millennia by people of higher awareness. In her trilogy, *Healing with Life Force*, Nayaswami Shivani explores the uses of subtle energy to heal us as individuals and rebuild the world as a whole.

In this third and last volume of the series, she explores how to build harmonious relationships, how to achieve prosperity and success, how to use vibratory healing, and the art of transitioning from the body at the time of death. Knowing how to work effectively in these areas brings not only health and happiness, but peace and fulfillment into our lives.

What makes these books exceptional are the countless personal accounts of how people have successfully used these techniques and attitudes. *Healing with Life Force* is a gift to the world at a time when the teachings it shares are desperately needed. We are most grateful to Shivani for this great offering which can bring healing to all those who read and practice its teachings.

–*Nayaswami Devi*, author, recipient of the United Nations Global Ambassador Peace Award; co-spiritual director of Ananda Worldwide

Brace yourself as you delve into this literary masterpiece, for its words possess an undeniable ability to unearth the hidden depths of your soul and reveal secrets of self-healing from one of the great masters of our times, Paramhansa Yogananda. The author seamlessly weaves together intricate threads of wisdom in such a way as to reshape the perception of our relationship to ourselves, to others, and to the divine healing power that lies within. –*Dr Ruchi Matta*, *physical therapist, acupuncturist*

Covering the vast spectrum of health from the moment of our conception, through the journey of life, to the soul's passing through the portals of death, *Healing with Life Force* is a clear, in-depth, and engaging practical guide to health and self-healing. Shivani has beautifully explored and elaborated on the teachings of Paramhansa Yogananda. Embellished with real-life stories that aptly illustrate the principles, and examples on how to apply the teachings and techniques, Shivani draws from over fifty years of experience of sharing these teachings around the world. The result is deeply moving and inspiring.

–*Dr Aditya Gait,* MBBS DNB (I)

With more than five decades of spiritual knowledge and experience, the renowned author of the *Healing with Life Force* trilogy shares pearls of wisdom in a lucid, uplifting, easy-to-understand manner, welcoming to any individual exploring the journey of self-healing and soul freedom! In these pages you find step-by-step guidelines for achieving more dynamism in your physical, mental and spiritual health, in your relationships, and in your creative and economic endeavors—health at 360 degrees!

–*Dr Noopur Gupta,* MS, MNAMS, PhD, *additional professor of ophthalmology, AIIMS, Delhi*

What you are holding is not just a book: it is a treasure chest of wisdom that will make you healthier, happier, more confident in yourself, and enthusiastic about your life. Like everything that Shivani creates, this compendium of Yogananda's teachings broadens our perspective so that we see ourselves as creators of our destiny. The personal stories of people's struggles and victories included throughout the books hearten us to make every circumstance in our life a springboard for greater success.

–*Andrey Skakodub,* *business operation advisor, Baku, Azerbaijan*

In both its concept and scope, *Healing with Life Force* is a veritable *magnum opus*. It should and will become a valuable reference book for those interested in spiritual well-being and self-healing and, more generally, in the teachings of Paramhansa Yogananda. Those who already follow his teachings, and those who will come to follow them as a result of reading this book, owe an immense debt of gratitude to the author.

–*Sanjaya David Connolly,* *author, retired professor of translation studies, University of Salonica, Greece*

HEALING WITH LIFE FORCE

HEALING WITH LIFE FORCE

TEACHINGS AND TECHNIQUES
OF PARAMHANSA YOGANANDA

VOLUME 3 MAGNETISM

SHIVANI LUCKI

Healing with Life Force

Volume Three: Magnetism

©2024 by Shivani Lucki
All rights reserved. Published 2024
Printed in the United States of America

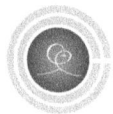

CRYSTAL CLARITY PUBLISHERS
1123 Goodrich Blvd. | Commerce, California
crystalclarity.com | clarity@crystalclarity.com
800.424.1055

ISBN 978-1-56589-049-7 (print)
ISBN 978-1-56589-532-4 (e-book)
Library of Congress Data available.

Cover layout and interior design by
Tejindra Scott Tully

Cover image by Apace on Freepik

Please be advised: The content in this book is not intended to be a substitute for professional medical advice, diagnosis or treatment. Always consult with a qualified and licensed physician or other medical care provider, and follow their advice without delay.

The Magnetism of
DIVINE LOVE

*Magnetism of every kind is born of
the magnetic power of God's love…*

*Divine love, though perhaps the least-known
force in the universe, and the one most apt to be
scoffed at by men as "impractical, unrelated
to mundane affairs, ineffective," is in fact the
most powerful—indeed, in the last analysis
the only—force in the universe.*

*By the magnetic power of divine love,
all things can be accomplished—
even that most seemingly impossible of
all tasks, our salvation from delusion.*

*What man by his own power alone
cannot accomplish, divine love accomplishes easily.
And its task, once accomplished, is accomplished
forever. The most important thing, therefore, is
for us by meditation to attune ourselves to that
subtlest ray.…God's love flows to you always.*

*It is you, by your love, who must complete
the circuit, thereby generating the magnetism
that can draw to yourself the very
consciousness of Infinity.*[26]

Swami Kriyananda, *The Art and Science of Raja Yoga*, 298

TABLE OF CONTENTS

VOLUME III | MAGNETISM

THE MAGNETISM OF DIVINE LOVE | 3
FOREWORD | 7
INTRODUCTION | 9

PART X: HEALTHY RELATIONSHIPS | 17

CHAPTER ONE: The Relationships Challenge | 19
CHAPTER TWO: Friendship | 23
CHAPTER THREE: Healthy and Unhealthy Relationships | 35
CHAPTER FOUR: Soulmates | 47
CHAPTER FIVE: Advice for Committed Couples | 63
CHAPTER SIX: How Healthy Are Your Relationships? | 67
CHAPTER SEVEN: Dissolution: Separation and Divorce | 69
CHAPTER EIGHT: Loss and Love Eternal | 79

PART XI: PROSPERITY AND SUCCESS | 89

CHAPTER ONE: Why Seek Prosperity? | 91
CHAPTER TWO: Poverty or Prosperity? | 97
CHAPTER THREE: The Law of Magnetism | 105
CHAPTER FOUR: Money Magnetism | 121
CHAPTER FIVE: Tithing Magic | 145
CHAPTER SIX: Secrets of Success | 155

PART XII: VIBRATORY HEALING | 173

CHAPTER ONE: The Vibratory Structure of the Universe | 175
CHAPTER TWO: The Three *Gunas* | 181
CHAPTER THREE: Mantra | 205

CHAPTER FOUR: The Sound of Music | 223
CHAPTER FIVE: Songs of the Soul | 241
CHAPTER SIX: Nature Therapy | 267
CHAPTER SEVEN: Colors Communicate | 275
CHAPTER EIGHT: Healing Habitats | 283
CHAPTER NINE: Pilgrimage: Sacred Shrines and Saintly Souls | 291
CHAPTER TEN: The Power of Ceremonies and Rituals | 307
CHAPTER ELEVEN: Protection | 323
CHAPTER TWELVE: Points to Remember about Vibratory Healing | 343

EPILOGUE:
TRANSITION AND TRANSCENDENCE | 355

CHAPTER ONE: Overcoming the Fear of Death | 357
CHAPTER TWO: Give Up or Fight? | 363
CHAPTER THREE: Letting Go | 369
CHAPTER FOUR: Helping a Dying Friend | 379

GLOSSARY | 392
BIBLIOGRAPHY | 395
PHOTOS & ILLUSTRATIONS | 399
ABOUT THE AUTHORS | 400-402
IN APPRECIATION | 403

FOREWORD

LATHA EMMATTY GUPTA

Years ago, when I first attended Shivani's seminars on meditation, prosperity, and healing, I found her to be an exceptional teacher and guide. Since then, she has influenced me deeply through her wisdom, and the immense body of practical knowledge and spiritual inspiration which she has assembled here in *Healing with Life Force*. Insights contained in these three volumes have given me invaluable guidance and practical solutions for my life and career.

How we approach success and fulfilment in our work life and career must be counted as a major contributor to our health profile. Having served for three decades in leadership and executive positions with multinational corporations, and now as an independent coach for global technology and consulting firms, I resonate deeply with the importance Shivani gives to the Laws of Magnetism. Readers will doubtless be aware of the increasing challenges and stresses of the modern workplace. These teachings empower us to attract inspiration, opportunities, and collaborators that can make the real difference between success and failure for ourselves and for our businesses.

Shivani skilfully blends Western scientific methods with Eastern wisdom to help us heal ourselves on all levels of our lives. Her many decades of devoted study and practice of the teachings of her guru, Paramhansa Yogananda, add deep authenticity and authority to these volumes. She has a wonderful way of blending scientific practicality with intuitive wisdom to reveal how we can transform ourselves and become dynamic co-creators of our destiny, instead of helpless victims of our circumstances.

In this increasingly busy, scary, pushy and insecure world – as robots and AI threaten to deprive us of our livelihood – mental health concerns are spiralling, and depression and anxiety are precipitously increasing. There is an urgent need for the practical wisdom of these volumes. Like a sturdy raft, this work can rescue us from confusion and suffering and carry us safely over the stormy seas of our modern lives.

Latha Gupta, MBA, is an executive and life coach, PCC International Coaching Federation, USA, and Director of the Ananda Yoga School of India

INTRODUCTION

The book you have in hand is the third volume in the *Life Force* trilogy—*Prana, Mind, Magnetism*—three guidebooks for your journey to better health. Together they represent an overarching view of Paramhansa Yogananda's teachings and techniques for self-healing and Self-realization.

Volume One, *Prana*, takes us back to the very beginning, when Life Force becomes the power that fashions creation. Yogananda shows us how to harness that power and use it to infuse our bodies with vitality. That force also gives rise to the eternal struggle between the soul and the ego, the root cause of all disease. Through the pages and practices of this book, you will learn how to reconcile these two protagonists through techniques of meditation; how to regenerate the cells and organs of your body with Yogananda's Energization Exercises; and how to nourish yourself and keep your body free from impurities with his dietary and detox recipes. A fascinating section in this volume presents Yogananda's techniques for utilizing the sun's power for self-healing.

Volume Two, *Mind*, highlights the superpowers of the conscious, subconscious, and superconscious dimensions of the mind. It offers extensive advice for breaking the stranglehold of negative habits, for using affirmations to carve new thought habits in the brain, and for learning to cooperate with the highest source of healing—Divine Love.

Volume Three, *Magnetism*, reveals how the Law of Attraction affects our lives and influences our health: how it draws us into contact with friends from past lives; and how we can use it to attract the economic and human resources for a successful career.

The final Part of the trilogy demonstrates how we can attune ourselves to the subtle, vibratory healing frequencies of mantra and music; of nature, holy places, and inspiring people. Important techniques are given to reinforce the magnetic aura which protects us from negative influences that threaten our physical, mental, emotional, and spiritual health and well-being.

We are not alone in this quest. Some of those who have come before us, in ages past and in our times, those who have reached the summit of what it means to be a fully Self-realized being, have left for us guidelines for our own achievements.

One such recent guide is Paramhansa Yogananda.

Paramhansa Yogananda

Author of the enduring spiritual classic, *Autobiography of a Yogi*,[1] Yogananda is universally regarded as an enlightened spiritual master of modern times. He had the remarkable gift of distilling the essential wisdom of India's great scriptures and presenting them in what he called "how-to-live teachings," useful and accessible to us today.

Yogananda was born in India in 1893, near the beginning of Dwapara Yuga, the Age of Energy. The start of this era made possible the discoveries of Albert Einstein and Nikola Tesla about the nature of energy, and the numerous inventions that have freed humanity from the confines of matter.

In the first decade of the twentieth century alone, the landmark inventions included radio, radar, and the electrocardiogram, to name a few. Energy now powers all our systems of transportation, communication, and the countless gadgets that simplify and enhance our daily lives.

When Yogananda arrived on the shores of the New World in 1920, around the time the Wright brothers had taken flight and Henry Ford had produced the Model T, the timing was right and people were eager to learn techniques of self-improvement that were based on principles of energy.

Although Yogananda is not remembered primarily as a miracle healer, in his early lecture tours across America he gave many public demonstrations of the power of self-healing. On October 21, 1924, he held a first "public divine healing meeting" in Portland, Oregon. During a healing program at his headquarters at Mt. Washington in Los Angeles on November 1, 1925, he healed a woman of crippling neuritis, after which she was able to walk without crutches.

In Washington, D.C. in 1927, a reported 5,000 people attended his healing program. It was at this time that he was invited to the White House where he met with President Calvin Coolidge.

Titles of his public talks reflect the scientific spirit of the new age:

"Practicing Religion Scientifically"
«Scientific Spiritual Healing»
"Law of Attracting Abundance and Health Consciously"
"The Mind: Repository of Infinite Power"
"Physical, Mental, and Spiritual Methods of Healing"

When divinely guided, Yogananda would occasionally perform a healing, but his intention as a spiritual guide was to teach others the methods by which they could draw upon the inexhaustible Life Force to heal themselves. The gift that Yogananda gives us in these pages is the key to unlock the mysteries of life.

In addition to the five million copies of his *Autobiography* in circulation, his other books are widely read. Included in these volumes are important writings about health and healing which are not easily available. Of special note are his early correspondence lessons, written by his own hand between 1923 and 1935; the articles he wrote for his organization's magazines (*East-West* and *Inner Culture*), including his "Health, Intellectual and Spiritual Recipes," and his parallel commentaries on the Bhagavad Gita and the Christian Bible.

I draw on these sources abundantly in these books. It is Yogananda's wisdom, in his voice and his words that I strived to convey as compiler, organizer, and annotator. All of his quotations are indicated in the text with a symbol of the spiritual eye.

Swami Kriyananda

J. Donald Walters, later to become Swami Kriyananda, was accepted by Yogananda as a monastic disciple in 1948. On the master's request, Kriyananda carefully studied his writings, especially his commentaries on the Bhagavad Gita and the Christian Bible. He took copious notes of the master's public talks and their private 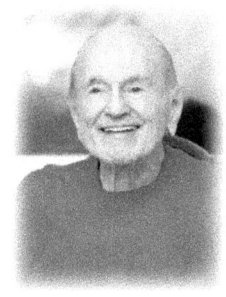 conversations, which he later incorporated in his books *The New Path* and *Conversations with Yogananda*. Yogananda designated him as head of the monks, authorized him as a minister and teacher, and gave him the authority to initiate people into the science of Kriya Yoga. His life work, Yogananda told him, would involve teaching and writing.

During his sixty-five years as a disciple (1948-2013), Kriyananda gave lectures around the world, including daily talks on major Indian television channels. He published approximately 140 books in which he showed how his guru's teachings can be applied to improve and elevate our daily life activities—in business and leadership, relationships, education, music and the arts, and for achieving dynamic health and well-being.[2] Excerpts from these and unpublished articles and letters are included in the text, the Endnotes, and the Appendices.

I was trained by Kriyananda from 1969 until his passing, and have been practicing and sharing these teachings for the past fifty years. In addition to those of Yogananda, I have drawn profusely from Kriyananda's writings. Each of his quotations in the text is indicated with this Joy Symbol.

Interactive

Throughout the three volumes you will find exercises to help you practice what you are learning. Your own experience of the techniques will give you an immediate awareness of their benefits.

Each exercise is aligned with a self-improvement goal, such as identifying our positive and negative, helpful and harmful habits. Doing the exercises at the points indicated will help you bring their benefits into your daily life.

Most of the exercises can be done, at your choosing, as you move through the book. Some of them are writing exercises that you will find in the online Appendices to download and complete electronically, or print and complete on paper.

Appendixes: A treasure trove of more inspiration!

Available exclusively for readers of this volume is access to an online site: www.healinglifeforces.com/volume-3/ (or scan this QR code below) where you will find:

- Paramhansa Yogananda's original lessons from the 1920s and 1930s

- Articles by Yogananda and Kriyananda on material and spiritual success, death, rebirth, and life after death

- Guidelines for helping those who are gravely ill, and preparing for our own transition
- Twenty musical compositions by Swami Kriyananda. An mp3 downloadable playlist with twenty musical compositions by Swami Kriyananda to be used for vibratory healing
- And much more!

> **You're also invited to join the Online Healing Community** for regular healing tips, interactive sessions, and seminars with the author. Come visit us at *www.healinglifeforces.com*.

Stories

Especially engaging, inspiring, and instructive are the stories that I have included throughout the books from people who have used these techniques for their own healing. Most of the stories are of real-life experiences, although some are allegorical or drawn from mythology.

Terminology

Because this is a handbook of spiritually based practices for improving health and finding healing, the central importance of **"Spirit"** cannot be overstated. Regardless of how we personally conceptualize and relate to the Supreme Reality, it must occupy a central position if we hope to understand and make effective use of these principles and practices.

Can an atheist find value in these teachings? Yes, because they are thoroughly grounded in the way human beings are made. Even if we reject the concept of "God," we may recognize the presence of a higher source of wisdom and inspiration. Many scientists, including physicist and cosmologist Stephen Hawking, and science-fiction writers like Isaac Asimov, have denied the existence of God while endorsing and popularizing cosmological principles that touch on the spiritual.

Yogananda urged us to be "spiritual scientists." He said that wheras the scientist approaches the Infinite from the outside, the spiritual scientist approaches it from the inside.[3]

Psychologist and researcher David DeSteno writes about "the science behind the benefits of religion."

> "I've come to see a nuanced relationship between science and religion. I now view them as two approaches to improving people's lives that frequently complement each other…If we ignore that body of knowledge, if we refuse to take these spiritual technologies seriously as a source of ideas and inspiration to study, we slow the progress of science itself and limit its potential to benefit humanity." [4]

Whether we think of ourselves as scientists, technologists, or believers, we can all experience the practical results of these scientific healing practices.

Energy

Yogananda uses a variety of phrases to refer to energy in its varied forms. His term "Cosmic Energy" refers to the universal energy by which all creation is manifested, and that is the source of all life. He describes this source also as the "Cosmic Electric Force," and the "Cosmic Intelligent Energy." [5]

As cosmic energy descends through the three universes and the three bodies that the soul inhabits (see Part I), it becomes what Yogananda termed "Life Force" or "Life Energy." When it enters the physical body, it becomes the "Lifetronic Force," synonymous with the Sanskrit term *prana*.

When quoting Yogananda directly, I have always used his exact words. In my commentaries and explanations, I generally refer to the healing force in the body as Life Force; interchangeably as *prana*.

Energization Exercises

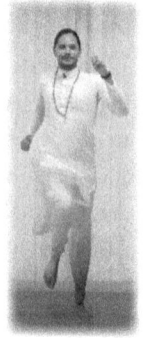

The primary Life Force healing technique described in these books is a practice that Yogananda developed in the 1920s that he originally called Yogoda Exercises. He later referred to them as Energization Exercises. Citations from Yogananda in the 1920s and 1930s use the term Yogoda, but I refer to them as Life Force Energization Exercises, and often simply as "energization exercises." Instruction in the practice of these exercises, in easy-to-follow videos, is included in the Appendices.

Sanskrit words appear sparingly throughout the text, usually when they capture a concept that is difficult to render in other languages. A glossary of Sanskrit terms is included at the back of each volume.

LEGEND OF CITATIONS

Each citation is referenced in the Endnotes. These are the symbols used within the text.

PARAMHANSA
YOGANANDA

HOLY BIBLE
(*King James*)

SWAMI
KRIYANANDA

SWAMI SRI
YUKTESWAR

BHAGAVAD
GITA

MAHAVATAR
BABAJI

Now it's time to start your journey of self-healing. May you make steady progress as you strive to become what Yogananda describes as
"the master of your destiny."

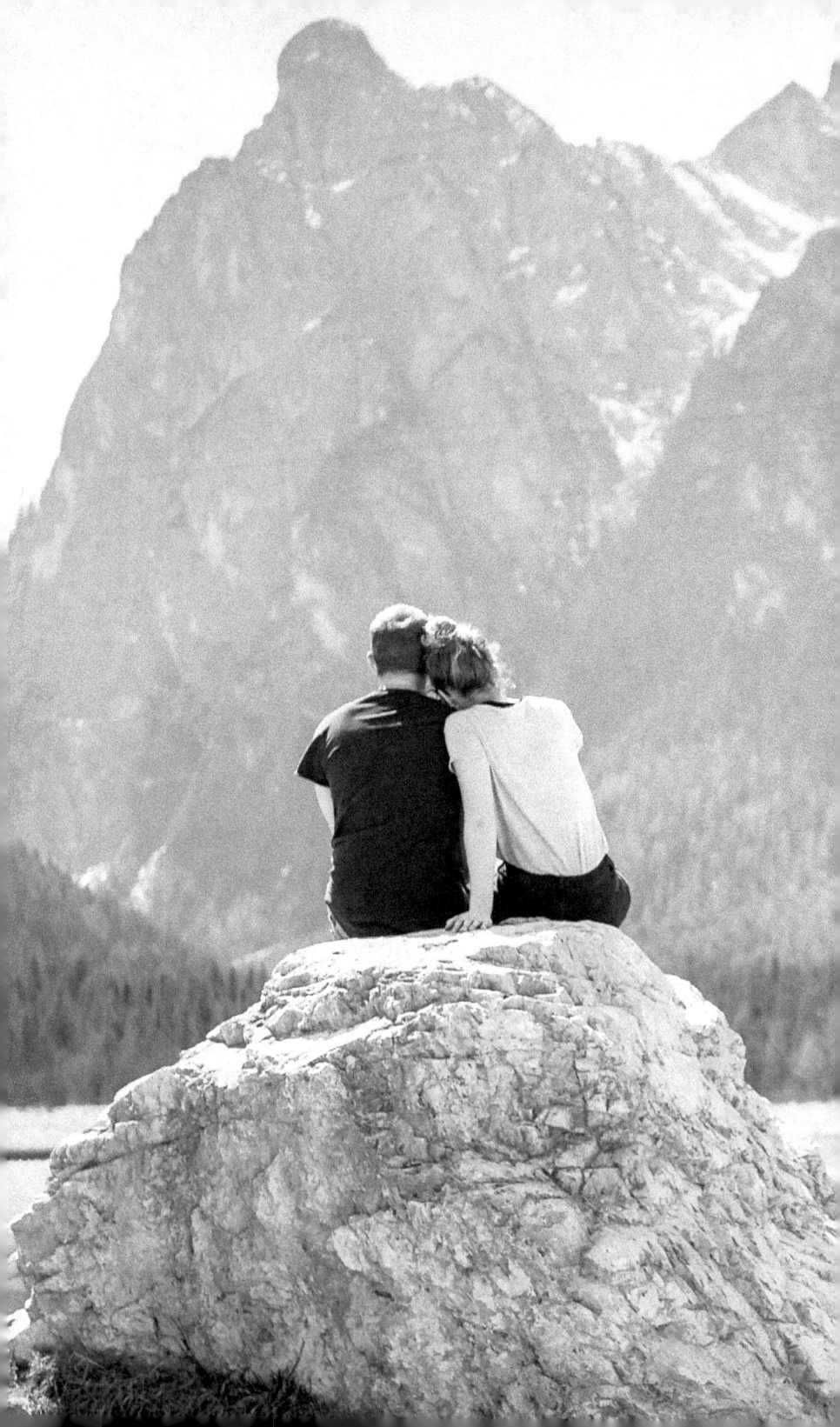

PART X
HEALTHY RELATIONSHIPS

Countless are the forms in which God comes to man. In each, He seeks to teach man something of His infinite nature. Through your parents He cares for you, supports you, and protects you. Through your friends He shows you that love is a free sharing, without any hint of compulsion. Through the beloved He helps one to find the selfless intensity of divine love. Through people's children He helps them to understand love as something precious, as a thing to be protected from harmful influences and nourished with devotion.... The lessons are there, for anyone whose heart is open to receive them.[1]

—YOGANANDA

✵ The Rabbi's Advice ✵

The monastery was ancient, and the few remaining monks were well along in years. The monastery had seen better times when a host of young men waited eagerly to be admitted and the chapel resounded with angelic voices at Vespers.

Those times had since passed, and the handful of elderly monks were no longer robust in their devotions. The abbot had struggled to attract novices, but to no avail. He fretted that the monastery would not survive after its residents had passed on.

The abbot was good friends with a rabbi who lived nearby, and who, rumor had it, talked with God daily. At their next visit, the abbot told the rabbi about his concerns and pleaded, "The next time you talk with God, please ask Him what can be done to save the monastery?"

The rabbi agreed, and at their next meeting he greeted the abbot with surprising news. "God has told me that Jesus Christ is living among you."

The abbot was flabbergasted. "If it's true," he stammered, "who could it be?"

"That is for you to discover," the rabbi said.

As he walked back to the monastery, the abbot thought of each of the monks. "It can't be Brother Joseph, the gardener. He is a simple soul, not good with his Latin, and irritatingly tone-deaf at Vespers."

"Could it be Brother Francis, the cook?" he pondered. "Doubtful," he decided. "Jesus would give us better fare."

That evening, he gathered the brothers and told them what the rabbi had said, whereupon they immediately began to treat each other with great respect and reverence. Brother Joseph the gardener expressed the common thought: "If my brother is Jesus, I want Him to know that I love Him."

As the brothers continued to look for Jesus in each other, the atmosphere in the monastery became vibrant with devotion, and it wasn't long until the cells were filled with dedicated young novices, their voices sweetly adding to the glorious harmony at Vespers.

✵ ✵ ✵

PART X   CHAPTER ONE

The Relationships Challenge

> You must love everyone. You love those who are dear to you so that you may give that love to the whole world. On the soil of your heart the seeds of love are grown, and you must cultivate those seeds with the water of universal love and universal sympathy. As soon as you love all people with the intensity of the love that you have for your family, then you express Divine love.[1] —YOGANANDA

From the moment we are born, we are surrounded by people – during our first years, primarily parents, siblings, and close relatives. But as we grow, we acquire friends, classmates, colleagues, and others with whom we share common interests.

The social exchange of ideas and energy is important for our health and happiness. Dr. Emma Seppala of the Yale School of Management, summarizes the results of studies on the links between health and social connectedness:

> Social connection improves physical health and mental and emotional well-being....One landmark study showed that lack of social connection is a greater detriment to health than obesity, smoking and high blood pressure. On the other hand, strong social connection:
> - leads to a 50% increased chance of longevity,
> - strengthens your immune system, and
> - helps you recover from disease faster.

People who feel more connected to others have lower levels of anxiety and depression. Moreover, studies show they also have higher self-esteem, greater empathy for others, are more trusting and cooperative and, as a consequence, others are more open to trusting and cooperating with them. In other words, social connectedness generates a positive feedback loop of social, emotional and physical well-being.[2]

Wide-ranging research suggests that strong social ties are linked to a longer life. In stark contrast, loneliness and social isolation are linked to poorer health, depression, and increased risk of early death. Researchers have found that having a variety of social relationships may help reduce stress and heart-related health risks. These connections may improve our ability to fight off infection and give us a more positive outlook on life.

Dr. Sheldon Cohen, a psychologist at Carnegie Mellon University, has explored the links between relationships and health for more than three decades. "It's generally healthy for people to try to belong to different groups, to volunteer in different ways, and be involved with a church or involved in their neighborhood," Cohen says. "Involvement with other people across diverse situations clearly can have a very potent, very positive effect on health."

In a study, Cohen's team exposed more than 200 healthy volunteers to the common cold virus and observed them for a week in a controlled setting. "We found that the more diverse people's social networks – the more types of connections they had – the less likely they were to develop a cold after exposure to the virus," Cohen said. His team has since found evidence that people with a greater diversity of connections also tend to have better health behaviors (such as not smoking or drinking) and more positive emotions.[3]

Social interaction, especially with people of varied ages, combined with physical movement such as dancing, is effective in warding off the onset of dementia.[4]

Our health is also strongly affected by the atmosphere in the home. Home life can nourish all family members, giving them strength to weather life's storms; but when the home becomes a battlefield, physical and mental health will suffer.

Workplace environments that are dominated by ambition and competition can be severely detrimental to health and unfavorable to creativity. Mutual respect, support, and collaboration create a workplace dynamic that encourages initiative and stimulates productivity.

In addition to improving our physical and mental health, meaningful contact with others contributes to our spiritual well-being. For it is God's love that calls to us through our human friendships.

> God ... Himself took the form of parents in order to protect the baby .... Not satisfied with only protecting man through the compelling instincts of parents, God also took the form of unlimited friends in order to extend unlimited love to [them]. Thus God's Love is playing hide-and-seek in human hearts.[5]

In our human relationships, we have an opportunity to discover God's unconditional love, and to develop our ability to love Him in others.

In his ground-breaking research into what he dubbed the "near-death experience," Dr. Raymond Moody interviewed 150 patients who were able to recall the events they experienced while in a state of clinical death. Although each person's experiences were unique, there were nine common themes. They included a "life review" during which the dying saw everything they had done, and every one of their interactions with others. The purpose of the review, they were led to understand intuitively, was to examine what they had learned in their most recent life, and to observe how much or how little they had loved.[6]

In Part X we consider how our interactions with other people can provide either a healing balm for our human distress, or contribute to mental and physical illness. When our relationships are loving and supportive, we are far better equipped to survive life's storms, but when our relationships are a battleground, there are bound to be casualties.

My current relationships

Before we continue, it may help to list the names of these five people:

1. **Someone with whom you have an intimate relationship**
2. **A family member**
3. **A friend**
4. **A colleague**
5. **Someone with whom you have a conflict**

Keep these people in mind as you read on. Recalling your personal experiences will help make the concepts clearer. In Chapter Five, we will consider an exercise that can help us improve these relationships.

PART X   CHAPTER TWO

Friendship

> Friendship is God's trumpet call, bidding the soul to destroy the partitions which separate it from all other souls and from Him .... Friendship is God's love shining through the eyes of your loved ones, calling you home to drink His nectar of all differences-and selfishness-dissolving unity .... When Divine Friendship reigns supreme in the temple of your heart, your Soul will merge with the vast Cosmic Soul, leaving far behind the confining bonds which separated it from all of God's animate and inanimate Creation. [1] –YOGANANDA
>
> Friendship is the purest of all love. In the love of parents for their children there is compulsion; in filial love there is compulsion; in the love of lovers there is compulsion; but in true friendship there is no compulsion. [2] –YOGANANDA

In this chapter we will discover God's healing love hidden in all of our relationships. We will explore ways to develop qualities of friendship that can make our home life and our work more nourishing, and we will look at the ego's evolutionary progress through many lives as it relates to our human relationships. It takes many lifetimes for the ego to evolve to a point where we can enjoy mature, loving friendships.

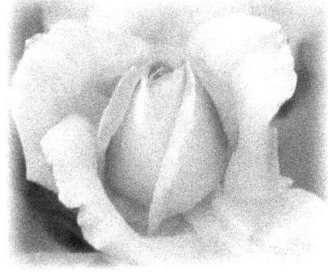

Karmic relationships

"You can't take it with you," as the old saying admonishes us. We cannot bring our material possessions and accomplishments with us as we transition from this life to the hereafter. Our human relationships, however, extend over many lives — we return to them again and again until we have perfected our love.

We have been many things to many people. In our circle of human relationships, we have been a parent, a child, a spouse, a grandparent, a business partner, and a competitor. We have loved faithfully, and we've strayed. We have trusted, and we have been betrayed. Strong feelings have bound our souls to certain others, and we've found ourselves connected in some fashion to those people again and again, in life after life.

> Make every effort to rediscover your friends of past incarnations, whom you may recognize through familiar physical, mental and spiritual qualities. Rising above considerations of material or even spiritual gain, perfect your friendship, begun in a preceding incarnation, into Divine Friendship.[3]

We have formed bonds of love with many souls, not all of whom we could possibly be destined to marry in this life. Love can grow between fast friends, business partners, and the members of close-knit groups who share a common interest, such as happens in service organizations, on sports teams, with training partners, and in spiritual groups.

The challenge in each lifetime is to understand the kinds of relationships that will offer us the best opportunities to expand our hearts from a narrow, exclusively personal kind of love, to serve as a channel for a divine universal love that embraces everyone in its healing rays.[4]

> There are (those) who give you the instantaneous feeling that you have known them always. This indicates that they are your friends of previous incarnations. Do not neglect them,

but strengthen the friendship existing between you. Be on the lookout for them always, as your restless mind may fail to recognize them. Often they are very near you, drawn by the friendship born in the dim, distant past. They constitute your shining collection of soul jewels; add to it constantly. In these bright soul galaxies you will behold the one Great Friend smiling at you radiantly and clearly. It is God who comes to you in the guise of a noble, true Friend, to serve, inspire, and guide you.[5]

Evolving relationships

In Part II of Volume One we explored the cycles of human evolution and how the ego expands its sense of self-identity over many lives. While evaluating our relationships with a desire to make them more reciprocally nourishing, it's helpful to be aware of our own and others' current stage of spiritual awareness.

Growth is a gradual process, and we should not expect ourselves or others to make great strides quickly, or even in a single life. Each of the four stages of evolution can take hundreds or even thousands of lives during which we are propelled by the overarching, universal desire of all created beings to avoid pain and suffering and to experience increasing happiness and well-being.

Let's look at the qualities of our human relationships as our awareness expands through each stage of evolution.

Shudra relationships. At the stage when the soul first inhabits a physical body, the shudra phase, the individual relates to others in terms of how they can help him satisfy his physical need for food, shelter, and sex. There is no attempt, or even a possibility, for the shudra to relate meaningfully to others. As evolution slowly proceeds throughout this stage, and the shudra's awareness begins to expand, he realizes that he can gain more of what he desires by putting out energy. Thus the individual will evolve from being passive and indolent to becoming unpleasantly and even violently demanding.

Shudras are a burden to their families and leeches on society. A relationship of give-and-take is nearly impossible at this stage of spiritual awareness, and there is little we can do but accept them as they are, with compassion for the spark of divinity in them. At a practical level, we can help them engage their energy productively by employing them for manual labor.

We can see traces of the selfish shudra mentality even in those who have become successful and powerful. The tell-tale attitude of the shudras is that they seek to fulfill their own desires without the slightest consideration for others. Their evolution depends on the law of karma. As they experience the consequences of their selfish attitudes and actions, they become tired of the loneliness and isolation that these attitudes bring, and they begin to desire meaningful relationships.

Vaishya relationships. These are associations characterized by an attitude of reciprocity: "I'll scratch your back if you scratch mine." Vaishyas value their relationships with others for what 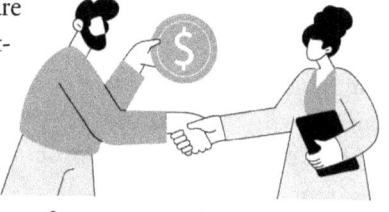 they can get from them in the form of money, prestige, and power.

At work, the vaishya's attitude is competitive – it can be cutthroat, when the stakes are high. At this stage, pure, selfless friendship is rare. In their pursuit of wealth and position, vaishyas are prone to betray their friends, colleagues, and even their relatives. "Nothing personal — it's just business," we hear the vaishya smugly proclaim. The voice of the soul that quietly whispers, "It *is* personal: people matter," is drowned out by the vaishya's self-seeking ego.

Whereas shudras rarely create their own family, and often make terrible decisions when they do, the vaishya ego broadens its self-identity to include a life partner and children. The desire to provide for a family is a very real step forward in the soul's long journey of self-expansion. With the passing incarnations, the vaishya is drawn to enlarge its definition of family beyond its original narrow identification with "us four and no more," as Yogananda put it.

If we attempt to motivate people of vaishya mentality with altruistic lures, we will find that they rarely work. Without pandering to the typical vaishya's mindset of "What's in it for me?" an effective strategy might be to highlight the more intangible rewards. In personal relationships, especially where there's a deep karmic bond, if the vaishya ego is at least minimally mature, it may be possible to introduce the idea of mutual benefit, with a "win-win" model replacing "I-win-you-lose."

For example, more evolved vaishyas may be persuaded that creating a scheme of benefits and services for their employees will increase their own bottom line by improving productivity, employee retention, and profits. As in the story of "The Typewriter King,"* when the vaishya begins to look beyond his own egoic boundaries, the intangible returns of inner satisfaction, recognition, and the esteem and affection of others begin to impel him to grow toward the next stage of spiritual evolution: the *kshatriya*.

Kshaytriya relationships are where selfless friendship and divine, unconditional love are able to blossom fully. Kshatriyas are aware of and sensitive to realities beyond themselves and their own family and work. Swami Kriyananda's definition of maturity aptly describes the level of consciousness that the kshatriya has reached: "*Maturity is the ability to relate appropriately to other realities than one's own.*" [6]

No longer focused on material gain or obsessed with outwitting competitors, the kshatriya ego has progressed to a point where it is capable of finding satisfaction in helping others, and is motivated by the pure joy of giving and the internal rewards of sacrificing his own comfort for their well-being.

Kshatriya parents will willingly make sacrifices for their children. In the earlier stages of their kshatriya evolution, they may complain, but in the latter stages they will not count the cost, or even mention it. This same selfless attitude characterizes the kshatriya doctor, business manager, politician, public service worker, sports coach, teacher, counsellor, military leader, and so on.

The kshatriya mentality is respectful and compassionate when interacting with the vaishya or shudra. It will make no attempt to convert them to a broader perspective. The kshatriya influences others by the example of his own actions and his expression of unconditional love. Relationships between kshatriyas afford a blessed opportunity for mutual growth.

---

* See page 52 in Volume One.

Brahmin relationships. As kshatriya friendships evolve to the stage of the brahmin, they become less personal and more oriented toward a loving relationship with God, and with the God who dwells in all beings. For the person of brahmin consciousness, all human relationships are divine. The brahmin sees and relates to God in everyone and consciously tries to channel His divine love impersonally to them.

> Those who live in ego-consciousness think of impersonal love as cold and abstract. But divine love is all-absorbing, and infinitely comforting. It is impersonal only in the sense that it is utterly untainted by selfish desire. The unity one finds in divine love is possible only to the soul. It cannot be experienced by the ego.[7]

It is in the brahmin stage that human love reaches its perfection, as divine love.

> Once the love of all human beings and all living things shall have entered into your heart, your heart will be the One Heart of God. Feeling all hearts as one, you will feel the One Cosmic Heart beating behind all hearts. Recognizing no individual selfish love, feeling the same love for all, you will feel the One Great Love which is everlasting and forever burns as pure white flame on the universal altar of all hearts.[8]

Ego expansion

The ego prefers to associate with a limited group of people who think and behave according to its own private standards and values. In contrast, the soul wants to extend its love by reaching out to include all of God's children.

> True friendship is broad and inclusive. Selfish attachment to a single individual, excluding all others, inhibits the development of divine friendship. Extend the boundaries of the glowing kingdom of your love, gradually including within them you family, your neighbors, your community, your country, all countries– in short, all living sentient creatures. Be also a cosmic friend, imbued with kindness and affection for all of God's creation, scattering love everywhere....
>
> *Consider no one a stranger; learn to feel that everybody is your kin.* Family love is merely one of the first exercises in the divine Teacher's course in Friendliness, intended to prepare your heart for an all-inclusive love.... his does not mean that you must know and love all human beings and creatures *personally and individually.* All you need do is to be ready at all times to spread the light of friendly service over all living creatures which you happen to contact. This requires constant mental effort and preparedness; in other words, unselfishness.[9]

The greater the number and variety of interactions we have with others, the better the odds of our enjoying good health mentally, emotionally, physically, and spiritually. The research is abundant, and the conclusion is crystal clear: isolation breeds illness. Just as cross-pollination invigorates plant species, contact with a variety of people stimulates our intellect, expands our sympathies, and enriches our life. Having interactions only with people who share our own background can be debilitating, as is evident in plant, animal and human inbreeding.

Actively participating in a group gives us ample opportunities to give and receive friendship in dynamic ways. Belonging to a group offers no guarantee that reciprocal friendships will follow – in every group there are those who are satisfied to receive the social benefits without giving in return. These one-way relationships reflect a shudra mentality.

Others will participate to varying degrees – the greater the participation, the greater the potential for increasing satisfaction and happiness.

Spiritual communities

Friendships between people in a group that is dedicated to high ideals can progress more rapidly from limited human affinity to expansive, divine love.

> Friendship is the universal Spiritual attraction which unites souls in the bond of divine love and may manifest itself either in two or in many.... When perfect friendship exists either between two hearts or within a group of hearts in a spiritual organization, such friendship perfects each individual.[10]

A cherished ideal of Paramhansa Yogananda's was to establish self-sustaining communities based on "simple living and high thinking." These communities would provide a healthy environment for spiritual growth, and a laboratory for a model of group living that would be based on harmonious cooperation.

> Yogananda repeatedly urged his listeners to band together in cooperative spiritual communities, to buy land together out in the country and there to live simply, close to nature and to God, guided by the twofold principle of "plain living and high thinking."
> Such communities, he said, would serve as models for the new age, when countless similar, self-sustaining communities will popularize voluntary cooperation over competition as the true key to lasting prosperity and inner fulfillment.[11]

Swami Kriyananda founded the first such community in 1969: the Ananda World Brotherhood Community near Nevada City, California. Today, tens of thousands of people are spiritually connected with Ananda communities in the U.S., Europe, and India.[12]

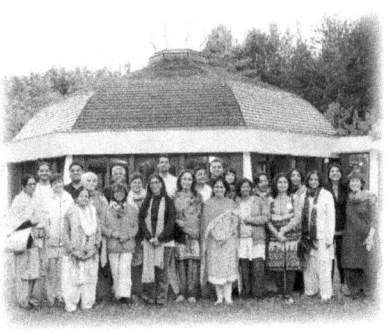

Relationships in a community that is dedicated to the ideal of living for God, and in God, are divine friendships in which each member seeks communion with God not only in his meditations, but also through his friends.... With mutual, divine respect for one another; sincere dedication to *what is* (as opposed to what they might be); a conditioned tendency, in any disagreement, to examine their own motives first; a commitment to the welfare of everyone; and, above all, with sincere love for God, it really is not difficult for a community of people to live in joyful harmony together.[13]

❈ Teamwork ❈

It started as a modest project that I felt I would be capable of handling. The Covid lockdown had pushed us toward offering online courses, and I was tasked with a variety of related assignments: training a pair of technicians, teaching them to operate Zoom and livestream courses, managing internet connections, and arranging locations, lights, cameras, recordings, and any additional media requirements during the classes. I knew how to do these things, and I was confident that my past teaching experience would enable me to make sure the courses had adequate technical support.

When the second Covid lockdown was announced, the project suddenly expanded, requiring a much larger permanent technical team to support the increased number of online activities. There would be days with four online programs running from early morning until evening. It was at this point that I stumbled into a role for which I had no experience at all: building a team. I had never held that particular responsibility in the community, and no one else was available. I alone could be involved full time, and I was willing, but I was worried. And then I remembered that I was not alone.

A friend taught me to build and manage a team, and from others I received spiritual guidance for how I could view the work as a service and not be stubbornly goal-oriented. My "boss" was a close friend and we overcame the challenges together. Meanwhile, a large team of technicians was formed, and a positive energy field developed as we moved into uncharted areas together.

What I remember most about this time is not the pressure of getting each program online at the announced time. Rather, I remember how our team became a group of joyful friends who supported each other and were always there when we were needed. Working together toward a shared goal, and seeing the goal as a service to many people who were home-bound, deepened our friendship and gave me a more profound understanding of the meaning of teamwork. –**Durga**, *Ananda Assisi*

Divine Friendship with God and Guru

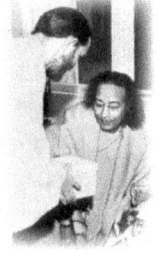

No human relationship is perfect. Even our best friends may occasionally misunderstand us, or be unable to help when we need them. They may even betray us. But the *satguru*, the person whom God has charged with the responsibility of guiding us individually to our ultimate freedom, is always present and is the one person who is best able to help us in every situation.

> My Master said to me, "I will be your friend from now until Eternity, no matter whether you are on the lowest mental plane or on the highest plane of wisdom. I will be your friend if ever you should err, for then you will need my friendship more than at any other time.[14]

God and the guru are bound by the sanctity of our free will, thus they will not impose their guidance unless we ask for it; nor will they intervene in our lives without being invited.

> God loves His human creations, and wants them to live in harmony, peace, and happiness. He will not impose His wishes on them, however, not even for their own welfare.[15]

The Indian scriptures describe in detail the various ways in which the individual soul can have a personal relationship with the infinite Spirit. These are called *rasas*, or "sentimental qualities," and they include *vatsalya rasa*, the loving, protective attitude of a parent for the child.

Saint Anthony of Padua had a mystical vision of Jesus in his form as a baby. This tender relationship is depicted in nearly every painting and statue of the saint. Saint Teresa of Avila, who personally founded sixteen Carmelite convents in Spain, had a vision of Jesus in his form as a child. She always carried a statue of the infant Jesus when she traveled to establish a new convent.

Hindus worship Lord Krishna in his form as the baby Gopal. Statues of the infant Bala Gopala are worshipped in elaborate rituals that depict a day in his life, from his awaking until he falls asleep at night. The idea behind these practices is that the devotee will make the transition from the parent's feelings of unconditional love for the child, to unconditional love for God.

The *rasa* that Jesus encouraged in his disciples is known in the Hindu tradition as *sakya rasa*, a relationship of friendship.

> Henceforth I call you not servants; for the servant knoweth not what his lord doeth: but I have called you friends; for all things that I have heard of my Father I have made known unto you. (JOHN 15:15)

Yogananda referred to the various rasas in the opening phrase of his well-known invocation:

"Heavenly Father, Divine Mother, Friend, Beloved God."

Thou and I are One
Excerpts from a poem by Paramhansa Yogananda

Thou art the Father, and I am Thy child;
We are one.
Thou art the Beloved, and I am the lover;
We are one.
Thou art the Lover, and I am the beloved;
We are one.
Thou art my Friend, I am Thy friend;
We are one.
Thou art the Master, and I am Thy servant;
We are one.
Thou art my Mother, I am Thy son;
We are one.
Thou art my Master, I am Thy disciple;
We are one.
Thou art the Ocean, and I am the drop;
We are one. [16]

PART X CHAPTER THREE

Healthy and unhealthy relationships

> Respect keeps a relationship non-invasive.
> Excessive familiarity, on the other hand,
> is demeaning to true friendship.[1]
> —KRIYANANDA

Visualize the people you chose in the first chapter. We will now consider each of them and consider how we can express the following virtues within those relationships.

HEALTHY RELATIONSHIPS

Respect and acceptance

Respect is fundamental to all healthy relationships – we could even say that it is more important than human love. In a respectful relationship, our love can grow, but without respect love has little to no chance of thriving.

To truly respect others means to accept them as they are, and not as we might wish them to be. In his booklet, *Secrets of Friendship*, Swami Kriyananda writes:

> The secret of friendship is accepting your friends
> as they are, and not trying to re-create them in your
> own image, or according to your own desires.[2]

A true friend may be able to see the potentials in others, but will hold no expectations about how they ought to develop them. A true friend will respect others' free will to act as they see fit. We can observe this in wise mothers and fathers who respect their children's wish not to follow in their parents' footsteps.

Swami Kriyananda wrote wedding vows in which one vow in particular captures the essence of true friendship.

> I will respect your right to see truth as you perceive it, and to be guided as you feel deeply within yourself.

Respecting another's free will means that we accept that all human beings make mistakes, although it does not mean that we will encourage or affirm a friend's self-harming behavior.

> Do not agree with him when he is wrong. Real friendship cannot witness with indifference the false, harmful pleasures of a friend. This does not mean that you must quarrel. Suggest mentally, or if your advice is asked, give it gently and lovingly.[3]

Diverse opinions need not stand between true friends. True friendship can exist even between rivals and adversaries. For example, U.S. Supreme Court justices Antonin Scalia and Ruth Bader-Ginsburg espoused diametrically opposite legal perspectives. They were rarely on the same side of an issue, yet they were such fast friends that they and their spouses vacationed and celebrated New Year's together. Similarly, world champion athletes often train together, respecting each other and enjoying healthy off-court friendships. Friendly rivalries can often help bring out the best in each one.

We also need to respect our friends' privacy.

> Out of respect...refrain from intruding unless they themselves extend an invitation....To preserve a certain mental distance, based on respect, makes communication easier. This is as true for communication between friends as between strangers. Respect keeps a relationship non-invasive. Excessive familiarity, on the other hand, is demeaning to true friendship.[4]

Loyalty and trust

One of the greatest traumas of adolescence is the experience of being abandoned by a friend to whom we have given our love and loyalty.

> Don't be fickle. Don't look about restlessly for alternatives. One-pointed loyalty is the highest virtue.[5]

When disappointments arise, the easy solution is to look for a new best friend, or as we grow older, a new partner. However, the capacity to be a loyal friend is a major step in the ego's progress from the indifference of the shudra and the selfishness of the vaishya to the altruism of the kshatriya, who is willing to sacrifice his own comfort to help others. Loyalty opens doors to higher levels of spiritual evolution.

> Develop loyalty—to your family, your friends, your chosen path in life. Loyalty, like a rudder, will hold your ship true to its course. Be loyal above all to the truth as you yourself best understand it.[6]

Loyalty means being available in times of need.

> True friendship consists in...
> offering your friends good cheer in distress, sympathy in sorrow, advice in trouble, and material help in times of real need. Friendship consists in rejoicing in your friends' good fortune and sympathizing with them in adversity. Friendship gladly forgoes selfish pleasures or self-interest for the sake of a friend's happiness, without consciousness of loss or sacrifice; without counting the cost.... [7]

When a loyal friend is disappointed in another's behavior, instead of assuming bad intentions or weakness of character, the loyal friend will assume that the other person is in some kind of difficulty, and offer his help.

Loyalty means standing up for our friends when they are under attack, neither adding fuel to the fire or remaining passively on the sidelines when others disparage them, even if what the others are saying about them has merit.

> When you believe in something, stand by it!
> When you believe in someone, stand by him!
> Such loyal self-commitment is a higher law
> than "seeing all sides". [8]

Kriyananda recounts this conversation with Yogananda.

> Some people had been speaking against
> Dr. Lewis (Yogananda's first disciple in America),
> saying that he had let the Master down in
> certain important ways. The criticisms were valid,
> and I spoke to the Master about them.
> The highest value to him, however, was loyalty.
> He was deeply loyal to his friends, even when they
> disappointed him. Thus I, as the messenger,
> had to bear his indignant response:
>
> "When you have been tested through
> many years, as he has, *then* you will have
> earned the right to speak these things!"....
> He then went upstairs and telephoned Dr. Lewis,
> simply to affirm his deep friendship for him.[9]

When our loyalty is able to survive the test of time, our friendships become truly mature and consolidated, and provide a solid basis for deeper, more intimate relationships.

Sincerity

Sincerity is the soil in which love and harmony flourish. In the ancient scripture *Yoga Sutras*, sage Patanjali highlights truthfulness as one of the ten important virtues, each of which is vital for the cultivation of healthy relationships.*

To what extent should we be truthful with our friends? It is difficult to be completely truthful even with ourselves! We are not constrained by spiritual duty to reveal everything to our closest friends and loved ones. At the same time, we must not be false with them, telling them things we know to be untrue, or withholding from them information that they have a right to know. To be able to exercise their free will, they must know how things truly stand.

Misunderstandings can arise even between the closest friends, despite our best intentions. Words can be inadequate, even treacherous vehicles to express our true feelings. In all languages, words have subtle shades of meanings that will depend on the context, the inflection of the voice, and the understanding of the person receiving them. Thus our words can easily belie our true intentions.

In our verbal and written communications, therefore, we will want to be thoughtful and considerate of our friends' situation and state of mind. Reactive, emotionally charged communications can be hurtful to others and ourselves. When we are hurt or confused by a friend's words or actions, instead of escalating the situation with self-justifications or a counter-attack, a calm, loving suggestion might set things right and restore friendship and harmony: "I don't quite understand your remarks (or actions). Let's talk about it so we can both have more clarity."

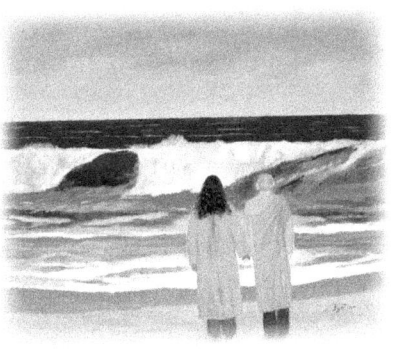

We want to see our friend's higher Self by appropriately encouraging them to embrace that potential. We can do this also for people who are antagonistic toward us and see themselves as our enemies.

---

* The *yamas* and *niyamas* are mentioned in Part II of Volume One.

> Practice loving those who do not love you.
> Feel for those who do not feel for you. Be generous
> to those who are generous only to themselves.
> If you heap hatred on your enemy, neither he
> nor you are able to perceive the inherent beauty
> of your soul.... Silently love [your enemy].
> Silently be of service to him whenever he is in need,
> *for love is real only when it is useful and expresses
> itself through action.* Thus will you rend the
> veils of hate and of narrow-mindedness
> which hide God from your sight.[9]

If you know that your friend's partner is unfaithful, does loyalty require you tell them? As a friend, you have no obligation to intervene in the karma of two other people, especially since doing so could involve you needlessly in the karmic consequences. You can pray for the situation to resolve beneficially for those involved, and be ready to offer your unbiased spiritual support if you are asked to. All relationships are multi-faceted and karmically complicated.

How candid should we be in sharing our problems with friends? On the one hand, that's what friends are for, isn't it – to help us in our times of need. It can be very helpful to ask for the counsel of a wise and trusted friend who will support our efforts to improve.

> Ask your friends for guidance,
> especially those you trust who've proved their
> sense of good judgment over time.[11]

On the other hand, it's important to discern which friends will actually be able to help us, practically and spiritually. Not every friend will have the wisdom and impartiality to offer good advice. While confessing your faults may momentarily relieve you of a burden, discrimination is needed, lest they later, in a fit of pique, use our faults against us.

> The Master used to say, "Don't tell your faults
> to others, unless they have spiritual wisdom,
> lest they hoard up that memory and use it against
> you sometime out of displeasure with you."[12]

We can and should be utterly open and sincere in discussing our problems and weaknesses with God, who is our most trusted, wise and loyal friend. We should trust that He will love us unfailingly in all the conditions and circumstances of our inner and outer lives.

> "God will never let you down," (Yogananda) assured
> his disciples, "so long as you make the effort. If ever
> you tell yourself, 'I am lost,' it will be so — at least for
> this incarnation. But if you keep on trying, the Lord
> will never stop trying on His part to help you."[13]

Cooperation and support

Every relationship is like a beautiful flower that needs to be cultivated and cared for according to its special requirements. Roses need different care than dahlias or peonies. Each friendship, too, is unique. There is no single way to be a friend that will be appropriate in every situation.

All friendships, however, are nourished by doing things together. We often hear the lament, "We've grown apart!" Surely we would rather grow together in our relationships, and participating together in activities that will broaden our horizons can help — whether our mutual interests are intellectual, cultural, athletic, spiritual, etc. It's also important to spend time relaxing together with our friends, family, or colleagues. With spiritual friends, we will want to look for, or create opportunities to meditate and pray together.

Our relationships are strengthened also by taking on challenges together. Collaborating on working toward a goal, regardless of whether we achieve the goal, can bring out our hidden individual strengths and tighten our bonds of friendship.

Years ago, my husband and I trained for a marathon. It was an experience that we still remember fondly. We often recall and discuss the challenges of our months-long training and completing the marathon race. I vividly remember how my energy took a nosedive in the later miles, and how he talked me all the way to the finish. "Working together to win together" is an exhilarating way to nurture a friendship.

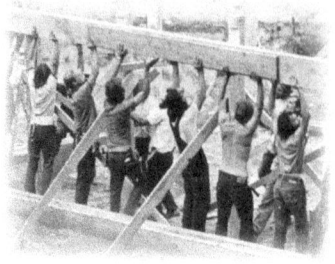

Learning to cooperate and support others is an important element of the ego's evolution. Shared activities loosen our hold on the ego, whose first instinct is to want to take credit for every accomplishment.

"Ensemble" activities such as team sports, singing in a choir, playing in an orchestra, acting, or serving on the support team for a play, concert, or other artistic event can help us loosen the vaishya mentality – "What's in it for me? – and replace it with the kshatriya's motto: "What's in it for everyone?"

❈ People before projects ❈

Our website urgently needed a new design that would make it more user-friendly and intelligent. Our team members were fully on board, but we hadn't been able to agree on how to achieve our goals.

As managing director, I proposed a solution that my years of experience told me was the obvious one: we would hire the consulting company that was already managing our other sites. But the company's communications coordinator and her team had a different idea: we would do all of the work in-house.

Given that the team had no programming experience, my rational mind told me that the problems would be legion, yet my intuition seemed to be telling me that it was the right thing to do, so I approved the project and the budget.

Today, I consider the project a huge success, even though we exceeded our budget long ago and we have yet to achieve all our goals. The site is working well enough, but the overarching benefit has been how facing the challenge together united our team, making us more consciously collaborative and capable of taking on responsibility. The team members have developed stamina and resilience, and the coordinator has learned a great deal about managing resources, and how to work compassionately and creatively with others.

For my part, I learned that the journey we traveled together was far more important than the result. It taught us to listen and support each other, to be grateful for each other, and to trust one another. We are not here primarily for the projects we do, but to help each other to grow. Thanks to our new synergy, we now have the experience and courage to take on challenges that we would formerly have considered unattainable. –**Fulvia**, *Milano*

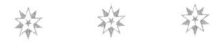

UNHEALTHY RELATIONSHIPS

In a healthy relationship, harmony prevails – harmony between the participants, and just as important, a sense of inner harmony with the laws of divine friendship (discussed above). Like a choir in which every voice is in harmony with all the others, beautiful melodies can flow through a relationship that is built on divine friendship. Using the worksheet in Chapter Six, you can observe the extent to which you are contributing to healthy, harmonious relationships.

Unhealthy relationships are marked by the absence of respect and acceptance, at home and at work. Unpleasant words and behavior, a lack of consideration, jealousy and competitiveness, bullying, shaming, mobbing, manipulation, oppression, and suppression are more likely to follow when there is insufficient respect and tolerance.

The quality of our relationships has a profound impact on our mental and emotional health. Gail M. Saltz, MD [14] reports:

> Lack of relationships, leading to loneliness, causes depression and anxiety, while tumultuous and disturbing relationships lead to chronic stress and lower mood and higher anxiety.[15]

Toxic relationships have a greater immediate impact on our health than any environmental pollutant. A relationship that is fraught with conflict, tension, and a dearth of mutual support is a breeding ground for illness.

The Whitehall II study,[16] a landmark body of research that followed more than 10,000 people for over 12 years, confirmed that the link between toxic relationships, stress, and health is real. According to this study, those who were in toxic relationships were at greater risk of developing heart problems, including dying from heart attacks and strokes, than those whose close relationships were not negative.[17]

What can you do if you find yourself in an unwholesome or toxic relationship? There are too many individual factors to offer detailed advice. In general:

- If you feel that significant long-term improvement is not possible, it might be necessary to consider removing yourself permanently or temporarily from the harmful environment.
- If distancing yourself from the relationship isn't an option, there are spiritual techniques for strengthening yourself physically and emotionally. These are discussed in detail in Chapter Eleven of Part XII.

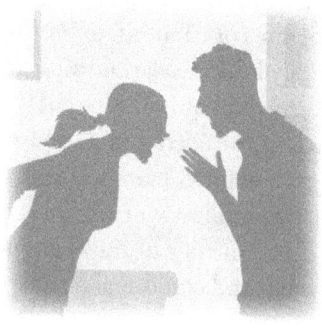

Each partner in a relationship is a key player, a main actor, a protagonist – even if one partner appears to be the victim. Whether to endure in an unhealthy relationship while continuing to try to improve it, or to leave when it seems there is no possibility of change, is a choice that only you can make.

Look again at each of the relationships you chose to consider at the beginning of this chapter to determine if your attitudes or behaviors are a cause of disharmony.

ADVICE FROM SWAMI KRIYANANDA
for living in harmony with others [18]

The following suggestions can help you in two ways. As you adopt them in your daily interactions with others, your understanding of yourself and others will deepen. Secondly, as you begin to understand others more deeply as extensions of your own self, harmony follows automatically. These suggestions are therefore also helpful as a checklist for how well you are succeeding in your current efforts to live in harmony with others.

- Be ever truthful and sincere — first of all with yourself, and then with everyone you meet.

- Look upon other people as friends and acquaintances of yours whom you may have known in past incarnations, and some of them perhaps closely and dearly. It is, indeed, probable that you have known many of them before.

- Whether or not they are your friends from before, God in His infinity is omnipresent. He therefore resides in everyone – *as* everyone! See all whom you meet as expressions of our one common Father/Mother God.

- Never judge anyone. Accept all as they are. Love them as extensions of your own self. We may think of each person as specializing, on behalf of the whole human race, in being, simply, himself!

- Never view anyone with the thought of needing or desiring anything from him. Give him perfect freedom, mentally, simply to be himself, and to be complete in himself.

- Develop a sense of humor, first as regards your own foibles, and second as regards the foibles of others.

- Don't accept error when you see it, but accept simply that people do make mistakes. Thus, love people not *for* their faults, but in spite of them, and because everyone is trying, each in his own way, to find his way around or out of his own pits of error. Then, if you are so inspired, *encourage them from their own point of view* to change and improve themselves. Realize that each person has a duty to change and improve himself. To do so is not *your* responsibility.

• Dismiss from your mind the thought of personal attachment to anything. Thus, when dealing with others, you will find you have no ulterior motives to warp your understanding of them.

• Live in the thought of God's loving, blissful presence within you....When in the company of others, try to share with them His inner bliss.

PART X   CHAPTER FOUR

Soulmates

> When true friendship exists between two souls and they seek spiritual love and God's love together, when their only wish is to be of service to each other, their friendship produces the flame of the Spirit. Through perfected Divine Friendship, mutually seeking spiritual perfection, you will find the one Great Friend.[1] —YOGANANDA

When we meet someone for the first time, there may be an immediate feeling of affinity. Yogananda said that these feelings are an indication that we've known each other in a past life. Although not all such sparks need to lead to marriage, these instant recognitions may hint that our soul's evolution could be aided by a closer relationship.

Do the instant feelings of familiarity indicate that you are "soulmates"? Whereas you may have been soul friends or spiritual companions in a past life (perhaps even spiritual partners), encountering our true soul mate is rare.

The idea of soulmates goes back to the dawn of creation. Yogananda tells us that the Spirit beyond creation represents the masculine principle and that the created universe, including all souls, express the female principle. In a parable, Jesus refers to God as a "bridegroom" and the beloved ones as the "wise virgins." (MATTHEW 25:1-13)

In Hindu lore, we find God manifesting Himself in the form of Lord Krishna and playing irresistible divine melodies on His flute to draw all souls to find their freedom in Him. In Hindu art we see Krishna's female disciples, the Gopis, dancing with him in ecstasy on the banks of the Yamuna River, representing the eternal dance of masculine and feminine, or Spirit and Nature. (SRIMAD BHAGAVATAM 10:30)

Yogananda says that in this manifested creation in which the law of duality applies, we can think of souls as male or female "half souls," the male half predominantly expressing reason, and the female half-soul expressing feeling.

> In the original plan of creation, man and woman, ideal soul mates, were to lead a heavenly life by keeping their minds in the Heavenly region of Bliss-Will in the forehead. The spiritual marriage consisted in woman or feeling, uniting with the knowledge or masculine force, and thus becoming one in God.[2]

Ordinarily, the two half-souls need to reunite by "spiritual marriage" in order to then find final liberation in God. The desire for such a refined level of companionship develops over many lifetimes during which we experience countless disappointments in search of a more earthly kind of love. We will look more closely at Yogananda's descriptions of "spiritual marriage" a little further along.

We must be highly advanced spiritually to attract our true soul mate. At this level of Self-realization, we will have transcended our limiting self-identity as a man or woman, and we will no longer live on the plane of gender differences. Soulmates can, in fact, meet on the physical, astral, or causal plane. Even if they are not in the same place, Yogananda said, they can unite in superconscious visions or dreams.

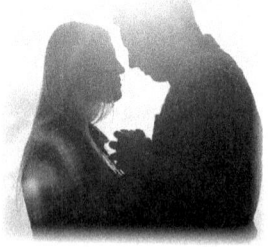

The English novelist Marie Corelli (1855-1924) penned a fascinating novel about the journey of soulmates, *The Life Everlasting*. In Corelli's book, the lovers are united after many lifetimes of tribulations and sail off into the sunset on his private yacht. Swami Kriyananda rewrote the novel, giving it a more uplifted vision in which, on being reunited, the soulmates dedicate their lives to serving humanity together. He titled the rewritten version *Love Perfected, Life Divine*.*

---

*Available from Ananda Sangha Publications, https://anandapublications.com.

Spiritual companions

Not all couples are soulmates. There are many kinds of relationships that help us in our spiritual evolution. Spiritual companions are those whose partnership is dedicated to helping each other experience God's unconditional love. Yogananda offers this practical advice on seeking a spiritual companion.

> You cannot attract a spiritual soul through animal magnetism. Too much living on the sex plane causes health and happiness to fly away.... If you attract a person by spiritual magnetism, then you will meet your soul companion.... When you have formed a tremendous friendship with a person that nothing can destroy, a friendship that has no compulsion in it and that increases constantly, you have found a true mate.[3]
>
> The spiritual way to choose the right companion is to affirm deeply after meditation: **'Heavenly Father, bless me that I choose my life companion according to Thy law of perfect soul union.'** If you practice this affirmation for six months with deep faith, you will marry your right companion, or the Divine Father will bring about sudden unfavorable circumstances which completely prevent your wrong marriage.[4]

I recently attended a wedding of someone who had used this prayer to find a spiritual companion, as her story reveals.

✵ FINDING MY SOUL COMPANION ✵

It's rare nowadays for a relationship to last nine years. For us, they were good years and our relationship might have continued, had I not committed myself to meditation and the spiritual path. Our life goals had diverged, and we amicably bade each other adieu, whereupon I gave my full attention to developing my relationship with God and Guru.

My first attempt at a spiritual relationship was short-lived. I realized that I wasn't ready to find a spiritual companion. Someone had told me about a special prayer that Yogananda recommended for those seeking a spiritual partner, and I began repeating it with great sincerity after every meditation:

"Heavenly Father, bless me that I choose my life companion according to Thy law of perfect soul union."

I made a list of the characteristics I imaged my future soul companion would possess and placed it on my altar.

After the suggested period of six months for offering the prayer, there was still no one on the horizon who fit the profile. I continued with my spiritual practices, trusting that if my spiritual growth required a companion we would be drawn together. I felt complete in myself, and content in my deepening relationship with God and Guru.

I remained single for the next nine years, during which I visited the Ananda spiritual community near Assisi often. I admired the sweet and simple friendships there, and I met couples who had been together as spiritual companions for decades.

During the Covid lockdown, when I was isolated at home for several months, I was able to go deeper in meditation and in the practice of introspection. I asked myself whether the life I was leading, however creative and financially rewarding it was, was helping me fulfill my spiritual goals.

During my next visit to Ananda, I knew that my future lay there. When I met my future husband, it was clear to both of us that our paths would continue together. We married a year and a half later, and although it took years instead of months for the prayer to work (the list of characteristics of my ideal mate had been a long one), the wait was well worth it. –*Jayita*, *Ananda Assisi*

Mighty Karma

The bonds of love between companion souls are strengthened and refined over many lives. When two souls incarnate at the same time on the same planet, the magnetism of their love will draw them together again, even in the unlikeliest circumstances.

I recently read the story[5] of a dedicated Catholic nun who had lived in a cloistered order for more than twenty years, utterly content with her spiritual life and her relationship with Jesus.

One day, a priest from an affiliated monastery visited the convent, and at the end of his visit he had dinner served to him before he departed. The nun helped the prioress during the dinner, and when the priest was preparing to leave and the prioress was called away, the nun opened the door for him. It was a brief encounter that resulted in the nun and priest marrying and continuing to serve God together – the former priest as a vicar of the Church of England, and the former nun as a hospital chaplain.

The priest and nun in the story were mature in their spiritual dedication when they met. It may also happen that soul companions will be drawn together earlier in their lives.

✻ Growing Together ✻

The fact that we met at a discotheque says a lot about how we were living forty years ago – just a pair of carefree, fun-loving young people dancing into the wee hours most summer evenings.

The spark was there, and we quickly became a steady couple. Within a year we had found a house and had begun to live together. We enjoyed doing things together, and we both had a strong sense of curiosity.

We decided to try a yoga class. At the gym we saw a poster for a meditation class, and we thought, "Why not?" That was the point when our lives evolved from fun-loving kids with only the foggiest notion of the meaning of life, to more serious spiritual endeavors.

The meditation teacher became our first spiritual guide. His discipline was very strict, and while many of his students ran away, we stuck it out, helping each other to grow into new realities. We are grateful to our first teacher for two additional reasons: because he introduced us to the writings of Paramhansa Yogananda, and because he encouraged us to marry. The fog had begun to clear, and we had found a new direction for our lives.

In those early years there were many fundamental changes, inwardly and outwardly. We did eventually marry, and we had two children, all the while continuing our spiritual practices. The cohesion we enjoyed at home extended to our work, which was challenging and fraught with difficulties, since we worked in the local outdoor markets. There were ups and downs, at home, at work, and with the children, but our spiritual path kept us united.

After thirty years, life decided that it was time for us to make yet another discovery. Through Ananda Assisi we acquired a large and joyful spiritual family, and in time we became disciples of Paramhansa Yogananda. We traveled together on pilgrimages to India and California, we prepared for and received Kriya initiation, and most recently we entered the new Nayaswami renunciate order as a couple.

We know that it is a rare blessing to share this life with a spiritual companion. We are certain that further spiritual adventures await us, and we continue untiringly determined to reach the final victory of Self-realization.

—Stefano and Emanuela, Rimini, Italy

Spiritual marriage

Yogananda uses the term "spiritual marriage" in three contexts. First, in the context of soulmates, where two half-souls unite in divine love. This is spiritual marriage in its perfected form, where the paired souls are liberated forever from the wheel of birth and death.

> When two souls are ideally mated,
> their love becomes spiritualized and is registered
> in eternity as the one love of God.[6]

Yogananda said that such freedom can also be attained without a need to unite with our soul mate. In this case, spiritual marriage refers to the union between the individual soul, the *jivatman*, and the infinite Spirit, the *paramatman*. Patanjali refers to this re-union in his *Yoga Sutras* as "samadhi." 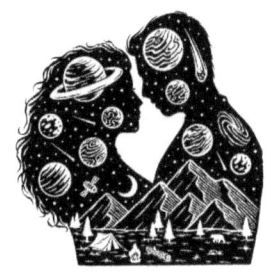 Through deep meditation and ecstasy, the awakened *kundalini*, the female principle lodged at the base of the astral spine, rises upward through the sushumna, the central passageway in the subtle astral spine, to unite completely with the masculine pole at the spiritual eye, the *kutastha*. These reunited forces then awaken the *sahasrara* chakra, the thousand-petaled lotus at the crown of the head.*

Yogananda refers to "spiritual marriage" more generally as a union that is dedicated to the partners' mutual spiritual growth, in which they live together as soul companions – as distinct from "soulmates."

Spiritual interests and activities may not occupy center stage in an ordinary harmonious relationship, but in a spiritual marriage the partners are committed to growing together toward Self-realization, and to transforming their exclusive and personal human love into expansive, universal divine love.

> The purpose of marriage is to know God, and to be together in God.[7] People who rise above the physical plane and continuously strengthen the love of their souls find their oneness in God. When the love of two persons burns as one flame, above the physical plane, then it has intoxicating eternal qualities. The marriage that is lived in self-control and intense spiritual preparation becomes emancipated.[8]

In a wedding ceremony written by Swami Kriyananda, the couple begin their vows by committing their life together to God.

---

* See Part III in Volume One for a discussion of the chakras.

> ***Beloved Lord,***
> *We dedicate to Thee our lives, our service, and the love we share.*
> *May the communion we find with one another lead us to inner communion with Thee.*
> *May the service we render one another perfect in us our service of Thee.*
> *May we behold Thee always enshrined in one another's forms.*
> *In every test of love, may we see Thy loving hand.*
> *In any disagreement, may we seek Thy hidden guidance.*
> *May our love not be confined by selfish needs, but give us strength ever to expand our hearts until we see all human beings, all creatures as our own.*
> *Teach us to love all beings equally, in Thee.*

After offering their union to God, the partners vow to spiritualize their relationship with one another:

> ***Dear Beloved,***
> *I will be true to you as I pray always to be true to God.*
> *I will love you without condition, as I would be loved by you—and as we are ever loved by God.*
> *I will never compete with you; I will cooperate for our own, and for all others', highest good.*
> *I will forgive you always and under all circumstances.*
> *I will respect your right to see truth as you perceive it, and to be guided as you feel deeply within yourself,*
> *And I will work with you always, in freedom, to arrive at a common understanding.*
> *All that we do, may we do for God's glory.*
> *May we live and grow together in His love and joy.*
> *And may the offspring of our union—whether human children or creative deeds—be doorways for the inspiration that we feel from Him, through each other.*
> *May our love grow ever deeper, purer, more expansive, until, in our perfected love, we find the perfect love of God.*

In his book *Self-Expansion Through Marriage*, Kriyananda cautions the reader about the need for a clear understanding of the role of marriage as an aid to spiritual growth.

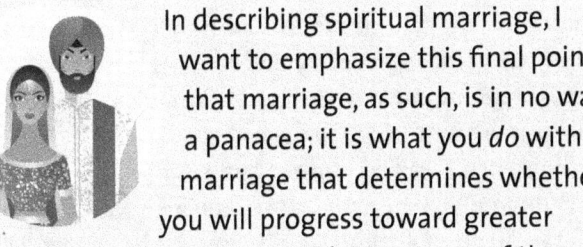

In describing spiritual marriage, I want to emphasize this final point: that marriage, as such, is in no way a panacea; it is what you *do* with marriage that determines whether you will progress toward greater freedom, or regress toward an increase of those delusions which, all your life, have brought you pain. The greater your inner freedom, the greater will be your happiness, and the deeper and more fulfilling your love.[9]

Are wedding ceremonies important?

People nowadays are often heard to ask, "Why should one get married? If two people love each other, why shouldn't they simply live together? What difference does a piece of paper make?"

The simple answer is that, when a marriage is sincerely entered into before God, with a ceremony performed in a spirit of blessing by a priest or a minister, there is a grace that can be felt almost tangibly in the air. This sense of blessing can carry a couple through many crises in the years to come, crises which, in less spiritually based marriages, would cause an irreparable rift.[10]

❊ Not just for the ❊
Bride and Groom

I was glad that I had made the effort to have an official wedding ceremony. My family had come all the way from England, and his family had traveled from Croatia. All of our friends were gathered here to celebrate and witness our commitment to each other. I thought, "This wedding is more for them than for us."

But when I walked into the temple, I became aware of something much greater – it was a divine presence, a feeling of sacredness. I felt that our union was being blessed by a higher power than the human love of family and friends.

When we made our vows, first to God and then to each other, the words were like a doorway into a luminous future: "May our love grow ever deeper, purer, more expansive, until, in our perfected love, we find the perfect love of God."

From the beginning, ours had always been a spiritual relationship; but the wedding ceremony was transformative, elevating it into a higher dimension. It also transformed the course of my sister's life. Months after our wedding, she told me that she had had a spiritual awakening during the ceremony, and that she had felt a peace and divine love that had turned her life in a new direction.

And so it ensued that the ceremony was indeed, for them and also for us, a sacred moment that changed our lives. –**Mahiya** (wife of Arudra), *Ananda Assisi*

❊ The Promises We Made ❊

The promises we made to each other on our wedding day set us on a journey toward the highest possible goal for a marriage: that our love be perfected in the perfect love of God.

Phrases from the vows come to mind often. When we are moving in harmony together, I remind myself that there is even more to experience: "May our love grow ever deeper, purer, more expansive…"

When we see things differently, I hear these words: "I will respect your right to see truth as you perceive it."

When we become irritated with each other: "May we behold Thee (God) always enshrined in one another's forms."

Our wedding vows were truly memorable, and they have been our lighthouse for these past ten years. —**Arudra** (husband of Mahiya), *Ananda Assisi*

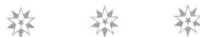

Do spiritual couples have an obligation to have children?

In the Bhagavad Gita, Arjuna asks his guru, Lord Krishna, to reveal to him the fate of advanced souls who have failed to attain liberation even after much spiritual effort. Krishna replies:

> He may reincarnate on earth in a family of enlightened yogis. Such a birth in this world, however, is difficult to attain. (In his new family) he recovers the yogic discrimination he attained formerly, and sets himself with even greater zeal to achieve (final) spiritual liberation.
> (BHAGAVAD GITA 6:42-43)*

Referring to this verse, Swami Kriyananda writes:

> Rebirth in the home of advanced yogis is difficult to attain, for such people seldom marry, and those who do so may prefer not to have children.[11]

The purpose of marriage concerns primarily the two individuals directly involved: **"Marriage is meant for spiritual re-union of souls."**[12] If a spiritual couple feel inwardly guided to welcome children into their home, Yogananda offers the following advice for attracting an advanced soul:

---

* This and all such Gita citations are from Yogananda, *The Bhagavad Gita According to Paramhansa Yogananda*.

> For couples desiring spiritual children...it is important that they keep their consciousness uplifted when coming together in physical union. For their vibrations at that moment will determine the quality of the flash of light in the astral world.[13] Parents should prepare their minds months in advance if they want to create a spiritual child. During the specific period, thoughts of invoking a noble Soul into the temple by uniting sperm and ovum cells must predominate. At this time, thought should remain in between the eyebrows, directing the holy work of creation, and never should be allowed to run down and become identified with the passion.[14]

While spiritual couples are not obligated to have children, when souls do join them, they have a sacred responsibility to take care of the child as a trust assigned to them by God.

> Children are not possessions: they are sacred charges. A couple's responsibility to their children is a responsibility in God, and must be discharged in truth, love, and divine respect. They must seek ever to touch the children at their highest level of reality.[15]

Parenthood is not the only way couples can honor their karmic relationships with other souls and fulfill our responsibility to them. Childless couples also can serve as channels for divine love.

> If you have no children of your own, adopt or teach the children of someone else, live an ideal life, and instill soul qualities into them. What you instill in the souls of children is imperishable. Anything you do that perpetuates your life, such as creative deeds, is, in a sense, your child. Thus fulfill your own true purpose in life.[16]

Spiritualizing a current relationship

If you would like to bring greater spirituality into your relationship, or deepen it, it will be important that you both be committed to this direction.

> **True growth in marriage is possible only if each partner assumes personal responsibility for their growth together.**[17]

The following are some suggestions from Yogananda and Kriyananda that you may find useful for the spiritual evolution of your relationship.*

People are more important than things

> **Don't make situations, or material things, or *anything* more important in your relationship than the love and respect you have for each other. Our circumstances change continually, but our outer circumstances are fleeting compared to the long-term relationship we are building together. If you nurture your relationship sensitively and wisely, it may carry you past the portals of this life into eternity.**[18]

Make time for shared spiritual experiences

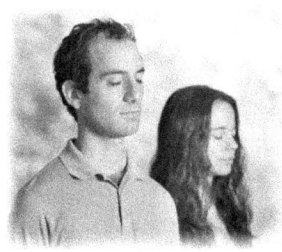

To bring your relationship onto a spiritual level, it is necessary to dedicate time to doing spiritual practices together. There is a magnetic exchange that happens when people meditate and pray together that silently develops deep bonds of love.

---

* Many other suggestions for couples who wish to broaden the scope of their relationship can be found in Yogananda's book *Spiritual Relationships* and Kriyananda's book *Self-Expansion through Marriage*.

Meditating together increases the degree of Self-realization of each (person) by the law of invisible vibratory exchange of spiritual magnetism.[19]

Be of service to one another

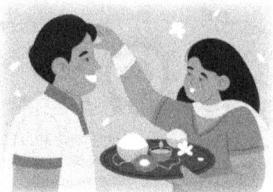

In most human relationships — especially those of the passive, low-energy shudra and self-centered vaishya kind — the ego is focused on how its own needs and desires will be met. In a spiritual relationship, the unselfish kshatriya mindset takes over, finding inner fulfillment and happiness by serving the other, instead of always wanting to be served.

> In marriage, love also grows through service to each other. When a husband and wife serve each other with the eternal inspiration of God, that is spiritual marriage.[20]

Keep your relationship fresh

> Marriage should be treated as an art.... To be so, it must be creative. Creativity implies a positive outflow of energy; lack of it implies passive receptivity to other people's energy, and to life. Passivity in marriage is like a slow-acting poison. Creativity is a tonic. The energy in marriage is like flowing water: As long as there is creative input, it will retain its freshness. But if it remains idle for too long, the marriage will grow stagnant .... Hence ... marriage should be ever-expansive.

Life Force / 60

> One suggestion for bringing creativity to your
> marriage is to try to do one thing every day that
> will give extra pleasure to your beloved: the gift
> of a flower, perhaps; a telephone call; a special
> smile—not with the lips, but *with the eyes*.[21]

Spend time apart

While time spent together in spiritual pursuits profoundly helps to consolidate and deepen the relationship, each soul's relationship with God is unique, and is best explored alone.

> The devotee must take time occasionally
> to be alone with God. Only as his awareness
> deepens of God's silent inner presence can the
> waves of his mental and emotional restlessness
> be stilled, and the boat of his life be steered
> serenely to the divine shores.[22]
>
> Couples need some time to themselves—
> both as a couple, and also apart from one another—
> for everyone needs some space of his own ....
> Only in a state of inner freedom can we preserve
> that creative joy which is the highest promise of
> any relationship.... Mutual growth is possible only
> from the soil of mutual respect. And respect
> flourishes best when a degree of distance,
> mutually agreed upon, is maintained.[23]

PART X CHAPTER FIVE

Advice for committed couples

YOGANANDA'S ADVICE [1]

- Husbands and wives must both develop their love for true ideals, then their love will continually increase, until the love of their hearts burns as a single divine flame.

- Married couples who continuously become more idealistic at home, in society, and in the world, find their love ever growing and changing, until that love becomes the idealistic love of God.

- No marriage can achieve its true purpose unless the husband and wife seek God first together.

- Meditate [together] every morning and especially at night.

- If husbands and wives are to live in friendship and harmony, they must be of spiritual service to each other... True love is based on unselfish mutual service and friendship soon.

- Have a little family altar where you...and your children gather to offer deep devotion to God, that your souls may be united forever in ever-joyous cosmic consciousness.

- Do not remain in the same room with [each other] all the time.

- Do not encroach upon your [partner's] independence.

- Do not disturb [the other person] when [they are] busy with important work or personal friends.

- Do not insult or be sarcastic...at any time.

- Do not argue... especially before others.

- Go out often...and frequently with your children as well.
- Study wholesome books and moral literature....Talk ... about literature, music, and higher spiritual truths.
- Make your home life simple and your spiritual life deep.
- Never lie to your partner.
- Never insult [the other's] parents.
- Never use harsh language, but always, instead, use sweet language.
- Address [each other] sweetly, with dignity and attention
- Thank [your partner] for every courtesy.
- Remember...birthdays and your wedding anniversary. Frequently offer ... presents.
- Give [each other] freedom to choose...friends. Learn to respect and, if possible, to like [them].
- Live a simple, inexpensive life... Save more; do not spend too much for luxuries.

Advice from Swami Kriyananda[2]

Shared ideals. To choose the right marriage partner, seek someone, above all, who shares your ideals.

Growing together. True growth in marriage is possible only if each partner assumes personal responsibility for their growth together.

Never criticize. *Offer* your ideas–tentatively, as a friend– mentally leaving the other person entirely free to accept or reject them.

An important guideline for married couples is to strive always to give one another *strength,* and not to contribute to one another's weaknesses.

Facing difficulties. Look on every difficulty as an opportunity – not for changing the other person, but for self-improvement.

Free will. Marriage is such a sensitive relationship that if in any way you try to coerce your partner to follow your ways, you risk damaging your relationship irretrievably.... Respect one another's free will. Instead of issuing emotional commands and ultimatums, *offer* your suggestions kindly–even humbly–for your partner's free consideration.

Respect.

- Respect and consideration are the simple kindnesses in human relationships that, like oil, keep the machinery of life flowing smoothly.... Without these, love never grows to become a healthy plant, capable of surviving the storms of life and of shifting fortunes.

- Respect for one another should include giving each other the freedom to grow and to change, each at his own pace.

- Respect flourishes best when a degree of distance, mutually agreed upon, is maintained.

- It is good, even in the intimacy of marriage, for couples to appreciate each other's need for privacy, for everyone needs some space of his own. Couples need some time to themselves—both as a couple, and also apart from one another—that they may return to the challenges of life refreshed and with renewed enthusiasm. Only in a state of inner freedom can we preserve that creative joy which is the highest promise of any relationship.

PART X CHAPTER SIX

How Healthy Are Your Relationships?

> **This exercise will help you evaluate any relationship –** with family members, friends, colleagues, intimate partners, and people with whom you find yourself in conflict. In the online Appendices for Part X (see p. 12) you will find the "Relationship Analysis" exercise formatted for easy printing. If you feel it might be helpful, use this exercise to evaluate your relationships with the people you identified in the first chapter, as well as others.

My relationship with _____

- What do I admire about this person?
- What irritates me about this person?
- What experiences and activities do we share?
- What do I receive from this relationship?
- What do I contribute to this relationship in terms of:
  - *Respect*
  - *Acceptance*
  - *Loyalty*
  - *Trust*
  - *Sincerity*
  - *Support: physical, psychological, spiritual*
  - *Cooperation/collaboration*
  - *Other important areas – add you own*
- What are three ways I can nourish this relationship?
- How do I see this relationship five years from now?
- Other important areas—add your own

PART X   CHAPTER SEVEN

Dissolution: Separation and Divorce

> If your love experiment in matrimony proves unsuccessful, then bid each other farewell in a kindly, gentle spirit, as befits true children of God.[1] —YOGANANDA

The ultimate purpose of our human relationships is to help us experience divine love and share it with others. This is, of course, a lofty goal, one that would be unrealistic to expect to attain and perfect quickly. Unconditional love develops over many lives. Each type of relationship — marriage, friendship, colleagues, etc. — will offer us unique opportunities to expand our love. Each type of relationship will offer us opportunities to grow, lessons to learn, and attainments that we can accomplish together.

Backing out of a marriage at the first sign of discord could result in merely postponing needed lessons until a later incarnation, although in some circumstances it may be the only reasonable course.

When a relationship has filled its purpose, or when mutual growth is no longer possible, the relationship may dissolve naturally. For example, circumstances may take the two people in separate directions. School friends who have been inseparable may drift apart as they gain greater clarity about their goals. Work colleagues who have enjoyed the pleasures of collaboration may be reassigned or transferred, and never meet again.

Relationships roles sometimes transform their nature. As a child matures into adulthood, the parent-child relationship may transition into one of adult friends. Later, the son or daughter may assume the role of a loving caretaker for the parents.

In this chapter our focus is on relationships that are inimical to spiritual well-being. When all our attempts to spiritualize a relationship fail, it may be spiritually appropriate to consider how we can dissolve it — in the best case, amicably and consciously.

Can divorce be justified spiritually?

Couples usually start their journey together with shared likes, goals, and aspirations, in the hope that these affinities will continue to sustain the relationship over the long term. But because every individual will have a unique arc of spiritual evolution, it is challenging for both partners to grow at the same pace throughout a lifetime, and often even to remain respectful and supportive of each other's development.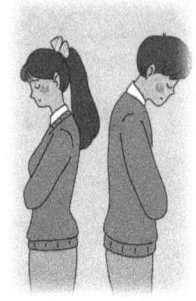

There are many couples whose love and respect are so strong that the spiritual pursuits of one partner will pose no threat to the other. There are also many couples who can maintain their inner bonds while following different spiritual paths. True love – that is, love that is based on mutual inner devotion to truth– can bridge all differences.

> A husband and wife should be loyal to each other, and try to make each other happy in every way. The spiritual wife should not forsake the unspiritual husband, nor should the spiritual husband forsake the unspiritual wife— they should try to influence and help each other as long as it is possible to do so.[2]

> Do your very best to make it work. Try to help your spouse, even if you do not see that you yourself are being helped. For in giving we often gain more than we realize. Marriage is an important commitment, and ought not to be abandoned until every other avenue has been tried.[3]

A situation that often arises is that one partner will begin to pursue an interest that isn't shared by the other – in this case, a spiritual interest.

If one partner actively impedes the other in his or her spiritual search, divorce may be a spiritually valid option.

> Divorce, the Master felt, is not necessarily in conflict with spiritual law .... If marriage obstructs a person's spiritual development, it may be his spiritual duty to leave it.[4]

Divorce is a momentous decision that is bound to have positive or negative karmic repercussions. Thus, it requires honest self-inquiry.

> Spiritual merit often lies in doing one's best under difficult circumstances; in this case, in living with someone who is not supportive of one's spiritual efforts. Nevertheless, the merit of sincere effort can also be overshadowed by the impossibility of success. In such cases, friendly separation may, sometimes, be a better solution than increasingly discouraging attempts at forging an unnatural bond together. There is no spiritual gain in a loving relationship that ends in bitterness.
>
> For not every marriage is made in heaven, theological claims to the contrary notwithstanding. When a duty conflicts with a higher duty, it ceases to be a duty. Mankind's highest duty is to seek God, and truth. A marriage that gives this ideal a secondary place, in the name of a merely human compromise, is destined for failure on both levels, human and divine.[5]

This is not a decision to be made emotionally, or to be taken alone. If we ask for God's help, He will guide our thoughts and actions. Yogananda suggests the following prayer:

> Father, we came together, teach us to
> live together in love, or if it is Thy will, teach us
> to part in love and understanding.[6]

Dissolving a relationship consciously and lovingly, with gratitude for its blessings, will enable us to move forward with a sense of freedom.

> If separate you must, do so with dignity.
> Better that than to get drawn downward into
> decreasing attunement with that principle,
> through bickering and misunderstandings.
> If you must separate, part with respect,
> and with love.[7]

❋ Friendly Divorce ❋

Who knows where our desires come from? We had known each other just three months, during two of which he was vacationing in Australia.

When we saw each other again, we had the same thought: Let's have a child together. I had my independence, having worked for eight years in a bank while living on my own. It seemed a good direction to marry and have a family. After all, it was what most women my age wanted. Nine months later we had our baby and our own house, and for a while I was happy to be a stay-at-home wife and mother.

After three years, my inner direction began to change and I began to want more from life. We spoke sincerely, as the good friends we were, and he understood why I wanted to go forward in another, spiritual direction.

As we had come together and lived together peacefully, so we separated peacefully. No arguments, no big dramas. We went shopping together to buy furnishings for his new apartment, and our son moved freely between our homes without a need for a formal legal arrangement. We would vacation together as a family, and we continued to be good friends.

Our son was living with me, when he decided that he would like to live with his father. They had a good year together, after which he returned to my home, content with his experience.

Although we were separated, we hadn't formalized our new situation. Then, after five years, he asked for a divorce, because he had found a compatible partner. They are very well-suited, and I am happy for him.

On our son's eighteenth birthday, we happily and harmoniously celebrated together: aunts and uncles on my side, and a new wife and child on my son's father's side. We keep in touch as we go our separate ways.

My husband and I had our moment together in time, and when the moment was over we moved on with love and respect for each other. –**Sonya**, *Switzerland*

❄ AN UNFRIENDLY DIVORCE ❄
WITH A HAPPY ENDING

We were too young to marry and to understand the hard work and sacrifices that would be required. We were also very different, which might have been a good thing, except that it drove us apart over time, eventually leading to divorce. I can see these things more clearly now, but at the time, and for many years after, I was very angry, blaming him for our lack of compatibility.

My daughter and I moved to the Ananda community near Assisi, and our son stayed with his father in Rome. I began to build a new life of meditation and service, but whenever I thought about my ex-husband in those early years, it was with lingering bitterness.

One day my daughter told me that her father's partner had expressed a desire to visit Ananda. I wasn't sure I could handle it, because even though she'd had no role in our separation, she had been emotionally involved in the divorce process.

Through meditation and honest introspection, I had been able to see my shortcomings in the marriage, and I thought, "Why should I stand in her way?" I talked with her by phone and told her that she should feel free to come with my ex-husband any time they wanted.

When they came, I realized that I had become a different person. When I saw them in the temple on Sunday morning, receiving the blessing during the Festival of Light, I felt an impersonal love blossom inside me toward them. I shed tears of happiness for them and for myself, feeling that the old karma was extinguished.

Today the three of us have an entirely different relationship: I regard him as a brother, and her as if she were my sister-in-law. We sincerely love each other. I often host them in my house when they come to Ananda, and they host me when I go to Rome.

I take no credit for this transformation. It was my Guru's gift through the power of meditation and selfless service that the ego could loosen its grip on me sufficiently to allow me to step back and see my responsibility in our situation, and to dispel the egoic veils of anger and open my heart to true love. –**Clarita**, *Ananda Assisi*

❋ THE GIFT OF UNCONDITIONAL LOVE ❋

It doesn't matter how far we've journeyed together; when the time comes to part ways, it is useless to hold on. Companions, children, friends – none of these belong to us; they are fellow travelers who may need to get off at different stations, not to hurt us but because the stretch of the journey we were meant to travel together has ended.

It took considerable suffering, pain, confusion, and heartache before I could experience the wisdom of the words I've just shared above. We were together for forty years, with two children, a grandchild, and a shared spiritual path. But none of those were sufficient to overcome our problems.

I kept asking God and my Master to help me resolve the problems and keep our relationship together, mostly from fear of change and worries about how I would get along on my own. But no help appeared to come, at least not in a way I could perceive, until I asked a different question: "What do I need to do to stop suffering like this?" Then the answer came quickly, and it was impossible to misunderstand: "Take back your dignity, and move on." And I did. I was the one who finally could say that enough was enough.

Having reached that decision, I was able to understand my husband's difficulties – his not knowing how to accept the passing of years, his regrets over not having had certain mundane experiences, his misunderstanding of the concept of freedom. At that point, forgiveness blessed my heart with understanding and a calm acceptance of what was happening.

I reconnected with my husband with an open heart. What had seemed the greatest, most insurmountable pain and difficulty of my life had instead brought a great gift, the greatest we can ever receive: the ability to love, above all else, with unconditional love. Even if my husband had stopped loving me, my heart continued to love him, and if he could be happy with his choices, I would be happy, too – just as if he were touched by suffering, I would have suffered with him while working to help him get better.

He has since passed on, and I was there by his side, wishing him well with all my heart as his soul continues its journey to true freedom in God's love. –***Ornella***, *Biela*

❄ Journey to Forgiveness ❄

When my husband left me for another woman, I reacted in different phases.

Phase 1: "How could he do this to me!!?!!" I was angry and deeply hurt.

Phase 2: "It's not my place to forgive him. It's up to God whether he is forgiven or not!" I said to myself, in righteous indignation, washing my hands of any responsibility in the matter of forgiveness.

Phase 3: Aware in my meditations of the pain and heaviness in my heart, and the tendency to contract my heart to avoid feeling that pain, I realized: "I know God doesn't want me to close my heart." I began to spend time during meditation with all my fingers touching each other at my heart and physically moving them apart repeatedly as if to open a sliding door, saying mentally "Open! Open! Open!" The result was palpable: an opening and a definite release of the pain and contraction of the heart.

Phase 4: I realized that forgiveness was not as important to my ex as it was for me; for my spiritual expansion and freedom, and for my capacity to be a channel for ever-deepening, ever purer, unconditional love. I would end my meditations with affirmations of Divine Love, offering that love up to God and outward to include all creatures, all human beings…and yes, also my ex.

Phase 5: It took some time to realize, in the natural flow of my meditation practice and service, that there really was nothing to forgive. That all that had happened was also my karma, and that those difficult, painful circumstances led me to the greater blessing of fulfilling my life's *dharma* in serving Yogananda's work, and of a deeper, more loving and lasting marriage. –*Anonymous*

Post-divorce recovery

An unexpected and undesired divorce can cause serious physical reactions, what to speak of the emotional and mental devastation it can bring. These words of solace and advice were offered by a friend of mine.

- The intensity of a divorce creates extreme reactions, both consciously and unconsciously. These emotional reactions cause severe imbalances that can result in undereating or overeating, not sleeping or sleeping too much. In my case, it felt as though the intensity would never end — but, of course, it did. I asked a doctor what to do, and he said that it was natural, in the circumstances, and that it would get better. He advised soups and broth, to stay away from caffeine and sugar, and to exercise a lot. I religiously followed his advice, and it helped me very much.

- These mood swings don't last too long, and it is good to make an effort to re-establish a balance. At the time, I didn't want to repress my emotions, so I would go through them — I let myself cry and express my rage. Sometimes I wanted to curl up and not move. The intensity of these emotions eventually decreases, and there will come a time to release them and go on. I kept repeating to myself: Acknowledge the emotions, work with them, and move on.

- I found that keeping busy helped me a great deal, not as an emotional escape, but to keep moving, even incrementally, in a positive direction. When I needed to cry, I would go to the bathroom or find a quiet place and do some pranayama or meditation. When the wave abated, I would return to my work. This turned out to be far better than staying home and being depressed. Sometimes, when I felt a wave of desperation approaching, I would go for a walk or run, or just keep busy with an engaging task.

- My spiritual practices were a great solace, when I could manage them. I had some of my deepest, and some of my worst meditations. It was a roller coaster, but it eventually slowed down, and then at a certain point it stopped. I spent a lot of time talking with God and my Gurus, I did lots of affirmations, and I prayed. It was good to remember that I was not alone.

- Although painful, this period in many ways strengthened me and enriched my life. It gave me deep insights that I can now use to help others.

Closure

How a relationship ends in this life will set its course for the future, because our human relationships continue from life to life. Just as the beginning of your relationship may have been inspired by love letters, Yogananda suggests that we write a letter to bring our relationship to a loving close.

> If you must part, write the following love letter: "Very dear one, we loved each other once. Let us remember that love again, and since we entered into a marriage-partnership in good-will and we meant well, and since we failed to make our marriage a success, let us part in kindness and in the memory of that 'old love.' I am leaving in order to preserve my kind thoughts of you forever, for I shall ever hold our past love as very sacred in the vault of memory." [8]

PART X   CHAPTER EIGHT

Loss and love eternal

> At death our loved ones leave with us a spark of undying heart-pang in order that we may fan it into a flame of wisdom, in the light of which we may behold all our lost loved ones....
>
> Love plays hide-and-seek in life and hides behind death, so that we may seek it still and find its secret bower in Omnipresence. Love races through the mazes of life and death to lead us to the land where it shines in all its brilliancy; for even in death, love lives on.[1] –YOGANANDA

The death of a loved one is a heart-wrenching event, and unless we are able to understand it on a deep level and integrate the fact of their passing into our life, the loss can lead to actual physical and mental pathologies, including heart disease, cancer, depression, and a higher risk of the death for the survivor during the first six months of bereavement.[2]

Our lives become intricately intertwined with the lives of our loved ones, as we come to rely on their continued presence as essential to our existence. No matter how well and wisely we have prepared for their passing, their permanent absence will be deeply saddening. It can be a comfort to realize that, for them, physical death is just a brief step in their passage to a more luminous world.

> Let us not bury the Soul in the grave and call death annihilation, but let us see it as a door through which bravely-marching Souls of earthly Life can enter to find the all-alluring, all-charming region of our ever-luminous, ever-peaceful Common Cosmic Home.

> Mortal fears, heartaches, dreams, and
> illusions fade, and the darkness of death
> changes into another infinitely more
> beautiful universe.[3]

Although our physical bodies are perishable, true love is eternal. **"We shall meet again,"** Swami Kriyananda says in his Astral Ascension Ceremony. **"Once more we shall laugh together, rejoice together, and share in the joy of seeking Him."***

In a letter, Swami Kriyananda counseled a grieving widower.

> Her passing is only an emigration to
> another country. What she had to do here was
> finished; now she has other things to accomplish
> elsewhere. But wherever there is true love,
> the great masters of all religions say that
> human parting always is only temporary.
> Love forms a magnet, drawing souls together
> even after the separation of death....
> The thread of love continue(s) through eternity,
> forever consistent, forming its own
> divine purpose. Divine love is indeed the
> only truly consistent fact in creation.[4]

In *Autobiography of a Yogi*, Yogananda tells how the passing of his guru, Swami Sri Yukteswar, left him deeply bereaved, and how the master appeared to him in his physical body and spent a long time with him, consoling him and telling him about the astral world:

> "Friends of other lives easily recognize
> one another in the astral world," Sri Yukteswar
> went on in his beautiful, flutelike voice.

---

* See the Astral Ascension Ceremony in the online Appendices for Vol. 3, Part X.

> "Rejoicing at the immortality of friendship, they realize the indestructibility of love, often doubted at the time of the sad, delusive partings of earthly life." *

If, at the death of a loved one, we allow grief to overwhelm us, it will not only be unhealthy for us, but it will also be detrimental to the soul of the departed.

> If we love souls, we must not try to keep them near us for our pleasure and comfort. If we really love them, we will continue to love them, particularly when they are taken away from us to advance on their path of reincarnation, or when they are called to rest in the bosom of the Father.[5]

Even as we have supported our loved ones in our life together, we can continue to support them with our loving thoughts and prayers for their well-being. The Astral Ascension Ceremony addresses the departed soul directly.

> Dear Friend,
> You, who have gone before us, have entered a realm which our souls remember:
> A place of freedom, light, and laughter.
> Take with you on your journey our blessings, and our love.
> We shall miss you!
> Our desire is not to hold you back, but only to tell you:
> Friend, we are yours; our love and support are ever yours, and our prayers for your highest happiness.

---

* Sri Yukteswar's thrilling description of the astral realms from which we incarnate and to which we return is worth reading multiple times to dispel the fear of death. –*Autobiography of a Yogi*, Chapter Forty-Three.

A period of adjustment

Over the long years of our lives together, we have formed certain roles, responsibilities, and dependencies. We have come to rely on our loved one in innumerable ways for their practical, emotional, and spiritual support. A period of adjustment will be unavoidable, during which we will need to take many of these responsibilities onto ourselves and seek the support of trusted friends and counselors.

As our grief wanes and the period of adjustment comes to an end, the next chapter of life begins to unfold and come into focus.

❈ TRANSCENDENT LOVE ❈

We were seekers. He was the scientist, I was the devotee. We were strong, determined personalities with differing points of view, but we both were seeking truth in ancient writings and cultures.

We married, and in time we each became a perfect complement to the other. Our life together was a challenging but glorious shared adventure, in which love and respect were forever uppermost, enabling us to overcome the difficult trials that our life often called us to face.

We discovered *Autobiography of a Yogi,* where Spirit and Science meet. How good it was to read the Master's teachings together and spend hours talking about them. With Yogananda's arrival in our home, it became a temple dedicated to Him. My husband and I were one; there was no need for words, because we understood each other by thought.

When he became gravely ill, we spent hours together daily in the hospital. We filled his room with spiritual music and mantras, listening to the voices of Yogananda and Swami Kriyananda. I would bring a book by Master and read it to him. We talked often about death, and he would try to prepare me for the event of his passing, always in a positive way. We would imagine the astral realm, where there is no suffering and the Masters are waiting to welcome us.

Yogananda was tangibly with us, helping my husband to see his forthcoming transition as a liberation. He would say: "I will go to a beautiful place where I will be well, where I will be with Yogananda, and together we will stand by you and guide you." His certainty was staggering to me!

After thirty-five years together, it was his time to leave. I would have preferred to live many years more with him, but I have since learned that love does not end with death. I am often sad because I feel his physical absence, and a nostalgia for our life together. Every day I face that void and fill it with the divine presence, while seeking my own connection with the divine plan. This is where faith, the guru's presence, and the spiritual path have helped me.

As I have learned to rely on that presence, a new world has opened for me. At seventy years young, I have been granted the courage to start new activities in a place far from our mutual home. I work with a group of young spiritual seekers, teaching them the path of Self-realization. My husband was perfectly right: he and Yogananda are guiding me from that other world. I feel my beloved husband always with me, as we continue our service to the Guru together. –**Lucilla**, *Monte Visconti, Italy*

The act of lovingly offering our service to others is deeply fulfilling. After the passing of her husband, Lucilla embraced the opportunity to redefine her life, even leaving her home to move to a distant region. Another widowed devotee, found meaning through service.

> When my husband passed, the best cure that helped me overcome the sadness was to work hard physically in the garden, to clean house, and to serve others. Each evening, I asked myself: What did I do today for another person? When I didn't know how to help someone, I would just make cookies and bring them to the neighbors.
>
> –***Gordana***, *Rijeka, Croatia*

Contacting your departed loved one

The love and support that two or more souls have shared during their earthly life can continue as strongly as ever, even after one partner has passed on to a higher realm. When our loved ones are in a physical body, a hug, a caress, or a glance of loving compassion can comfort them; but when they are no longer physically present, we will need to seek other ways. The bridge that connects us to our loved ones is love itself. When we are able to keep this feeling alive in our hearts and broadcast it to them in meditation and prayer, the departed souls are sure to perceive it, wherever they are, whether on the astral plane, and even if they have been reborn.

> If time cannot make you forget a departed friend, then try to contact him. A continuous desire to know about a departed soul is the best astral broadcasting that you can send forth... If you carry the feeling of the presence of your departed friend, and then try to concentrate with closed eyes upon the spot between the eyebrows and visualize him, he will appear to you after some time. It may take months, or even years, but if you are patient and keep on every increasing the depth of the astral call of meditation, you will succeed.
>
> Every night, with closed eyes, concentrate in the Christ Center, or the astral broadcasting microphone of the spiritual eye, and broadcast your good will to your departed ones by mentally saying: "Resurrect, and be quickened in God." They will get your message. Then sit in silence and try to feel their love, and when you feel exhilarated, know that they have answered you.[6]

CHAPTER 8: *Points to Remember*

- Our meaningful interactions with others improve our physical health and our mental and emotional well-being.
- Our close relationships will span many lives – the people who are known to us now are souls we have known before.
- Sensitivity to the realities of others becomes more refined through the stages of human evolution: from the dull shudra, to the active vaishya, the noble kshatriya, and the God-inspired brahmin. Meaningful, reciprocal relationships are more possible as human consciousness evolves.
- Friendship is the purest kind of relationship, for in friendship, love is given voluntarily.
- Friendship gives us opportunities to express and experience God's unconditional love.
- Accepting and respecting others exactly as they are is the basis for all health-enhancing relationships.
- Relationships that are fraught with conflict and oppression are a major cause of illness.
- Each person in a relationship is a key player, and each is responsible for the quality of the relationship.
- A spiritual partnership is one in which both parties commit to help each other grow in unconditional divine love.
- It may be necessary for our own health and that of our partner to end a relationship.
- How a relationship ends will set its course for the future, for relationships continue from life to life.
- Loving relationships transcend death.

NOTES | PART X

Title Page
1 Yogananda, *The Essence of Self-Realization*, 16:7.

Chapter One
1 Yogananda, "Vibration," *Inner Culture*, July 1936.
2 Dr. Seppala, Emma, "Connectedness & Health: The Science of Social Connection," Stanford Medicine Center for Compassion and Altruism Research and Education, May 8, 2014, http://ccare.stanford.edu/uncategorized/connectedness-health -the-science-of-social-connection-infographic/.
3 "Do Social Ties Affect our Health? National Institute of Health News, February 2017, https://newsinhealth.nih.gov/2017/02/do-social-ties-affect-our-health.
4 "Life," CNN Health, https://edition.cnn.com/videos/health/2023/03/28/dementia-prevention-tips-lbb-orig.cnn.
5 Yogananda, "Why Our Loved Ones Die," *Inner Culture*, August 1934.
6 Moody, Raymond, *Life After Life*, https://www.goodreads.com/book/show/28790866-life-after-life;* https://near-death.com/raymond-moody/.

Chapter Two
1 Yogananda, "The Art of Gaining Friends," *Inner Culture*, March 1936.
2 Yogananda, "True Friendship," *Inner Culture*, March 1940.
3 Yogananda, *Super-Advanced Course No. 1*, Lesson 4.
4 To the likely disappointment of many of their fans, Olympic ice dance gold medalists Tessa Virtue and Scott Moir were not romantically involved. Their twenty-year friendship and collaboration on and off the ice is an exquisite example of how close friends can grow together personally and professionally.
5 Yogananda, *Super-Advanced Course No. 1*, Lesson 4.
6 Kriyananda, *Education for Life*, 35.
7 Yogananda, *The Essence of Self-Realization*, 16:12.
8 Yogananda, *Advanced Course No. 1*, Lesson 12.
9 Yogananda, *Super Advanced Course No. 1*, Lesson 4.
10 Yogananda, Lesson 4.
11 Kriyananda, *The Road Ahead*, 79-80.
12 www.ananda.org; www.anandaeurope.org; www.anandaindia.org.
13 Kriyananda, "Clarity in Relationships," *Cities of Light*, 60.
14 Yogananda, "Spiritual Interpretations of the Scriptures," *East-West*, April 1932.
15 Kriyananda, "Attunement," *Sadhu, Beware!*, 126.
16 Yogananda, "Poems," *Whispers from Eternity*, 199.

Chapter Three
1 Kriyananda, *Hope for a Better World*, 188-189.
2 Kriyananda, *Secrets of Friendship*, Day Nine.
3 Yogananda, "The Art of Gaining Friends," *Inner Culture*, May 1936.
4 Kriyananda, *Hope for a Better World*, 188-189.
5 Kriyananda, *Hindu Way of Awakening*, 228.
6 Kriyananda, *Do It NOW!*, November 27.
7 Yogananda, *Super Advanced Course No. 1*, Lesson 4.
8 Kriyananda, "Moral Vigor," *Affirmations for Self-Healing*, 110.
9 Kriyananda, *Conversations with Yogananda* No. 457.
10 Yogananda, *Super Advanced Course No. 1*, Lesson 4.

11 Kriyananda, *Intuition for Starters*, 41.
12 Kriyananda, *Sadhu, Beware!*, IV:23, 29.
13 Kriyananda, *Conversations with Yogananda* No. 237.
14 Gail Saltz, MD, is a clinical associate professor of psychiatry at the NY Presbyterian Hospital Weill-Cornell School of Medicine.
15 Lindberg, Sara, M.Ed, "How Does Your Environment Affect Your Mental Health?," *verywell mind*, March 23, 2023, https://www.verywellmind.com/how-your-environment-affects-your-mental-health-5093687.
16 De Vogli R, Chandola T, Marmot MG. Negative Aspects of Close Relationships and Heart Disease. Arch Intern Med. 2007;167(18):1951–1957. doi:10.1001/archinte.167.18.1951.
17 Cole, Will, "The Science Behind How Toxic Relationships Affect Mental Health," Dr. Will Cole, https://drwillcole.com/mindful-living/the-science-behind-how-toxic-relationships-affect-your-health.
18 Kriyananda, "How Well Do You Get Along with Others?," *Clarity Magazine*, Winter 2011.

Chapter Four

1 Yogananda, *Super Advanced Course No. 1*, Lesson 4.
2 Yogananda, *Advanced Course on Practical Metaphysics*, Lesson 7.
3 Yogananda, "Spiritual Marriage," *Inner Culture*, May 1940. You will find the complete article in the online Appendices.
4 Yogananda, *Praecepta Lesson*s, Vol. 3:59.
5 Maqbook, Aleem, "The monk and the nun who fell in love and married," 2 January, 2023, BBC, https://www.bbc.com/news/uk-64125531. The ancient Hindu tradition, in accordance with the Laws of Manu, provided for a stage of monastic training before a young person would consider marrying.

During the *brahmacharya* stage, from approximately age six to twenty-four, the young person would study in the ashram of a spiritual master, leading a monastic life that emphasized self-control and spiritual discipline.

Most brahmacharis would then enter the *grihastha* stage, where the focus was on starting a family, supporting the family, and contributing to society. Other brahmacharis could decide to remain monastics for the rest of their lives.

At roughly age fifty, when their children had left home, the *grihastha* couple would retire from worldly activities to live in or near a spiritual ashram or community, focusing once again on their spiritual development. In modern times the couple might volunteer their time and resources to support spiritual and charitable causes, go on pilgrimages, and serve in a religious or spiritual organization as lay members.

In the final stage, known as *sannyasa*, the focus of the monastic would turn to attaining spiritual Self-realization, or in the case of those sufficiently advanced, serving as a spiritual guide to help others attain their liberation.

6 Yogananda, *Super-Advanced Course No. 1*, Lesson 4.
7 Yogananda, "Spiritual Marriage," *Inner Culture*, May 1940.
8 Yogananda, *Super-Advanced Course No. 1*, Lesson 4.
9 Kriyananda, *Self-Expansion Through Marriage*, 137.
10 Kriyananda, *Cities of Light*, 118.
11 Yogananda, *The Essence of the Bhagavad Gita*, Verse 6:43, 288.
12 Yogananda, *Yogoda Course*, Lesson 9.
13 Yogananda, *The Essence of Self-Realization*, 9:4.
14 Yogananda, *Yogoda Course*, Lesson 9.

15 Kriyananda, "Guidelines for Conduct of Members of Ananda Sevaka Order," Article 7.
16 Yogananda, "Spiritual Marriage," *Inner Culture*, May 1940.
17 Kriyananda, *Self-Expansion Through Marriage*, 62.
18 Kriyananda, 68.
19 Yogananda, "How to Keep the Church Steadfast, *East-West*, September 1933.
20 Yogananda, "Spiritual Marriage," *Inner Culture*, May, 1940.
21 Kriyananda, *Self-Expansion Through Marriage*, 61.
22 Kriyananda, *Rays of the Same Light*, Week 22, 62.
23 Kriyananda, *Self-Expansion Through Marriage*, 62-63.

Chapter Five

1 This compilation of advice from Yogananda for couples is drawn from the following three sources: *Spiritual Relationships*, Chapter Four; "Art of Finding True Friends of Past Incarnations"; *Super-Advanced Course No. 1*, Lesson 4 (which can be found in the online Appendices); *Praecepta Lessons*, Vol. 3:60.
2 This compilation is drawn from Chapters Six and Seven of Kriyananda's book *Self-Expanion Through Marriage*, and from his *In Divine Friendship, Letters of Counsel and Reflection*, Chapter Five.

Chapter Seven

1 Yogananda, *Praecepta Lessons*, Vol. 2:44.
2 Yogananda, *Yogoda Course*, Lesson 9.
3 Kriyananda, *Self-Expansion Through Marriage*, 78.
4 Kriyananda, *Conversations with Yogananda* No. 13.
5 Kriyananda, *Self-Expansion Through Marriage*, 153-154.
6 Yogananda, *Praecepta Lessons*, Vol. 3:61.
7 Kriyananda, *Self-Expansion Through Marriage*, 78.
8 Yogananda, *Praecepta Lessons*, Vol. 3:61.

Chapter Eight

1 Yogananda, "Why Our Loved Ones Die," *Inner Culture*, August 1934. You will find this article in the online Appendices.
2 The death of a loved one is recognized as one of life's greatest stresses and has long been associated with increased health risk, especially for the surviving spouse or parent.... In 1963, a follow-up of 4486 widowers, comparing their mortality to that of married men, reported a 40% increased mortality rate in the first 6 months of bereavement, with little differential thereafter....In a recent study bereaved participants had a higher risk than nonbereaved participants of dying from any cause...including cardiovascular disease, coronary heart disease, stroke, all cancer, smoking-related cancer, and accidents or violence. In one 10-year follow-up study, it was shown that increased health risk may continue for many years after bereavement, especially in surviving spouses. "Physiological correlates of bereavement and the impact of bereavement interventions," National Library of Medicine, https://www.ncbi.nlm.nih.gov/pmc/articles/PMC3384441/.
3 Yogananda, "Life Everlasting," *Inner Culture*, February 1936.
4 Kriyananda, "General Advice: Death," *Letters to Truthseekers*, 17-18.
5 Yogananda, "Solving the Mystery of This Cosmic Movie House," *East-West*, March 1933.
6 Yogananda, *Advanced Super Cosmic Science Course*, Lesson 5.

PART XI
PROSPERITY AND SUCCESS

Know at all times that *you, as God's child,* own everything that belongs to the Father… Your native endowment is perfection and prosperity…"[1]

—YOGANANDA

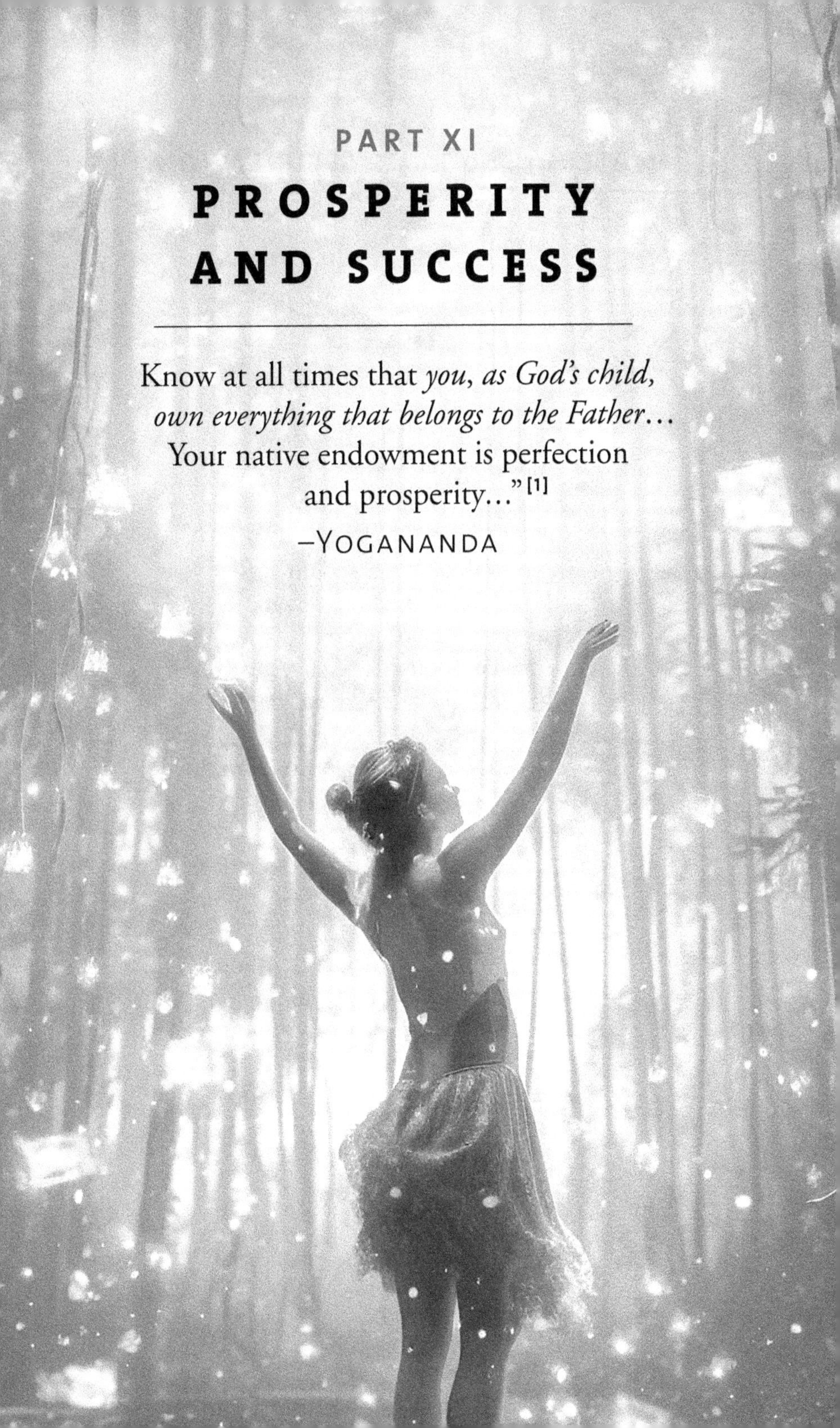

MATERIAL SUCCESS AFFIRMATION
by SWAMI YOGANANDA

Thou art my Father
Success and joy
I am Thy child
Success and joy
All the wealth of this earth
All the riches of the universe
Belong to Thee, belong to Thee.
I am Thy child
The wealth of earth and universe
Belongs to me, belongs to me
O belongs to me, belongs to me.
I lived in thoughts of poverty
And wrongly fancied I was poor
So I was poor.
Now I am home and Thy consciousness
Has made me wealthy, made me rich.
I am success, I am rich
Thou art my Treasure, I am rich, I am rich.
Thou art everything, Thou art everything
Thou art mine
I have everything, I have everything
I am wealthy, I am rich
I have everything, I have everything
I possess all and everything
Even as Thou dost, even as Thou dost
I possess everything, I possess everything.
Thou art my wealth
I have everything.

Scientific Healing Affirmations, 1924

PART XI CHAPTER ONE

Why seek prosperity

> Prosperity does not consist just in the making of money; it also consists in acquiring the mental efficiency by which man can uniformly acquire health, wealth, wisdom, and peace at will.[1] –YOGANANDA
>
> The goal of your material life should be maximum business efficiency, peace, health, and general success. Material prosperity consists in acquiring the mental efficiency by which you can gain all these things at will.[2] –YOGANANDA
>
> Every day strive to be healthy, wealthy [and] wise.[3] –YOGANANDA

How does our physical, emotional, mental, and spiritual health influence our prosperity and success? While it is self-evident that wealthy people aren't always healthy, a lack of economic resources can raise obstacles that make it more difficult to achieve a healthy, balanced, successful life.

> As human beings, we have been endowed with needs and we must meet their demands. As man is a physical, mental, spiritual being, he must look after his all-round welfare, avoiding one-sided, over-development. To possess wonderful health and a good appetite, with no money to maintain that health and to satisfy that hunger, is agonizing.[4]

"Prosperity" and "wealth" are not synonymous. A "prosperous" person will be content to possess whatever he requires to fulfill his material obligations and engage in creative and spiritual pursuits — whereas a "wealthy" person may be consumed by a voracious appetite for accumulating ever more wealth. In pursuing material riches, we may easily lose our true wealth — our inner peace, happiness, health, and friendships.

> Make contentment your criterion of prosperity...
> Be ever comfortable within your means.[5]

> If money-making for securing the material comforts of man is necessary, then making happiness is supremely necessary. For possession of material riches without inner peace is just like dying of thirst while bathing in a lake.[6]

Spiritual prosperity

Material prosperity flows naturally from spiritual prosperity, not the other way around.

> And seek not ye what ye shall eat,
> or what ye shall drink, neither be ye of
> doubtful mind. For all these things
> do the nations of the world seek after:
> and your Father knoweth that ye
> have need of these things.
> But rather seek ye the kingdom of God;
> and all these things shall be added
> unto you. (LUKE 12: 29-31)*

---

* This and all Bible citations are from the King James Bible.

> I will seek God first, and make sure of my actual contact with Him; then, if it is His will, all things – wisdom, abundance and health – will be added as part of my divine birthright, since He made me in His image. I want prosperity, health and wisdom without measure, not from earthly sources, but from God's abundant, all-possessing, all-powerful, all-bountiful hands.[7]

People who compromise their moral and spiritual principles to gain material security always end up feeling insecure. Stocks, bonds, and crypto-currencies are ephemeral – their value fluctuates whimsically. A lovely vacation house by the ocean can be swept away. But a home that is built on the bedrock of inner peace will weather any storm.

The astral law of prosperity

The eager accumulation of wealth will never bring us health, harmony, or happiness, as we often see in the lives of the rich and famous. Whatever abundance we have is meant to be shared.

> Those who seek prosperity for themselves only, are bound to be poor for some time, or to suffer from mental inharmony, but those who take the world as their home and who really think and work for group or world prosperity, start the Astral forces to work, leading them to the place where they can find their legitimate prosperity. This is the surest secret law. Prosperity is not dependent only upon creative ability, but upon your past actions, and also on the Astral law of cause and effect, which has the power to distribute prosperity equally to all without exception. Those who rouse this Astral power of positive prosperity succeed wherever they go, whether they are in prosperous or poverty-stricken environments.[8]

Circumstances as a springboard

Stories abound of children born to privilege who turn to drugs, crime, and even self-destruction. Children born into a wealthy home may not be strongly motivated to develop their character and talents, whereas others born into poverty may be highly motivated not only to lift themselves but to help others.

✺ THE NEWSPAPER BOY ✺
WHO BECAME PRESIDENT

His ancestors were wealthy Tamil Nadu traders, but by the time Abdul was born in 1931 the family had fallen into dire poverty. His mother often went hungry to ensure that her five children were fed, and Abdul sold newspapers to help provide his parents and siblings with food.

The school in his small fishing village offered little in the way of serious studies, yet Abdul had a burning desire to learn. He spent hours studying mathematics on his own. Watching the birds at the seashore, he knew that his destiny would be intimately related to flight.

Abdul's will to learn was so strong that he came to the notice of a teacher who arranged for him to study at a better high school in a nearby city. Abdul flourished, and after overcoming many obstacles, he received a degree in aerospace engineering from the prestigious Madras Institute of Technology.

In his 1998 book, *India 2020: A Vision for the New Millennium*, he proposed a nationwide plan for making India a developed country. The plan, used as a roadmap to this day, included designs for nuclear power improvements, technological innovations, and increased agricultural productivity.

After being named Principal Scientific Adviser to the Government of India in 1999, Abdul became India's president in 2002 with the support of 89% of the votes and the love and respect of his countrymen. His concern for education and culture had earned him the epithet "the people's president."

He was the perfect embodiment of a principle that Yogananda strongly endorsed: "simple living and high thinking." He remained humble and modest, owning no real estate, television, or air conditioner, and he never asked for money for his talks. Although a practicing Muslim, he regularly read the *Bhagavad Gita*. He became a friend and follower of Pramukh Swami, writing the book *Transcendence* about his experiences with the master.[9]

He said, "People think India is poor. It is only our thinking that is poor. If we think big, we can become big.... All of us do not have equal talent. But all of us have an equal opportunity to develop our talents."

After his term in office, he launched the "What Can I Give" movement to develop an expansive, generous attitude among India's youth, encouraging them to contribute toward nation building by taking manageable positive steps.

Abdul Kalam's dream to give his country wings encouraged him to take many small steps – facing poverty with hard work, overcoming meager educational resources with a resolve to learn, and meeting scientific challenges with determination. In the end, he earned a place of international prominence and respect for himself and his country.

In the following chapters, we will delve into the laws of success and discover spiritual secrets we can apply to become more healthy, prosperous, and wise.

PART XI CHAPTER TWO

Poverty or Prosperity

Wealth is the *consciousness* of abundance. And Poverty is the *consciousness* of lack. Wealth and poverty are both states of mind. You are as rich, or as poor, as you believe yourself to be.[1] –KRIYANANDA

You must eradicate from your mind all thought of lack or poverty. Universal Mind is perfect, it knows no lack; and to reach that never-failing supply, you must create a consciousness of abundance – even if you do not know where the next dollar is to come from. When you refuse to be apprehensive, when you do your part and rely on God to do His, you will find that mysterious forces will come to your aid and your constructive wishes will materialize.[2] –YOGANANDA

✸ PENURY TO PROSPERITY ✸
Told by Swami Yogananda, Abridged

As there are habitual criminals and also naturally successful people, so there are habitual failures. My friend and student, John, was such a born failure. He was young, intelligent, diligent, and painstaking in his pursuit of money-making, but it seemed that no matter what job or business he gave his attention to, it resulted in abject failure. Harassed, deserted, penniless, he sought the shelter of my advice.

I questioned John as to the cause of his troubles. He replied: "Sir, I am a great failure. For some mysterious reason, not only do I lose my job but usually my employer loses his business after employing me. I hate to seek a job for fear of destroying the business of my new employer through the deathly grip of my failure vibration."

Through my influence John got a job in a small business concern and I advised him to affirm daily, before going to bed and upon waking: "Day by day, in every way, I am succeeding more and more in my job."

A month passed and John returned: "Honored Sir, the business concern you got me into is starting to fail. Please take me out before it goes on the rocks completely. Perhaps my resignation will save the business from destruction.

I told John to keep up his affirmation of success and to hold on to his job. After a fortnight John came to me one evening, and with a sigh of relief exclaimed: "It happened: the business concern collapsed,"

I turned to John and remonstrated: "While you have been affirming 'Day by day I am getting better and better,' isn't it true that, way in the background of your mind a little octopus of obstinate mentality has kept on mentally saying: 'You little simpleton, day by day, in every way, you know that you are getting worse and worse, no matter how much you repeat that you are getting better?'" He admitted the truth of this.

I advised John to be sure to cast out all strong negative vibrations as soon as they visited his mind, because a convinced, conscious mind influences the subconsciousness, which in turn, through the law of inner psychological reciprocity, influences the conscious mind through the power of habit.

I told John that his success was conditioned by his creative ability, his environment, and his pre-natal and post-natal habits and tendencies, and that if he contacted the all-powerful, unlimited superconscious mind, then alone could he create a new cause for absolute success.

I succeeded in getting John into a bigger business and after six months he said to me: "Sir, this business has also failed." "John, never mind, I will get you another job." I secured for John a very good job in a very big concern.

A year passed and nothing untoward happened.

I asked John now to invest his money in a business of his own. He was beside himself with fear: "If I invest the money I have saved, I am sure to lose it." I firmly assured him: "You must invest your money and energy in some good project which requires no large investment nor overhead, and I am sure that you will succeed." In the course of a few years, John became the successful owner of a handful of chain stores.

Once he was thoroughly convinced of his success, he found himself succeeding in everything that he undertook. One day he laughingly said: "Through God and you I am now changed from a great failure to a great success. Pray tell me the reason? I can understand my own failure due to lack of understanding, but I cannot understand why I succeeded in demolishing other peoples' businesses."

I replied: "You were not the cause of their failure. The law of attraction which governs people of like vibrations operated in the case. Being a failure attracted you to a business about to fail, and vice versa. You were a failure and the business was about to fail too. By law of affinity, you went down the hill of failure together to explode at the same time."

Let it be remembered that absolute success signifies "the power to create at will what you need by developing your unlimited superconscious power." This superconscious power can be awakened by knowing the definite technique of meditation, as taught by the Master Minds of India in order to produce prosperity, health, success, wisdom, and God-contact at any time, at will, and without limitation.[3]

Some people appear to have the Midas touch – everything they attempt turns to gold – while others seem to be cursed with failure at every turn, even after putting forth their best efforts. Where is the justice? In the ever-just Law of Karma*, we find that the seeds of success or failure, prosperity or poverty, have been sown over long incarnations and merely blossom in this life. These tendencies are part of our metaphysical genetic makeup, telling of past history, but not of our future destiny.

> The failures and successes of everyday life become rooted in the mind. Unless they come to fruition or are worked out by wisdom, they bear seeds which the soul must carry over into another incarnation as tendencies and traits. These stubborn ghosts of the past are hiding in the recesses of your mind, emerging suddenly to help and inspire or hinder and discourage, according to the circumstances confronting you. It is for this reason that so many people fail in their undertakings, in spite of their conscious efforts.... Friendly success tendencies are ready to help an individual, and inimical failure tendencies to crush him, depending in the first cast on his unflinching efforts, and in the second on his attitude of resignation to "his fate." These are his invisible friends and also his unseen enemies....[4]

The tendencies toward poverty and failure that we have carried over from past lives are manifesting in this life as mental deficiencies that, unless we make an effort to address them here and now, will continue to plague us, and may in time become chronic psychological diseases.

* See Part I, Volume One for a discussion about the Law of Karma

> Most people fail and are not prosperous
> because they have hypnotized themselves with
> the consciousness of their failures and they do not
> make repeated, steady efforts to succeed.[5]

Even if our karmic seeds of success and prosperity are few, nevertheless they exist; and with proper spiritual gardening we can help them flourish and prevail over the toxic weeds of lack.

Where are these seed tendencies? Our memories of past failures and the related fears are stored in the subconscious. The conscious mind dwells on these memories and reinforces them with thoughts that we are poor or prosperous, a success-in-the-making or a chronic failure.

> All the successes and failures and troubles of
> many, many lives are packed as seed tendencies
> in your present brain of consciousness,
> subconsciousness, and superconsciousness.[6]

> If you are firmly convinced you are a failure,
> change your mental attitude at once;
> be unshakable in your conviction that you
> have all the potentialities of great success.[7]

The superconscious mind is able to see the whole picture, and how all of our past experiences, painful and positive, have been spiritually instructive and helpful to us.

> A man striving for permanent success must
> meditate every morning and night, and when the
> superconscious peace-and-concentration rays break
> through the nocturnal blackness of restlessness,
> he must concentrate these rays on the brain and mind,
> scorching out the lurking seeds of past failures and
> stimulating the success tendencies.[8]

Failure as a stepping stone to success

> I have not failed. I've just found 10,000 ways that won't work.... People are not remembered by how few times they fail, but by how often they succeed. Every wrong step is another step forward.
> —Thomas A. Edison

In his book for teachers and parents, *Education for Life,* Swami Kriyananda describes our failures as a necessary part of our journey to eventual success.

> Failure...is an instrument of learning. Every failure accepted, understood, then placed resolutely behind one can be an important stepping stone to higher achievement.
>
> It is never wise, then, to say, "I've failed." The courage that leads to achievement says, "I haven't yet succeeded." The repeated thought of failure acts as a negative affirmation; if it doesn't actually attract failure, it creates the conditions for failure by slowly weakening the will power. But the repeated thought of success, even in the face of repeated failures, is an affirmation that *must*, eventually, produce the achievement one desires.[9]

When we define a project as a failure, or worse, if we identify ourself as a failure, the subconscious mind is ready to supply us with negative feelings that will further imprison us in failure consciousness. But if we see the inevitable setbacks not as failures but as necessary stepping stones to success, we will be free to use our conscious powers of reason to reflect on our mistakes and ask the superconscious to tell us what we can improve.

> If failures invade you repeatedly, don't get discouraged. They should act as stimulants and not poisons to your material or spiritual growth.[10]
>
> The season of failure is the best time for sowing the seeds of success...Weed out the causes of failure by searching for them, and then with double vigor launch forth on whatever you wish to accomplish... Every new effort after failure brings true growth. But it must be well planned and charged with increasing intensity of attention and with dynamic will power....[11]

Although we may imagine in our moments of failure that we are unworthy of God's grace, Swami Kriyananda assures us that this is very far from true.

> God will often bless you more if you're unsuccessful, because you had the courage to try in the face of such obstacles.[12]

Recipe for transforming failure to success

- Instill thoughts of success at all levels of consciousness with this affirmation, on waking, before sleep, and during the day.

  > *"The sunshine of His prosperity has just burst through the dark sky of my limitation. I am God's child. What He has, I have."* [13]

- Accept and analyze each failure, and make a success plan that will avoid those failure traps – then act on your plan daily until you have achieved your goal.
- Use your willpower every day – make repeated, steady efforts to succeed in a realistic endeavor.
- Make repeated, judicious efforts in daily meditation to awaken your sleeping success tendencies.

PART XI CHAPTER THREE

The Law of Magnetism

> Success in any field depends more on magnetism...than on knowledge. For magnetism *attracts* success, whereas knowledge merely tells you how success has been achieved by others.[1] –KRIYANANDA
>
> The human magnet draws according to its power of attraction. Some people attract physical things, some attract mental things, and some attract spiritual things. It depends on what kind of a magnet one wishes to be. We must develop two kinds of magnetism–one to attract God and another to attract our material necessities. If we use all our magnetism to gain material things, sooner or later we shall be disillusioned. It is true that God gave us bodies, and we must look after them; but if we first develop spiritual magnetism, it will guide us in the proper ways to supply all our material needs.[2] –YOGANANDA

We are attracted to some people and repelled by others. Visiting a place for the first time, we may feel comfortable and at home, whereas other places will make us feel nervous and eager to leave. We feel drawn to certain teachers and speakers, and wary of others. Even without knowing how the law of magnetism works, we are affected by its power to attract and repel. When we know how the law operates, we can use it to obtain almost anything, more directly, quickly, and confidently than with a haphazard "trial-and-error" approach.

Prosperity and success are intricately linked to the Law of Magnetism on physical and metaphysical levels. Swami Kriyananda often gave the example of the molecules in a bar of iron. When the molecules are aligned randomly, the bar has no magnetism, but when the molecules are aligned, the bar emits a powerful magnetic field that attracts other iron-containing objects. The mind, he said, is like the iron bar. When our thoughts and efforts are aligned in a single, focused direction, we develop the magnetism to attract the resources we need to achieve our objective. But if our thoughts are vague and scattered or in conflict, success is unlikely.

Formula for success

Yogananda assures us that when are able to activate the various components of the Law of Magnetism and bring them to bear on our desired goal, prosperity and success will be ours. In this chapter, we will consider each of these components and learn how we can combine them to achieve our "legitimate prosperity."

We have considered these "ingredients" in past chapters, and now we are meeting them in a new context.

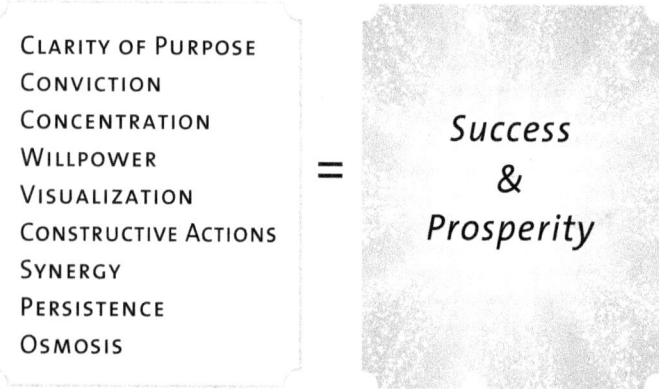

CLARITY OF PURPOSE
CONVICTION
CONCENTRATION
WILLPOWER
VISUALIZATION
CONSTRUCTIVE ACTIONS
SYNERGY
PERSISTENCE
OSMOSIS

= *Success & Prosperity*

Clarity of Purpose

The American comedian W. C. Fields said, "If you don't know where you're going, any road will take you there." In the context of magnetism, it's easy to imagine Yogananda responding: "Once you know where you're going and you are determined to get there, you will attract all of the resources you need."

First, then, form a clear idea in your mind of the kind of solution you want. Don't ask for an answer vaguely. At the same time, don't pray in the vague hope that the answer will suddenly appear. Rather, tell your superconscious specifically what you want.[3]

Go deep into the calm region where your inner Self reigns. As soon as you are attuned with your soul, you will be able to think correctly regarding everything you do, and if your thoughts or actions have gone astray they can be realigned.[4]

In our journey to prosperity and success, we can receive guidance most reliably from the calm region of the superconscious. In superconsciousness we see our projects and plans as part of the greater scheme of our spiritual evolution – something that will benefit us and possibly others, that will harm no one, including ourselves, and that has the support of the universe.

It's important also to have a clear idea of the *inner experience* we hope to achieve by our accomplishments. If your goal is to find a good job, you might not merely want a high salary, but also work that you can be passionate about, that challenges you, and that will allow you to make a worthwhile creative contribution.

Be aware that a too-specific goal such as "I want to earn x-amount of money per month" could prevent you from receiving all that the universe has in store for you.

A cautionary note: activating the Law of Magnetism can bring us whatever we desire, but if our desire isn't consistent with our highest good, obtaining it might take us in a dangerous direction that will only bring us suffering.

People of strong willpower and high energy can obtain wealth, success, and power to the detriment of their health and spiritual evolution. Famous people have suffered in this regard – perhaps you have known strong-minded people who have achieved results that failed to make them happy, healthy, or wise.

This is why it is vital to align our efforts with our *dharma* from the start – that we align ourselves with the directions that will be most consistent with our spiritual development. Yogananda said that we should **"not will and act first, but contact God first and thus harness [our] will and activity to the right goal.**"[5] Attunement with Spirit will align our efforts with a power and protection far greater than our limited human abilities and resources.

Conviction

Along with being clear about our purpose, we need to be confident that we are capable of achieving it.

> **Believe you are inherently healthy when you want good health; believe you are inherently prosperous when you want prosperity; believe you are inherently wise when you want wisdom – then health, prosperity, and wisdom will manifest themselves in you.**[6]

Strong clarity and conviction will help us set the Law of Magnetism in motion.

> **A person who believes in his own power and in the power of God continuously without doubt can accomplish everything, spiritual or material, whatever he wants.**[7]

We need to reinforce our initial conviction constantly in order to overcome the demotivators that are bound to try to turn us away from our goal. Affirmations are a powerful tool to help us keep the interlopers of negative thoughts and feelings at bay, especially affirmations that express a powerful statement of our intention, while at the same time consciously expressing our desire to align ourselves and our efforts with the power of the universe.

> "Father, I am Thy child, guide me
> to my right prosperity."[8]

Concentration

Once we have established a clear purpose, we should make it the target of every effort, keeping it strongly focused like a laser.

Whereas a light bulb casts a relatively weak and diffused light in many directions, in a laser beam the light waves are concentrated in a narrow linewidth that can traverse long distances and deliver a great deal of energy to a small area. Laser light has been beamed to the moon and back to measure the distance from earth. Lasers are used to cut through metals, and even diamonds, the hardest naturally occurring substance on earth.

Our thoughts can have the diffused power of a flashlight, or the concentrated power of a laser beam. When our thoughts are scattered, they lack the focus and power to achieve a successful result.

> On every level of mental activity, it is
> concentration that is the key to success...
> Concentration it is that awakens our powers
> and channels them, dissolving obstacles
> in our path, literally attracting opportunities,
> insights, and inspirations. In many ways,
> subtle as well as obvious, concentration is
> the single most important key to success.[9]

Whenever Swami Kriyananda was engaged in writing a book, it would become a major focus of his conversations, and often a centerpiece of his public talks. It can be tempting to let our thoughts wander, or to allow ourselves to be distracted or so mentally overwhelmed that we give up, relaxing with a sigh and putting the project on a shelf where it will shortly become stale. But tenacity, almost obsessive tenacity, and mental discipline are required in order to suceed.

> If you learn how to withdraw your attention from all objects of distraction and place it upon one object of concentration, then you will know how to attract at will what you need.[10]

> The deep power of concentration that comes through daily meditation enables a person to resolve an issue in minutes perhaps, where, otherwise, he might have fretted over it for weeks. Even more important, where the will is concerned, the concentration that comes due to regular meditation generates with perfect naturalness the strength of will that is necessary for success in any undertaking.[11]

For many years, I was a bit over-enamored of multitasking, considering it a mental strength. But I remember how in the course of a conversation with Swami Kriyananda, I mentioned my admiration for an Indian spiritual teacher who was able to dictate five books to five secretaries simultaneously – and how Swamiji was unimpressed. He reminded me how Yogananda had insisted that we should concentrate on one thing at a time, on doing it well and thoroughly.

> Devote your entire will power to accomplishing one thing at a time, do not scatter your energies or leave something half done to begin a new venture.[12]

> We can accomplish a great deal in life, if we can discipline ourselves to do one thing at a time, to do it wholeheartedly, and not to worry distractedly about all the things we'd like to accomplish, or wish we had accomplished in the past.[13]

Life Force / 110

Concentration exercises

Long periods of intense mental work requiring our full concentration can result in tension and fatigue. These simple exercises (also mentioned in Part VI of Volume One) will help you refresh your mental powers. You can do them in roughly a minute, before and during any work that calls for deep concentration. The exercises stimulate the blood circulation and help bring oxygen and energy to the brain.

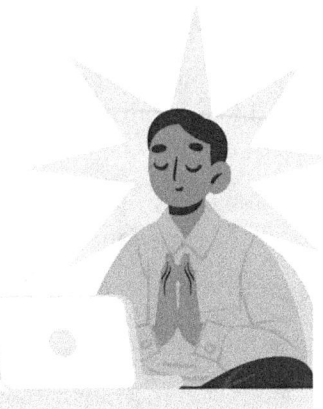

- *Massage the medulla oblongata.** Place the middle three fingers of both hands firmly in the indentation at the base of the skull, and with pressure, massage that point in all directions.

- *Skull tapping.* Vigorously strike the skull and forehead with the knuckles of both hands for at least 30 seconds. With closed eyes, imagine that each blow is stimulating the brain cells, flooding them with energy and intelligence.

- *Hair pulling.* Insert the fingers of both hands into your hair and pull the hair upward from the roots. If you have no hair, proceed to the next exercise.

- *Scalp massage.* Whereas the previous exercises stimulate the brain cells and head, this exercise relaxes physical and mental tension. Place your fingertips firmly on the scalp and move it backward and forward, side to side, and in a circular motion.

- *Herbal aids:* I've found that applying lavender oil to the forehead and a few drops of Brahmi oil to the crown of the head helps relax and focus my mind.

---

* The vital importance of the medulla oblongata is explained in Volume One, Part III, Chapter Three.

Willpower*

Whereas our thoughts give direction to our actions, willpower generates the energy that creates a magnetic field.

> Will power is the key to awakening energy. Yogananda used to say, 'The greater the will, the greater the flow of energy.' We can apply this principle to the task of keeping the body in good health and healing our illnesses. We can apply it also to drawing inspiration at will. For energy in the body, like electricity in a copper wire, generates a magnetic field, and that magnetism attracts to itself its own affinities, and repels that for which it has no affinity. A strong thought, when directed by will power, can generate the magnetism necessary to attract solutions to any problem one faces. That magnetism can attract true friends, hoped-for opportunities, and success in any undertaking.[14]

The start of a new project or direction is exciting and invigorating, but as time passes and the road to success turns out to be longer than we expected, our energy may flag. Success is a marathon, not a sprint. To keep our willpower strong and resilient, we need to exercise it daily, like a physical muscle. When the mind insists on saying "No," we need to forcefully and immediately say "Yes!" and act accordingly.

Another effective approach to strengthen our willpower is practicing the Full Body Life Force Recharge† several times every day. During long periods of concentration, it helps to practice it every hour.

The seat of willpower in the physical body is at the spiritual eye, at the point between the eyebrows. The spiritual eye is the positive pole of the sixth chakra. (The negative pole is at the medulla oblongata, at the base of the skull.) The following exercises will help you magnetize the spiritual eye – and your willpower.

* The importance of willpower is explained in Volume One, Part III, Chapter Four.
† See Volume One, Part IV, Chapter Two.

- While concentrating your vision and feeling between the eyebrows, close your eyes and repeat the following three times: **"I will, with my own will, which flows from the Divine Will, to be healthy, to be well, to be prosperous and spiritual, to be well, to be well."** [15]

- Carrying a thought with dynamic willpower means entertaining that thought until it becomes an outward form. When your will power develops that way, and when you can control your destiny by your willpower, then you can do tremendous things. Before you will to do a thing, reason about it. Make sure that you are directing your will toward accomplishing something good and helpful to yourself and others. [16]

- A tip from Swami Kriyananda: When you want to magnetize a thought, hold it at the spiritual eye and mentally rotate it three times in a clockwise direction.

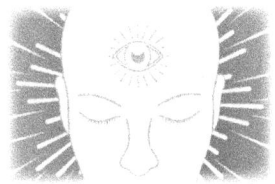

Enemies of will

Every positive attitude, including our eagerness to succeed, is likely to be resisted by subconscious habit-tendencies of reluctance, discouragement, and subtle memories of past failures. Be on the lookout for these enemies.

Unwillingness

> Certain attitudes are inherently more magnetic than others. Willingness, cheerfulness, kindness— all wholesome, spiritual attitudes are magnetic. Unwillingness, discouragement, and similar negative attitudes, on the other hand, are like iron molecules turned conflictingly—or like toxins in the nervous system; they impair the free flow of energy. [17]

Doubt

Doubt is perhaps the greatest obstacle to success. It tries insidiously to insert itself into our affairs in countless subtle ways.

> With too much reasoning comes hesitation, confusion, and doubt. In the end, you may find that your will power has become so paralyzed that you are incapable of acting at all.[18]

When we allow thoughts of doubt and unworthiness to enter the mind, we lose focus and motivation, and our magnetic power to attract success is weakened.

> Will power, combined with faith, directs a clear, unwavering flow of energy. Doubt, on the other hand, interferes with that flow, weakening it, for it creates vortices of indecision...[19] If you could put all your will into making something happen, and not have any conflicting doubt, you would find that your will is enormous.[20]

Procrastination

When we unduly delay an undertaking, the initial inspiration, enthusiasm, willpower – and magnetism – is dissipated and the psychological weight of the uncompleted tasks impedes our creativity.

Visualization

Self-doubt is one of the greatest impediments to success, sneakily inserting itself into the mind. We may think that we are moving toward our goal with full force, yet we could be harboring in our minds images of ourselves struggling to get there. An effective way to release these mental doubts and shore up our power is by strongly visualizing ourselves having already arrived at our goal.

Many champion athletes use visualization to prepare for competition. Research has shown that it can improve their performance as much as forty-five percent. Kayla Harrison, gold medalist in judo at the 2016 Olympics, used it regularly:

> Every night I visualize myself winning the Olympics.... I picture myself (defeating my opponent) in the final and standing on top of the podium and watching the flag go up and feeling the gold medal go around my neck and hugging my coach. I visualize all of that every night. [21]

Strong images and affirmations of success are a powerful aid to help us attain our life's goals. As I write this, I am visualizing these books already published and in your hands, and I am imagining my feelings of gratitude and relief.

Constructive actions

Once your goal is clear, your conviction is firm, and you've activated your willpower, the next step is to engage in energetic and unceasing actions toward your goal.

Whatever we undertake in life, the process is the same: we move from the causal plane – the realm of ideas, where we determine the purpose and construct a mental template – to the astral plane of energy, where we magnetize our thoughts with willpower to create a strong flow of energy and a powerful magnetic field – to the material plane, where we can create a plan of action and set it in motion.

There are any number of ways to achieve our goal, just as there are many paths up a mountainside. Of course, some paths are more direct, and some are less risky. Before we set out, we would do well to ask for guidance in meditation.* If you don't immediately perceive a clear direction, consider the various possibilities and inwardly try to feel which directions resonate with you, your temperament, your talents, and your past experiences.

If your project is substantial, the path to success will likely stretch out over time. It may pass through stages, each of which will give you a direction for the stages that follow. My approach, based on

---

* Techniques for obtaining inner guidance are discussed in Volume Two, Part IX, Chapter Four.

my particular temperament and mental makeup, is that once I have a goal clearly in mind and I feel an inward approval and blessing, I map out what I logically perceive as the various stages. From long experience, I know that I will have to modify this "first draft" many times – there will be course corrections, factors to eliminate, and others to be added.

Once I've recognized that there is a path to completion, I proceed one stage at a time, and within each stage I go forward one step at a time. Taking this book as an example, I set aside about six months for the project. In the first three days, I outlined the entire book, finding that it included three primary themes, each with a host of sub-topics.

Sixteen months later, the book has become a three-book trilogy, containing twelve themes, each of which includes many chapters. Each chapter begins with its own action plan and usually grows beyond it. For example, this chapter now includes double the number of subjects I originally intended to discuss. Like a newborn child, the book seems to have a mind and destiny of its own.

While it's important to have clarity about our goal, it's just as fundamental to be open to new inspirations, and to stay flexible to adapt to changing circumstances.

Any large project will require discipline. There will be temptations to become distracted, to slow down, to procrastinate, and to give up. Some stages will be easy, others will be harder. It's important to set out with a determination to work through the hard stages. When the flow of inspiration is hopelessly blocked, jumping ahead to an easier aspect can often reignite our enthusiasm, renew the inspiration, and bring a fresh flow of energy.

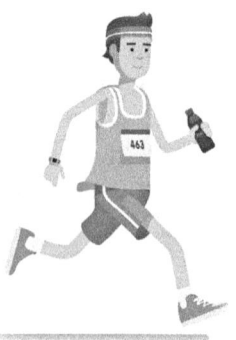

To maintain a magnetic flow of energy and inspiration, it's important to keep moving, but not necessarily at full speed. Pacing is important — periods of activity need to be balanced by periods of rest, just as the systolic contractions of the heart muscle alternate with the diastolic phase when the muscles relax and restore.

When my husband and I trained for the marathon, we followed a balanced and safe training schedule. The weekly recipe included an increasingly long run, three increasingly long medium runs, two short runs, and a day of rest. If we did too much on the short days, we had less energy to stretch the long run. The rest day was essential to let our muscles regenerate and relax the muscles of our mental strength and willpower. By keeping to the schedule, we were able to run a marathon after only three months of training.

In any long-distance project, it's essential to take substantial breaks. Otherwise we can easily get too close to the project and too tensely involved, to a point where we lose our perspective and can no longer see the forest for the trees. Several rest days might be enough to relax and restore our inspiration and enthusiasm so that we can clearly see the project in a new light.

Synergy

Synergy refers to an interaction or cooperation resulting in a whole that is greater than the sum of its parts. (From the Greek *synergos*: to work together; to cooperate.) In a theological sense, synergy refers to the cooperation between humans and God. Bringing divine wisdom and guidance into our plans is an essential step toward success.

> When you want to create something important, sit quietly, calm your senses and your thoughts, and meditate deeply upon what you want to do or acquire. You will then be guided by the great creative power of Spirit. After that you must use all material resources to bring about whatever you wish to accomplish.[22]

Choosing appropriate partners, coworkers, consultants, and mentors can boost the magnetism of a project by broadening our mental horizons and bringing in fresh talent and expertise.

Businesses employ consultants; athletes seek professional coaches, and people in all fields seek wise, experienced, magnetic mentors.

Ask people whom you know to be wise and discriminating when looking for corroboration of your intuition. When inviting collaboration, it is best to present at least a skeletal proposal as a point of reference for their input.

Although inspired projects are generally born of the creative intuition of a single mind, contact with others who share our interests can stimulate our creativity. Among famous authors, we find a fertile exchange of ideas between the Brontë sisters, Dostoyevsky and Turgenev, Hemingway and Gertrude Stein, and C.S. Lewis and J.R.R. Tolkien. Notable friendships between visual artists include Gauguin and Van Gogh, Degas and Manet, Pissarro and Cezanne. And while there were as many rivalries as friendships during the Renaissance, we see a fertile exchange of ideas between Leonardo and Michelangelo, Donatello and Raphael, Lippi and Botticelli, and Ghiberti and Brunelleschi.

*Persistence**

In nuclear physics, a certain amount of effort (fissile material) is required for self-sustaining results (fission). In everyday life, "critical mass" refers to the stage in a company's development where it can finally stand on its own and make a profit without further investment.

In any undertaking, attaining critical mass requires that we exert our willpower and resources until we have generated enough magnetism to launch an endeavor that will run smoothly and be self-sustaining. This is also referred to as a "tipping point," and it can happen unexpectedly, from one moment to the next. In physics, there's a formula to calculate how much material will be required for fission to occur. But in human activity there are too many variables to predict how much energy and time will be required. (From personal experience, I can attest that it's always more time and energy than we expected!)

It has been said that the last 20 percent of a project requires the same energy as the first 80 percent. As we draw closer to our goal, the scope of the project tends to expand. Unanticipated events are almost certain to occur: illness, changing priorities, unexpected setbacks. These are meant to test our commitment and challenge our staying power. We need to be like long-distance competitors who keep a certain power in reserve, ready for the final sprint.

On a metaphysical note, the closer we come to success, the more powerfully Maya resists. Many undertakings fail in the last lap. Thus persistence is a fundamental ingredient for success.

---

* An entertaining allegory, "The Shiny Pail," can be found on page 73 in Volume One.

> Our greatest weakness lies in giving up. The most certain way to succeed is always to try just one more time... Many of life's failures are people who did not realize how close they were to success when they gave up. –THOMAS EDISON

> When you get into a tight place and everything goes against you, till it seems as though you could not hold on a minute longer, never give up then, for that is just the place and time that the tide will turn. When you're down to nothing, God is up to something. The faithful see the invisible, believe the incredible and then receive the impossible. –BENJAMIN FRANKLIN

> Fight to the finish. Never turn back. Never say, "I could not find the way, so I give up." Ask the way if you have made mistakes, but never give up. Many give up when the difficult turns in the path come. Failures should consult and associate with the successful persons and not with failures. Make up your mind you will succeed.[23]

It is important in achieving success that even in the face of setbacks we persist. Although setbacks are inevitable, they can also serve as course corrections on the journey to success. As we move forward, there will be times when we need to adjust our direction. If we are too doggedly determined to continue in the present direction, or if we fail to check our superconscious intuition, a setback or an apparent failure may be exactly what's needed to make us pause, reflect, and get back on course.

Setbacks and failures can serve as opportunities to strengthen our willpower and raise our energy and awareness and find better solutions. It's worth repeating Yogananda's encouraging advice to those who want to succeed.

> Even failures should act as stimulants to your will power, and to your material and spiritual growth. The season of failure is the best time for sowing the seeds of success...Weed out the causes of failure by searching for them, and then with double vigor launch forth on whatever you wish to accomplish...Every new effort after failure brings true growth. But it must be well planned and charged with increasing intensity of attention and with dynamic will power....[24]

Magnetism by osmosis

It can greatly help us to associate with people who have achieved the kind of success we are seeking.

> To acquire strong magnetism oneself it is important to mix with people who already have the kind of magnetism that one wants to develop. To develop success-magnetism, mix with successful people, not with failures. Mix with artists to develop an artistic magnetism; with devotees, to develop spiritual magnetism....
>
> Mixing with others to acquire their magnetism requires not physical proximity so much as an attunement of consciousness. Without this attunement, physical nearness may result in little or no true exchange. If such attunement exists, on the other hand, a magnetic exchange may occur even at a distance. In every case the amount of the exchange will depend on one's own magnetic drawing power, which in turn depends, of course, on a deep, sincere effort of will.[25]

PART XI CHAPTER FOUR

Money Magnetism

> We must learn to view money
> not as a thing merely, but as an expression
> of energy–ultimately, as an expression
> of *our* energy.[1] –KRIYANANDA
>
> Money is not a curse. It is the manner in which you
> use money that is of importance.[2] –YOGANANDA
>
> To love money is to be lost. That is the snare.
> You must use it rightly. You must use the
> right voltage of prosperity to shine through
> the bulb of your life... [3] –YOGANANDA
>
> Business life need not be a material life:
> business ambition can be spiritualized. Business
> is nothing but serving others materially
> in the best possible way.[4] –YOGANANDA
>
> Divine Abundance follows the law of service
> and generosity. Give and then receive.
> Give to the world the best you have, and the
> best will come back to you.[5] –YOGANANDA

If you were a farmer in Mesopotamia in 3000 B.C., you would take a bag of grain to the temple, where you would exchange it for a clay token that you could use to pay your temple debts. If you were a trader in China in 1200 B.C., you would carry cowrie shells, conveniently small and light, as an accepted form of representative money in Africa, Asia, and Australia. The Native American Indians used shells, called *wampum,* as a medium of exchange that was adopted by the Dutch colonists in their New World dealings. Today, our wampum is a plastic card, or it's floating invisibly in cyberspace.

Whatever form it takes, money's value lies not in the object we use as a proxy, but in its power to obtain and exchange goods and services. The more shells or coins you possess, the more energy is at your command.

> It isn't only that we attract money to us:
> We attract energy, which then manifests itself
> in the form of money. And the supply
> of energy is cosmic in scope.[6]

Why is money sometimes considered evil? The Christian Bible says, **"For the love of money is the root of all evil."** (1 Timothy 6:10) It is our obsession for it that is unhealthy.

The pursuit and possession of money can become an addiction no less enslaving than alcohol, drugs, or sex. People obsess over money, they hoard it, and they use it to gratify their self-destructive desires. Money is "evil" only when it makes us its slave, overpowering us like any other addiction and imprisoning us in an ego-centric world. Those who are attached to their money and possessions are rarely content with what they have; they often live in fear of losing their perceived security, and lose their health in the relentless pursuit of even more.

The other side of the coin is that we can use money to help ourselves and others.

> Money-making is the next greatest art after the
> art of realizing God. All the good and philanthropic
> works of the world, all noble successes, have to be
> accomplished through money. No saint lived who
> directly or indirectly did not use money...
>
> To earn money abundantly, unselfishly, honestly,
> quickly, just for God and God's work and making

> others happy is to develop many sterling qualities of character that will aid one on the spiritual as well as the material path. Responsibility, knowledge of organization, efficiency, order, leadership, and practical usefulness are developed in business success and are necessary for the all-round growth of man.[7]

Before he met his guru, James Lynn (Rajarsi Janakananda), Yogananda's most advanced disciple and spiritual successor, built a multimillion-dollar business empire by his own prodigious effort. After meeting Yogananda, he devoted himself to achieving God-realization. This is his story.

✵ THE MILLIONAIRE WHO ✵ BECAME A SAINT

Born dirt-poor as the son of a tenant cotton farmer, he built a business empire that included three major insurance companies, oil fields, railroad and banking interests, vast citrus orchards, vineyards, and vegetable farms. James Lynn is an inspiring example of determination, hard work, intelligence, and wise intuition in investing his wealth.

At fourteen, James left school to earn money for his family. He studied late into the night to earn his high school diploma, then earned a law degree and accreditation as an accountant.

With all his success, he felt an inner emptiness. "I had thought that money could give me happiness, but nothing seemed to satisfy me. I lived in a state of nervousness, a state of strain, an inward state of uncertainty."

And then, in 1932, his life changed when he met his guru, Paramhansa Yogananda, who recognized his untapped spiritual greatness. With no previous instruction or experience, Mr. Lynn meditated for six hours with Yogananda at their first meeting, and the guru transmitted to him an experience of spiritual ecstasy.

The qualities and capabilities he had developed on the road to wealth now served him in his ascent to Self-realization – including the ability to focus his mind, apply his willpower, and persevere in the face of setbacks. As a result, in a relatively short time he attained high states of realization, including *samadhi*, cosmic ecstasy.

Yogananda counseled him to arrange his schedule so that he would have a daily period of meditation. He reminded him that unwillingness to meditate is *Maya's* strongest weapon.

Mr. Lynn continued with a full schedule of business activities that included serving on the boards of many companies while faithfully attending to his spiritual activities. Each morning he would shut his office door and meditate for several hours. His intuition became so keen that in a few short minutes he was able to resolve complex business problems that had stumped others for weeks.

His investments returned satisfying profits which he donated in large part to Yogananda's organizations in America and India. Thanks to his generosity, the guru's headquarters in Los Angeles were freed from debt, and his school for boys in Ranchi, India became financially independent. Rajarsi built a hermitage by the sea in Encinitas, California where Yogananda could retreat to meditate and write his books.

Yogananda fondly called him "Saint Lynn" and later bestowed on him the spiritual name Rajarsi Janakananda, which means "king of saints."

In this chapter we will consider the best ways to attract and use money for our overall happiness and well-being, and how to use money to uplift the consciousness of humanity.

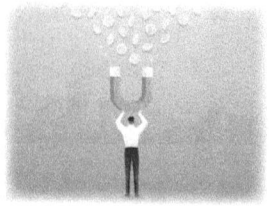

Earning money dharmically

The Sanskrit saying *"Jato dharma, tato jaya"* is repeated often in the Indian epic *Mahabharata*. In English it means, **"Where there is truth and righteous action, there is sure to be victory."** It is inscribed on the emblem of the Supreme Court of India, and is one of the mottos of Ananda worldwide.

Our personal *dharma* includes both material duties — providing for our family, fulfilling our work responsibilities, contributing to the wider community — as well as attending to our spiritual progress. When we are not able to attract the material resources that we need, it affects all areas of our life, creating anxiety, disharmony and weakening our natural immune defenses. It is important, then, to learn to apply the Law of Money Magnetism.

The money that comes into our possession has an important role to play in our spiritual destiny. When we use money in the pursuit of *dharma*, it fulfills its highest purpose and becomes increasingly magnetic.

The first principle of the Law of Money Magnetism is the need to earn money righteously.

> The great paradox and riddle of life lies in judiciously acquiring money.... It seems that making money honestly is the most difficult of all life's undertakings, next to finding God.[8]

"Making money honestly" is not easy, because the power of *adharma*, or unrighteousness, is particularly strong in our dealings with money. All of us have, doubtless, been tempted by money's allure, whether in this or former lives. Money's promise of power and material satisfactions has very likely led us astray repeatedly; it may even have lured us to leave the path of truth and righteousness.

> All moral business men must resist the temptation of making money by the unscrupulous, dishonest or treacherous means used by business men with blunt conscience and poor spiritual judgement.[9]

Although dishonesty is temptingly convenient in many situations, its fruits are inevitably, and often dramatically disappointing — even ruinous. Those who acquire money by means that harm the well-being and integrity of others, in the end harm themselves. Motivated by greed, dishonesty ends in ignominy.

Notorious are the names of those who have swindled others and ended in jail, or with grave illnesses, broken families, or by committing suicide. Ill-gotten gains do not attract long-term prosperity or happiness. We carry these tragic consequences with us as karmic *samskars* from one life to the next, where they subconsciously interfere with our ability to magnetize and use money properly now. Although we can't undo the past, we *can* choose our present attitudes and actions so as to align ourselves with the *dharma* of money.

In Part Two, we learned about the *vaishya* state of consciousness, where the ego wants to get more than it gives and has few qualms about taking advantage of others. In the early vaishya stages, theft, deceit, fraud, and extortion are common. The desire for maximum profit will manifest in endless devious ways, such as selling counterfeit goods, persuading customers to buy unnecessary services, charging exorbitant prices for life-saving medications, and countless other shady schemes.

The unrefined vaishya discovers only very slowly that taking advantage of the vulnerabilities and insecurities of others not only fails to attract lasting prosperity but incites the Law of Karma to even the scales.

✷ A HOUSE FIT FOR A KING

Although the king possessed a palace of stunning splendor, and vacation homes throughout the realm, he expressed a desire for a modest but well-appointed manor house in a tranquil setting not too far from the capital so that he could go there to rest on the weekends. He entrusted the project to one of his ministers, giving him an appropriate budget.

The minister considered the project plans too extravagant for a house that the king would use rarely, and so, rather than use the best materials and furnishings as the king had requested, the minister cut corners and put the savings in his own pocket for his upcoming retirement. He slyly reasoned that if the king discovered what he was doing, he would blame the suppliers, and in any case, he would soon be retired and no longer in the king's employ, so he would be safe from his wrath.

In due course the house was finished, and on the final day of his service the minister gave the keys to the king. Much to his surprise, the king handed them back. With a knowing smile, the king said, "This house is my gift to you, in gratitude for your years of service and as your retirement pension." Thus the minister was compelled to retire to a rapidly disintegrating house instead of a country estate fit for a king.

✻ ✻ ✻

How much money do we need?

Yogananda was practical in applying spiritual laws to daily life.

> Since God has given us hunger and since we have a physical body to look after, we must have money and earn it honestly and scientifically by serving the right needs of our fellow beings.[10]

He urged us to us this affirmation as our guidepost.

Affirmation

"I will pursue material prosperity, not for fanning the fires of ceaseless desires, for unnecessary necessities, but for satisfying the hunger of my real need."[11]

The "hunger of our real need" includes not only the basic necessities of life, but also whatever we need to fulfill our individual *dharma*. Among those necessities, we can include a good education and the tools of our trade. But a dignified life need not be a luxurious one that takes us out of harmony with the laws of nature.

> The Divine Spirit does not like the
> children who revel in luxury while some of
> His other children are suffering.[12]

How much money is actually available?

Money is an expression of energy and is therefore potentially limitless. Even though the value of money declines as governments print more, the reservoir of cosmic energy is always full. Droughts may plague the earth, but energy never dries up.

How much energy we are able to attract in the form of money will not be limited to our salary or the profits from a business. When we have a real need, and we invest our best efforts while appealing humbly and confidently to the divine Source, our need will be fulfilled in unexpected ways: through an unforeseen bonus at work, a long-forgotten tax reimbursement, an inheritance from a great-aunt we haven't seen in years, an overdue loan repayment, or a gift from a dear friend.

Truthfulness and integrity

To magnetize money effectively, we need to be scrupulously truthful in our dealings. Truth has power. Truth *is* power, because it is the fabric from which the universe is created – *Sat-chid-ananda*: truth, awareness, and bliss. Being honest and transparent in our business dealings creates a strong magnetism that attracts success, prosperity, and all the money we need to fulfill our dharmic obligations.

> Live by the truth, and it will serve you far better than you could ever serve yourself.[13] Be completely honest and truthful in all your dealings. Any corners you "cut" in this respect will only weaken your powers of accomplishment, and will also weaken your ability to persevere to final success in any worthwhile undertaking. Both honesty and truthfulness harness one's power to the infinitely greater power of the universe.[14]

When we find ourselves in financial straits, the universe will tempt us to compromise our values in the name of practicality. Yogananda told a story about such a situation.

> Years ago a rich man came here who thought to buy me with his wealth. Knowing we badly needed money just then, he tried in certain ways to get me to compromise my ideals. I refused. Finally he said, "You'll starve because you didn't listen." Leaving here, he talked against me to a rich acquaintance of his, a student of this work. And that was the man God chose to give us the help we needed! [15]

When we uphold *dharma*, the universe upholds us, placing its vast resources at our disposal. Whatever money comes our way we should consider a divine trust, given to us to be cared for and used wisely, rather than spent in acquiring possessions and pursuing endeavors that will not inwardly enrich our lives. Wisely used and invested, as Yogananda advises, money, like a healthy tree, will bear abundant fruit.

> Earn rightly, spend less than your income, invest your money in absolutely secure things, and prosperity will seek you. [16]

To spend or save?

An important secret of magnetizing money-energy is that money needs to circulate. When we set energy in motion, and focus it in a clearly defined channel, it creates a magnetic field that attracts even more energy. When we buy useful goods and services and pay promptly, we help create a magnetism around all the money in circulation. By keeping the flow of money moving, it adds to our own prosperity and to the cycle of prosperity of the micro-economy in which we participate.

When we invest money judiciously, it has the power to produce more money, like a seed planted in fertile soil and lovingly tended that produces an abundance of fruit and many seeds. The best investments are those that enable us to improve our skills, expand our knowledge and experience, and help us become well-rounded human beings. Invest in your future by pursuing your passions, preserving your health, and creating wealth for others.

Spending money we don't have engenders a consciousness of indebtedness, which weakens our money magnetism; and regularly paying bills late weakens the money magnetism of the local economy. People who are habitually in debt have no ability to magnetize fresh energy in any area of their life. They become trapped in their inner debtor's prison.

> From today onward, make it a principle to avoid debt. If for any reason you need to borrow, make a serious attempt to pay off that debt as soon as possible. It simply won't be worth the cost, in terms of your peace of mind, to have debt of any kind hanging over your head like the sword of Damocles. [17]

Building money magnetism requires that we achieve a subtle balance between judicious spending and wise saving: being neither penurious or profligate in its use.

> Remember that along with the art of money-making, it is well to learn the art of money-saving, for a large income is of no lasting good to you if it creates only habits of luxury and no reserve fund. Think for a moment. If you should get sick suddenly, how would you continue your luxurious habits, without the usual income, if you have no savings put away? It is a bad thing to cultivate luxurious habits if you have only a small income. Is it not better to live simply and frugally and grow rich in reality? [18]

Saving money and *hoarding* it are not the same. Hoarding means to hold on to money with the false notion that the money itself is our security. When money is locked away, its magnetism becomes stagnant and unproductive, even losing its face value and buying power. The Scrooges of the world are usually lonely, unhappy people who wind up never enjoying the benefits of their wealth.

The money magnetism of an organization

If you are responsible for the finances of an organization, do your utmost to ensure that the money is properly accounted for, that the records are accurate and transparent, and that financial information is communicated promptly, comprehensively, and understandably to those who must make decisions. Make sure your accountants and financial advisors are qualified, knowledgeable, and trustworthy.

Compensate the workers well, pay them promptly, and make all possible sacrifices elsewhere before you ask them to sacrifice. The workers are the main ingredient in the organization's success, and their well-being should be a paramount consideration.

The joy of giving

The most powerful and effective way to attract money is to share it. It may seem paradoxical, but the more we give of our money, the more the universe gives us in return.

> Money, ultimately, brings happiness only if it is shared. When it is used generously to help others, one feels happy in himself and finds his happiness expanding to include others' well-being. Money, in this case, can be a real blessing, not a misfortune....
>
> Whatever goodness a person, or a nation, offers to others will bring expansion of consciousness in return: an expansion of sympathy, understanding and success. When one helps others to achieve prosperity, he attracts greater prosperity to himself.

> When he helps others to grow in understanding,
> he finds understanding deepening in himself.
> When one helps others to grow spiritually, that
> action brings him closer, himself, to spiritual
> enlightenment. The law works infallibly.[19]

☀ Pray, Share, Rejoice ☀

Surely I'm not alone when I talk about the blessings that come from praying for others in need. I find it interesting that I experience the same joy and blessings when I donate money to a good cause. For me, praying for the well-being of others and donating for the well-being of a spiritual cause are one and the same.

Over the forty years that I have donated to the spiritual path that I follow, I have been blessed with inner guidance and increased financial resources. The times I have been most successful have been due to the blessings I have received by offering monetary support to help others.

Praying comes from the heart, with a desire to help, heal, and inspire. Donating also comes from the heart and is done for the same reasons. The only difference is that a donation is a healing prayer in physical form. –**Mark**, *Austria*

Mark's testimony suggests a perpetual loop of giving and receiving, with each cycle building magnetic power. What we receive goes far beyond any material returns. Doctors, dentists, and other health professionals experience the happiness of giving when they volunteer their vacation time with charitable medical groups. Actors, musicians, and other performers who travel to war-torn countries to bring a spark of beauty and grace to the injured and homeless, experience an inner spiritual reward.

The following is a personal story of a humble act of generosity that stands out strongly in my memory.

❋ Our Highway Angel ❋

My husband and I were on the freeway during the evening rush hour when our car suddenly began to sputter and shake and finally rolled to a complete stop. We pulled over and asked each other what we should do – this was long before cell phones.

Not a minute passed before a car stopped and a man got out and came over to offer his help. He had a friend who ran an auto repair shop not far from the freeway. Attaching a cable to our car, he pulled us all the way. The problem was minor, and the mechanic had the part to fix it. Our Good Samaritan insisted on remaining with us until the car was roadworthy again.

When we thanked him, he said, "No, it is I who must thank you." When we expressed surprise, he said, "I am a Christian, and I promised Jesus that every day this year I would help someone in need, in His name. The whole day had passed, and when I left work I hadn't had a chance to help anyone, so I was a little distraught. But then I saw your car on the side of the road, and I could only praise the Lord for giving me the chance to fulfill my promise. So, my thanks to you for being His instrument today."

Invest in the welfare of others

During the countless incarnations of the *vaishya* stage of our spiritual evolution, our attitude toward business and money-making very gradually and slowly becomes more refined. We begin to discover the inner joy and satisfaction of thinking not only of our own profit, but of how our efforts can be of service and benefit to others.

We activate the laws of magnetism and prosperity when we apply our energy, talents, and experience to serve others, and to help them in their development.

> It isn't really important what we do, so long as we see everything we do as an opportunity for service, for applying energy creatively, for working for the welfare of all, for expanding our sympathies and awareness, for attuning our consciousness to the Infinite Intelligence....Whatever we are given in this world, whether money, popularity, or talent, should be taken as an opportunity for service. We were not put here on earth merely to live for ourselves. We were given the blessing of a human body that we might enter into a greater awareness of all life.[20]

When our money-making endeavors include the happiness and well-being of others, the magnetism of our efforts is greatly enhanced.

> Make an effort to earn more so that you can be the means of helping others to help themselves, for one of the unwritten laws decrees that he who helps others to abundance and happiness always will be helped in return by them, and he will become more and more prosperous and happy himself. This is a law of happiness which cannot be broken.[21]

Just as some people are born with a prodigious talent for music, art, or sports, others are karmically endowed with an exceptional talent for making money. Speaking of such souls, Yogananda taught that those who have more money than they need have a moral obligation to offer their resources to help others.

> Man should make money not only by serving and getting something in return, but also for the sake of using money for creating philanthropic institutions

> which serve public needs. When one makes a great deal of money by making others prosperous and again uses that wealth for helping others to help themselves, that is spiritualizing ambition. [22]

Yogananda praised those industrialists of his day who looked out for the welfare of their employees – which was not at all common at the time. Most factory owners maximized their profits by using cheap immigrant or child labor, maintaining working conditions that were unhealthy and hazardous, and requiring their employees to work long hours. The Industrial Revolution brought out the worst in some entrepreneurs and the best in others. In the 1920s, for instance, manufacturing plants required a work week of six days and 74 hours. Speaking with the *New York Times*, Ford Company president Edsel Ford revealed a strikingly different corporate approach.

> "Every man needs more than one day a week for rest and recreation…. The Ford Company always has sought to promote an ideal home life for its employees. We believe that in order to live properly every man should have more time to spend with his family."

The Ford company was also a pioneer in involving the workers in production decisions and sharing some of the profits with them.

Yogananda wrote an article for his magazine in support of Ford's groundbreaking proposal for a five-day work week.

> I think Mr. Henry Ford has inaugurated a new era in spiritualizing business life by proposing a five-day week…. because the hard-working man could utilize all Saturday for relaxation, gardening and amusement, and use Sunday wholly and solely for church or temple or mosque…or self-discipline through the technique of concentration and meditation. [23]

✻ THE CHOCOLATE KING ✻

You have to be a special person to have a city named after you, and to have your name become synonymous with one of the most famous American products of the twentieth century.

Born in 1857 on a farm in central Pennsylvania, shortly before the American Civil War, Milton S. Hershey grew up speaking "Pennsylvania Dutch," the language of his Swiss and German ancestors. From them he inherited a propensity for hard work, diligence, and thriftiness.

Hershey was a candymaker, and in the beginning not a successful one. His first two businesses failed.

Undeterred, he tried a new direction. He visited the 1893 World's Fair in Chicago* where he bought two chocolate-making machines, and the next year he established the Hershey Chocolate Company. In 1900 he introduced the Hershey's Milk Chocolate Bar – to immediate success – and in 1907 he introduced the wildly popular Hershey's Kisses.† For Americans, Hershey is synonymous with milk chocolate, and Milton Hershey became a very, very wealthy man.

He believed that wealth should be used for the benefit of others. He established an industrial trade school for orphan boys where they were lodged, fed, clothed, and given training so that they could find gainful employment. Today known as the Milton Hershey School, it offers training to over two thousand boys and girls each year.

Hershey used his money to benefit his employees and the local residents, building an ideal town that provided a "natural setting, where healthy, right-living, and well-paid workers could live in safe, happy homes." Hershey, Pennsylvania today is, thanks to his vision and generosity, a tree-lined community that includes a trolley system for transporting the workers to and from work, public elementary

---

* The year 1893 is notable for two other reasons: It was the year that Paramhansa Yogananda was born in India, and the year when Swami Vivekananda gave a famous speech at the First World Parliament of Religions at the same Chicago fair.

† Perugina established its chocolate company in Italy in 1917 and introduced its "Baci" in 1922, similar to Hershey Kisses, with the addition of hazelnuts.

and high schools, churches, parks, a community theater, a sports arena, a bank, a hotel, a golf course, and a zoo.

In 1918, twenty-seven years before his passing, Mr. Hershey gave the majority of his fortune, valued at $670 million, as well as his shares in the Hersey company, to a trust fund that would provide educational and cultural opportunities for residents of the city of Hershey.

The Hershey company continues to operate in his philanthropic spirit, recently giving a $50 million endowment for the Penn State Medical Center and teaching hospital.

The inscription on a bronze bust of Hershey at the Hersey School reads: "His deeds are a monument. His life is our inspiration."[24]

Social responsibility

As the self-interested *vaishyas* transition further into the more refined *kshatriya* state, they begin to understand that wealth brings with it broader social responsibility.

The Father of Indian Industry

Corporate social responsibility (CSR)[25] is a self-regulating business model used by many companies as a means of contributing some of their profits to the welfare of society. In 2014, India became the first country to establish CSR as a legal mandate, requiring large corporations to give 2% of their net profits for social initiatives.

A hundred years before it had a name and an acronym, giving back to society was a way of life and a way of business for Jamsetji Tata, who is honored and revered in his native land as the "father of Indian industry."

Everywhere in India you will encounter the Tata name on cars, trucks, hotels, steel and cotton mills, electric generating companies, airplanes, agricultural equipment, information technology, cement, tea, and far more. Tata's empire stretches across one hundred countries on six continents. School children all over India know Jamsetji Tata's name and learn his story. The city he envisioned is named for him — Jamshedpur — and was built according to his designs, with "wide streets planted with shady trees… space for lawns and gardens, parks, and areas earmarked for Hindu temples, Mohammedan mosques and Christian churches."

Although the British Raj would eventually knight Tata's sons, they did not encourage Jamsetji's vision of developing homegrown Indian industry because they knew it would create an economic foundation for India's later independence. Tata's vision was to build an iron and steel company, a hydroelectric plant, cotton manufacturing mills, a world-class learning institution, and a unique hotel. All came to pass and would prove crucial to India's industrial development. The remarkable Taj Mahal Palace Hotel in Bombay was completed in his lifetime, the first to have elevators and electric lights in its six hundred rooms.

From the outset, Tata's entrepreneurial wizardry was accompanied by an altruistic desire to make India a proud and independent country. His earliest endowment, a fund for Indian scholars to study abroad, provided an education to an Indian president, as well as renowned scientists and artists. He is acclaimed as the world's premier philanthropist, having donated over $100 billion dollars to educational institutions, scientific research, and innumerable charitable foundations. At his death, the *Times of India* wrote:

> "He was not a man who cared to bask in the public eye. He disliked public gatherings, he did not care for making speeches, his sturdy strength of character prevented him from fawning on any man, however great, for he himself was great in his own way, greater than most people realized. He sought no honor and he claimed no privilege, but the advancement of India and her myriad peoples was with him an abiding passion."

His descendants have brought to fruition all of his visions and continue to carry forward his philanthropic ideals, ensuring the Tata legacy of industriousness and generosity.

The Giving Pledge

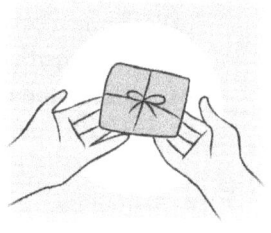

Titans of twenty-first-century enterprise are using their wealth to promote the welfare of humanity. The "Giving Pledge," initiated in 2010 by Warren Buffet and Bill and Melinda French Gates, challenges billionaires to make a commitment to give the majority of their wealth to philanthropic causes, either during their lifetimes or in their wills. The goal is to inspire the world's wealthiest people to give more, to give sooner, and to bring more social and environmental awareness to their giving.

Among the 230 signatories to the Pledge is J. K. Rowling, who was a single mother on welfare before Harry Potter came into her life. Thanks to Harry, she now earns approximately $1.6 million per day. By 2012 she had given away $160 million, supporting many charities, especially those in aid of women and children facing health or financial crises. She says, "You have a moral responsibility when you've been given far more than you need, to do wise things with it and give intelligently."

Gaia

Swami Sri Yukteswar maintained: "So long as you breathe the free air of earth, you are under obligation to render grateful service." [26] This is the story of a billionaire who is fulfilling his responsibility to his workers and to the planet that gives us life.

❋ THE CLIMATE PHILANTHROPIST ❋

A pioneering rock climber and environmental conservationist, Yvon Chouinard was not enamored of capitalism. Reluctantly he became a billionaire through the global success of his company, Patagonia.

In the 1960s, Yvon lived out of his car and could barely afford food. At an early age, he took to blacksmithing to make good quality pitons for his climbing adventures. They were of such good quality that his buddies eagerly bought them, and word spread in the rock-climbing community.

To serve the growing demand, he set up a small business in the backyard of his parents' home. With a partner, they redesigned and improved almost every known climbing tool, making them stronger, lighter, simpler, and more functional. By 1970, they were the largest suppliers of climbing hardware in the United States. They diversified and began to produce innovative, lightweight, efficiently insulating outdoor clothing and accessories for sports enthusiasts.

Chouinard and his wife, Malinda, make sure that Patagonia's employees have what they need to be healthy: a vegetarian cafeteria, childcare, sports facilities, and excellent wages. To help the employees remain inspired and committed to the company's ideals, Patagonia offers free trips to natural locations, particularly in areas they want to see preserved.

The company ensures that its ecological and energy footprint is as negligible as possible, producing much of its own energy and using certifiably organic materials. With the voluntary participation of the employees, Patagonia creates campaigns to educate people about the environment, and to influence governmental bodies to pass laws and regulations favorable to conservation.

From its earliest years, the company has given 1% of its total sales to grassroots environmental initiatives and activists. After activating the Laws of Prosperity the company's sales soared and the Chouinards' worth climbed robustly, putting them, embarrassingly, among the excessively wealthy. They began to dedicate 10% of yearly profits to small groups working to preserve the environment.

In 2013, Yvon Chouinard founded Tin Shed Ventures, a venture capital fund to help startup companies that place environmental and social responsibility on an equal footing with financial returns.

The Chouinard family recently divested themselves of their entire fortune, transferring ownership of Patagonia, valued at $3 billion, to the Patagonia Purpose Trust, that will continue to operate Patagonia as a socially responsible business and donate its profits to combat climate change. As other companies become inspired by the example of the Chouinards and the ethics of Patagonia, our home planet just might survive.

Toward a simpler life

Throughout his lifetime, especially in his later years, Yogananda frequently spoke about future economic upheavals on a global scale.[27] While there are regular, unpredictable economic cycles, Yogananda foresaw a massive economic breakdown that would affect every home in the world. Current world conditions indicate that such a collapse is within the realm of possibility. Yogananda offered a number of recommendations for how we can prepare.

One is that people begin to lead a simpler life by resisting rampant consumerism, taking stock of what they truly need to be healthy, happy, and wise, and become more self-sufficient in terms of food, clothing, shelter, and energy.

In pursuit of this simpler, more autonomous, healthier life, Yogananda recommended that people join together to form small cooperative communities, either where they are currently living in urban, suburban, and rural areas, or on land purchased in common, where they can grow their own food, and where the buildings will not be dependent on centralized government energy sources.

The first "world brotherhood colony" envisioned by Yogananda was founded in 1969 by his disciple Swami Kriyananda, with branch communities now in Europe and India.[28]

> It is evident that there is a danger of hard times ahead. If I am wrong, you will anyway have made a sensible investment. If a global depression does arrive, and perhaps even a global war of terrible proportions, you may be able with a little preparation not only to help yourself and your family, but also to save many friends as well as others. These are difficult thoughts to face, but surely it would be unwise to do nothing to prepare for them. There are at present too many signs pointing in the direction of disaster. On the other hand, if no disaster occurs, at least you will have the satisfaction of knowing that you took sensible precautions.[29]

Gratitude

Another essential principle of the Law of Magnetism is gratitude. While the universe doesn't need or demand our thanks, gratitude is, for us, a critically important attitude.

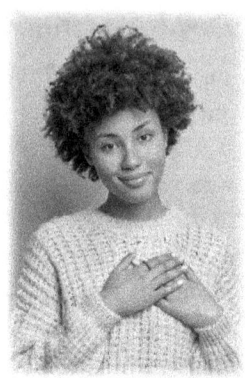

We can justifiably assume that the Source of all abundance will respond to our needs, but we should never presumptuously imagine that it will fulfill our every desire. When the Source of our being fulfills a need, answers a prayer, or responds to an innocent wish, and we humbly and lovingly offer our gratitude in return, we return the blessing to its Source, whereupon it comes back to us again. This is the dynamic that keeps the Law of Magnetism in motion.

> Gratitude is a way of returning energy for energy received. Only a thief takes without paying for what he gets. And one who accepts a kindness without returning gratitude, as though the kindness were his by right, demeans both the giver and himself. He demeans the giver, because by ingratitude he implies that the kindness was inspired by selfish motives. And he demeans himself, because by giving nothing in return he breaks the cycle of creativity, without which prosperity's flow, both materially and spiritually, is blocked.
>
> Accept nothing, inwardly, for yourself, but offer everything to God. Don't let yourself be bought by others' kindnesses. Be grateful to them above all in your soul, by blessing or praying for them. Give gratitude first of all to God, from Whom alone all blessings truly come.[30]

Affirmations for Divine Abundance [31]

I will use my creative thinking ability
to gain success in every worthwhile
project that I undertake.

I will help myself that I may bring into
proper use all my God-given powers.

I will strive for business success not only
for selfishly making money, but also that
I might serve my country and the world
well with some worthwhile things.

I will use my honestly acquired money
to live simply, doing away with luxury,
and I will try to use my money to make
the world-family better and happier,
according to the measure of my ability.

God will help me if I help myself,
and then pray to Him to help me to bring
my efforts to a successful issue.

CHAPTER 4: *Points to Remember*

- Money is a form of cosmic energy, and as such, it is limitless.
- To attract money, earn it honestly.
- Offer products and services that are useful and of good quality.
- Spend money judiciously for your material and spiritual needs.
- Pay bills promptly.
- Save money against difficult times.
- Be neither penurious or profligate in managing money.
- Invest money in a better future for yourself and others.
- Include others' well-being in your own happiness.
- Live a simple life, enjoying and being grateful for God's abundance and beneficence.
- Give regularly to causes that inspire you and that uplift humanity.

PART XI   CHAPTER FIVE

Tithing magic

> If you tithe a portion of your income to God, you will find that, far from depriving yourself, you will be blessed by the Source of all abundance, God. All real security comes from Him.[1]
>
> —KRIYANANDA

※ POEM BY RABINDRANATH TAGORE ※
from *Gitanjali*

I had gone a-begging from door to door in the village path, when thy golden chariot appeared in the distance like a gorgeous dream and I wondered who was this King of all kings!

My hopes rose high and me thought my evil days were at an end, and I stood waiting for alms to be given unasked and for wealth scattered on all sides in the dust.

The chariot stopped where I stood. Thy glance fell on me and thou camest down with a smile. I felt that the luck of my life had come at last. Then of a sudden thou didst hold out thy right hand and say "What hast thou to give to me?"

Ah, what a kingly jest was it to open thy palm to a beggar to beg! I was confused and stood undecided, and then from my wallet I slowly took out the least little grain of corn and gave it to thee.

But how great my surprise when at the day's end I emptied my bag on the floor to find a least little grain of gold among the poor heap. I bitterly wept and wished that I had had the heart to give thee my all.

The practice of tithing has its origins in the survival skills of ancient cultures. From the bird's nest of nine eggs, the hunter would perhaps take five, leaving the others to hatch. When nomadic tribes developed permanent settlements and began to farm, survival meant setting aside some of the harvest to seed the next year's crops.

This practice later took on religious significance and became a symbol of man's mutual relationship with a benevolent higher power. In the Christian Bible tithing is mentioned in this context.

> **A tenth shall be holy unto the Lord.** (LEV 27:32)
>
> **Give, and it shall be given unto you; good measure, pressed down, and shaken together, and running over.** (LUKE 6:38)

In Biblical times there were "tithe barns" where offerings from the harvest were stored as a reserve for times of need. Today, the "fruits of our labors" are monetary – tithing now means donating a portion of the money we earn to support a church or other spiritual institution, or a humanitarian work or other source of inspiration.

Tithing and charitable giving play a role in most religious traditions. Islam requires the *zakat* as one of its five main pillars, second in importance only to prayer. From the Qu'ran (34;39): "Whatever you spend for good, He replaces it, and He is the best of Providers." The Sikhs practice the *dasvanth*, the Jews honor the *ma'aser kesafim*, and Christians are committed to tithing.

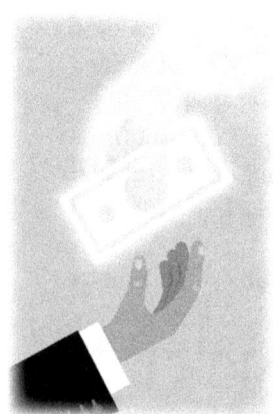

Many people ease into the practice by giving a small percentage of their income. As they reap the spiritual and practical rewards and grow confident in the divine providence, they may adopt the traditional practice of giving 10 percent of what they receive.

Some individuals have become so inspired by the practice that they've gone far beyond the standard ten percent.

Robert LeTourneau, a devout Christian who founded a highly successful company that manufactured 70 percent of World War II's Allied Forces earth-moving and engineering equipment, is an outstanding example. He gave 90 percent of his own salary and his company's profits to religious organizations.

The epitaph on his grave is from the Gospel of Matthew (6:33): "Seek ye first the kingdom of God and His righteousness and all these things shall be added unto you."

The reciprocal aspect of the Law of Tithing is a promise that the universe will reward those who give by supplying their needs in abundance.

> "Bring the whole tithe into the storehouse,
> that there may be food in my house.
> Test me in this," says the Lord Almighty,
> "and see if I will not throw open the
> floodgates of heaven and pour out
> so much blessing that you will not have
> room enough for it." (MALACHI 3:10)

Tithing is a wonderful means by which we can bring God into our lives in a practical, down-to-earth way. By tithing we enter into a synergistic relationship with the divine Giver, who lovingly, and often surprisingly, shows us that our ability to fulfill our earthly needs is never limited to our own human capacities.

> Share (your) wealth with others.
> This is how to find riches and success
> pouring out on you from all sides,
> like showers of gold.[2]

Tithing not only reliably attracts prosperity but can initiate a profound spiritual healing of our relationship with God, as our faith in His loving care grows strong, and our trust in the divine Providence is repeatedly justified.

✵ Replenishing the Spiritual ✵
Bank Account

Although Shanti was an orphan, she had been very lovingly cared for as a child and young girl by the convent sisters, especially Sister Thérèse, who raised and educated her as if she were her own daughter. Shanti admired Thérèse's deep inner communion with God, her lifelong dedication to Jesus, and her complete surrender to the divine will. Shanti was particularly amazed to observe how God always seemed to provide the funds required to run the convent.

Confident and well-prepared for life, Shanti moved from her native southern India first to France for her higher education, then to Switzerland for work. She found a good job and a good husband with whom she had two children. It was at this point that she discovered her spiritual path and became part of the Ananda family of Self-realization.

Shanti considers Ananda her "spiritual food bank" where she receives physical sustenance and soul nourishment daily. Recently, feeling that she had withdrawn a plentiful amount of spiritual funds from Ananda, she decided that it was time to start replenishing the account – tithing would be the conduit for her gratitude.

In the beginning, she feared that tithing might leave her with insufficient resources to support her children. But she interpreted these qualms as a challenge to place her trust in God and let go of the illusory security of money. Looking back over her life, she was comforted to remember how God had provided for her throughout her childhood.

And so she began to tithe a full 10 percent of her income. As the months passed, her devotion grew stronger than her initial fears. Her faith enabled her to experience the truth that her offspring were God's children first and foremost, and that He would care for them. Today, she continues to experience the countless ways God takes care of us. Shanti reflects:

"The river of superconsciousness is constantly flowing, but our fears create eddies that prevent the flow of clarity from reaching the higher Self. With deep faith and active surrender to God, these fearsome eddies begin to lose their grip on our consciousness.

"As devotees, we seek inner freedom and the power to pass through the portal of the final exam in shimmering colors. May we all pass our final exam spiritually rich, so as to lay our treasures at His holy feet, when He will come to greet us in the astral world."

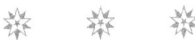

The practice of tithing is more than a ritual offering to be made just once, or when a generous mood strikes us. It is a way of life that enriches us in remarkable ways.

❋ I TRADED AN AUDI FOR INNER JOY ❋

In my work as an executive with a Fortune 500 company, I had to fight an endless battle to stay on top in the dog-eat-dog corporate world. I was strong, competitive, and delivered decent results on challenging global projects. I had earned a reputation as a no-nonsense go-getter. However, patience, flexibility, and a willingness to see things from a compassionate point of view were not my way of coping with the world.

I had begun to feel exhausted by the highly competitive pace that left hardly any time for relaxation or to enjoy the fruits of my labors. Maybe this was why I was attracted to the book *Material Success Through Yoga Principles,* which changed my life many times over.

As I studied the lessons, I was also learning to meditate, and finding new horizons appearing in terms of happiness and prosperity. Generosity was something I had not considered. Now, something shifted inside me, and I began to donate to the needy and disadvantaged. As my meditations and devotion deepened, I encountered some breakthrough ideas on how to relax in these high-tension environments.

I started to tithe by supporting a spiritual organization I had joined, and I became more actively involved in volunteering and serving others. It was then that a number of major changes began to happen in rapid succession.

Soon I received an attractive offer of a job that gave me a great deal more balance, peace of mind, and attractive benefits. I travelled business class for conferences and meetings to idyllic places around the world, and I was given a chauffeur-driven Audi, a golf course membership, a lucrative pension plan, and generous annual bonuses.

Tithing changed the quality and direction of my life. I was becoming a person I would never have imagined before – more sensitive, calm, kind, energetic, and courageous, in new ways. At age fifty, I moved out of the corporate rat race, and today I run a boutique coaching and leadership development company from my home. I am a sought-after consultant for industry associations, where I play strategic advisory roles.

The new work leaves me more time to meditate and volunteer. I lead the pan-India Yoga and Meditation Teacher Training Programs for Ananda Sangha, and I am on the board of an international non-profit charity that works with underprivileged children.

At times, I miss the comfortable Audi and chauffeur, but then I quickly remind myself of the pressures and stressors I've left behind, and of the joy I have found through sharing my life with God, a joy that increases with every tithe. – **Latha**, *Pune, India*

One need not be a billionaire to begin tithing. Milton Hershey, the "Chocolate King" mentioned earlier, was donating to charity at age sixteen. He began tithing to his church at twenty, even though he had very little money in those early years.

❊ BARELY ABLE TO MAKE ENDS MEET ❊

While working as a carpenter some years ago, I found myself deep in debt. Tithing was the last thing I thought I could afford. I donated a bit here and there, but I didn't tithe regularly, as I was barely able to keep afloat.

One Sunday the minister told a story about tithing that prompted me to give it a try. Even though I was flat broke, I gave a tithe from my next paycheck, and to my surprise, none of my checks bounced that pay period even though I was sure they would. No big financial windfalls came, and no huge amounts of money miraculously appeared, but after I began tithing I always seemed to have enough. Things stopped going wrong financially, and I eventually even turned down a pay raise simply because I had enough money and I didn't need more. – *E.G.*

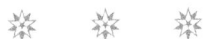

When business ventures become adventures

India's great scripture, the Bhagavad Gita, tells the story of the relationship between God in the form of Krishna and his foremost disciple, the young spiritual warrior Arjuna, who symbolically rep-

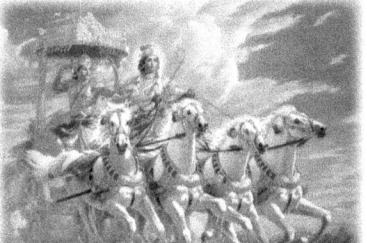

resents the individual soul that dwells in each of us.

At one point in the story, Arjuna is confronted with the challenge of leading his army in a battle where they will be greatly outnumbered. Offered a choice to have Krishna's many soldiers join his army in the fight, or to have Krishna alone by his side, Arjuna unhesitatingly chooses Krishna to drive his chariot, certain that he will be victorious. Arjuna knows that Krishna's wise counsel will ensure the victory, because He will unerringly guide him to fight the right battle, at the right time, and in the right way.

One of the ways tithing changes our lives is by giving us a chance, like Arjuna, to make God our partner. A friend of mine always referred to her business as a partnership, even though she was the sole proprietor. She included God in every detail of the business – together they made plans and projections, worked through challenges, and celebrated accomplishments. Her business was both personally fulfilling and prosperous. When we make space for God to be our Partner with all of the infinite resources at His command, miracles happen.

Tithe vs. donation

The Law of Tithing, like all laws, has precise demands. When we *donate*, we decide how much, when, and to whom we will give. Donating is a very good and healthy practice – for ourselves, for mankind, for the planet, and to open fresh channels for a higher energy to flow into our life and improve our health and well-being.

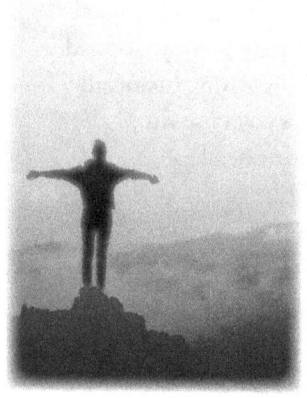

Once we decide to give a regular percentage of our income as a *tithe*, however, the dynamic changes. The tithe is always our first commitment — we tithe the moment we receive funds, not after our bills are paid. Thus tithing requires a deeper faith in God and His law than donating does.

> **People who give selflessly to God find that He sustains them. Whatever energy they put out flows back to them, reinforced by the power that sustains the universe.[3]**

The amount of the tithe isn't fixed: it is based on the amount of money God sends us. This aspect of tithing helps us realize that money isn't static, but that its flow will expand as needed when we leave the responsibility in God's hands. Tithing offers us the adventure of partnering with an infinitely wise, loving, and generous divine Providence.

Also unlike a donation, when we tithe we don't specify or place limits on how the tithe will be used. We give without conditions or expectations, trusting that God and His channels will wisely decide its destination. Those channels, of course, will have a divine responsibility to use the tithes for God's work. Our role is to invite God to inspire us where to give our tithes.

Personal experiences*

"Tithing did not come easily for me, but I found, bit by bit, that it helped me tune into the concept of money as a flow of energy, rather than a set amount that I receive and give every month. This helped tremendously to increase my faith in God and in the knowledge that He is taking care of me. Recently, when I found myself worrying about money, the first thing I did was write a tithing check. Tithing is such an effective way to stop holding on to things and stop affirming a sense of lack, when in truth I can have the feeling of abundance whenever I choose!"

"After several years of experimenting with tithing, I finally added it to my 'always do' spiritual practices. It is one of the most joyful and freeing practices I have. I am very grateful for how it has brought faith into the fearful realms of my practical day-to-day life."

"I must confess that until I had a series of financial failures, it never crossed my mind to donate money on a regular basis. I had been doing well with my properties, until the pandemic hit and it all fell apart. The tourist villas I had built became a financial burden, and I was no longer the young, successful entrepreneur.

"It was at this point that I learned about the practice of tithing, and I admit I initially saw it as a way to attract my lost prosperity. But that wasn't the immediate result – actually, things got worse before they began to get better. But I made a commitment to give ten percent of whatever money arrived, no matter how little or much it might be. For such a long time my sense of security had come from the amount of money I possessed, but these events taught me that things can change in an instant. Now my security is my faith in God, which is increasing month by month through this exciting experiment."

* Names are not included with these testimonials, by request.

"When I first started tithing, I was very, very shaky about it. There were often lean times when giving ten percent meant not going to a movie, or it meant giving the part of my income that was reserved for a little rest and relaxation. But I would tithe, even though I wasn't always a cheerful giver.

"In time, I found that I had enough money to go on vacation. The next thing I knew, I had a little money in the bank. These things came of themselves – I wasn't concentrating on them. Every once in a while, I would have a crisis in faith, when it was time to tithe and things were looking tight financially. I would then take out my list of all the ways tithing had worked for me. Or I would re-read my books on tithing, and it would lift my spirits. The most important thing I found about tithing was that it gave me a growing feeling that God is trustworthy, and that I can have faith in Him on all levels.

"It is very important to trust God, because it's a bond that creates a channel for great love. When that bond isn't there, one party is always suspect – it's hard to love somebody who is under suspicion for not providing enough. This bond of faith is the greatest thing tithing has given me, and I would happily tithe forever just for that bond."

In the words of the poet Tagore

But how great my surprise when at the day's end I emptied my bag on the floor to find a least little grain of gold among the poor heap. I bitterly wept and wished that I had had the heart to give thee my all.

PART XI CHAPTER SIX

Secrets of Success

> When wealth is lost, you have lost a little;
> when your health is lost, you have lost something,
> but when your peace of mind is lost, all is lost.
> Therefore, success must be measured
> by happiness – by your ability to remain in
> harmony with Cosmic laws.[1] –YOGANANDA

People who speak multiple languages often notice that once they became fluent in a first foreign language, the others came more easily. The brain adjusts, its memory areas are activated, and the insights that brought proficiency in the first language are helpful in the others.

So, too, with success – each achievement is a springboard to the next. In Chapter Three, we learned to activate the Law of Magnetism. In this chapter, we will consider some helpful hints for increasing the probability of success.

Follow your passion

During the Covid pandemic, a significant portion of the workforce had to work from home. When the restrictions were lifted, many workers didn't want to return to their former jobs because they had found more satisfying work. When we are passionate about what we're doing, the floodgates of creativity are opened. The great painter Vincent Van Gogh was never a financial or social success, but he was so passionate about his art that he produced more than eight hundred works. Van Gogh summed up his philosophy:

> "Love many things, for therein lies the true strength, and whosoever loves much performs much, and can accomplish much, and what is done in love is done well."

Yogananda offers similar advice.

> Perform little duties very well. Do you know that you have been using only five or six per cent of your attention in your vocation? You ought to use one hundred per cent concentration in doing your work henceforth... Be in love with your present work, but don't remain contented forever with what you are doing. You must progress, try to be the very best in your profession. You must express the limitless power of Soul, in anything you take up. Every position in life you hold, will be the stepping stone to a higher one if you strive to climb upward.[2]

If you believe you are giving your best at work, yet you feel inwardly unfulfilled, it may help to find a hobby, a pastime, or a volunteer activity that sparks your enthusiasm. The magnetism of the energy and love you invest may attract opportunities in line with your passion.

Yet "doing what we love" might not always be in the best interests of our spiritual growth. A talent or tendency may be a remnant of something we've done well in former lives. When a composer like Mozart is reborn, his soul may no longer need to compose music, though he will surely have a facility for it. More important than doing what comes easily, though, is to take the next step on our journey to Self-realization.

> Analyze what you are, what you wish to become...
> Decide what your deep and secret task is –
> your mission in life – so that you can make yourself what you should be and what you want to be.
> As you keep your mind on God and yourself attuned to His will, you will know more and more surely what your true mission in life is. Your ultimate purpose is to find your way back to God, but you have a task to perform in the outer world. Will power, combined with initiative, will help you recognize it.[3]

Initiative/Creativity

It takes little energy to do things as they have always been done. If security is the goal, then established protocols and tried-and-true routines are good sheepdogs that keep us corralled within the parameters we have set for ourselves. If, however, progress is the goal, we will need to break out of established patterns, as Yogananda recommends.

> Most of us follow the beaten track. It is the new energetic explorer on the pathway of success who succeeds. Initiative is the creative faculty within you, a spark of the Infinite Creator... It urges you to do things in new ways... Initiative enables you to stand on your own, free and independent.... The world is full of imitators; there are few creative workers.[4]

Initiative is born from a desire to set things in a new or better direction, or in some way to improve the human condition.

✷ THE PLANT WIZARD ✷

We often think of our circumstances as unchangeable. The following story introduces a man who showed us that *everything* can be improved – even Nature.

With only a high-school education, Luther Burbank trained himself so thoroughly in horticulture that he would achieve world fame as the "Plant Wizard."

He developed more than 800 strains and varieties of plants, including fruits, flowers, grains, grasses, and vegetables. He whispered to the cactus that it needn't be afraid, and it grew without thorns. He encouraged the walnut tree to produce an abundant harvest in half the time. Through cross-pollination, careful selection, and grafting, he invented the nectarine, the seedless peach, the Santa Rosa plum, and the Shasta daisy. The Burbank potato is now the global standard for baking and frying.

His creative initiative was boundless. He said: "Nothing worthwhile is possible without fearless experiments. At times the most daring experiments are needed to bring out the best in fruits and flowers."

His secret was love, as he revealed in his later years: "I love flowers, trees, animals, and all the works of Nature as they pass before us in time and space. What a joy life is when you have made a close working partnership with Nature, helping her to produce for the benefit of mankind new forms, colors, and perfumes in flowers which were never known before; fruits in form, size, and flavor never before seen on this globe; and grains of enormously increased productiveness, whose fat kernels are filled with more and better nourishment, a veritable storehouse of perfect food – new food for all the world's untold millions for all time to come." [5]

Burbank counted Thomas Edison, Henry Ford, and Paramhansa Yogananda among his friends, and they were frequent visitors to his gardens in Santa Rosa, California. Yogananda dedicated his *Autobiography of a Yogi*: "To the memory of Luther Burbank, an American Saint."

At Burbank's passing in 1926, Yogananda wrote this heartfelt tribute.

"He, who was so close to nature, so confidential and so understanding to her, is now part of her great spirit, whispering in her winds, shining in her stars, walking the dawn with her.

"I loved him very dearly. He was one of the saintliest men I have ever met. To look at his sensitive face with its compassionate eyes and kindly smile was to see a man bathed in a great spiritual radiance. I would not mind walking all the way from New York to Santa Rosa to meet him and discuss humanity and spiritual subjects with him once again." [6]

Opportunity/Vision

"Some people have all the luck" is an often-heard lament of those who believe themselves to be poorly favored. Successful people don't wait for good luck or depend on their good karma to motivate them.

> The one who creates does not wait for opportunity, blaming the fates, circumstances, and the gods. He seizes opportunities or creates them with the magic wand of his will, effort, and searching discrimination.[7]

Where others see misfortune, successful people see opportunity. As the popular saying goes: "When life gives you lemons, make lemonade."

> What comes to you is, generally, that for which you yourself are prepared! The most important thing, then, is to be *prepared* for the opportunities that come your way. In a way, you *create* them. Karma is certainly a part of that process, but even more important, because immediately useful to you, are right attitude, right expectations, right use of energy...
>
> The successful person is one who *looks*, and who *expects* opportunities to appear in his life. Many others receive countless opportunities in life, yet pass them by as though they wore blinders and dark glasses. They see what lies straight ahead of them, but see even that only dimly as far as opportunity is concerned....
>
> Face life with expectation. Wonderful adventure awaits you practically underfoot.[8]

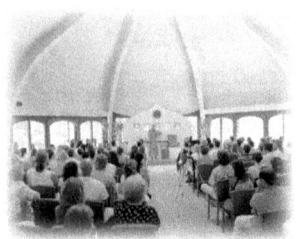 At Ananda Assisi, where I live, the guest facility had offered successful programs for more than thirty years. During the busy summer guest season we were able to accommodate up to a hundred people while offering five concurrent programs. From time to time we would talk about creating courses that people could study at home, but all of our energies were dedicated to expanding our successful in-residence offerings. Then, in March 2020, the world changed and suddenly no one could travel. Was it a tragedy or an opportunity?

It was an opportunity – of course! At long last we could devote ourselves to developing home-study courses, online live programs in real time, and remote yoga and meditation sessions that people around the world could attend together. Whereas people formerly could only participate in these activities only once or twice a year, or not at all due to issues of health, finances, etc., those barriers were now gone.

> **Your success in life does not altogether depend upon natural ability; it also depends upon determination to grasp the opportunity that is presented to you. Opportunities in life come by creation, not by chance.[9]**

In 1985, IBM owned the corporate market for computer hardware. IBM was the world's most profitable company, earning $6.6 billion that year. They had pioneered the portable computer in 1977, but they doubted that it would be of much commercial interest, believing that computers were meant to be in offices, doing office work. IBM needed an operating system for its small computers, and they licensed one from a nineteen-year-old college dropout named Bill Gates. Gates envisioned a day when everyone would have a computer, not only at work, but also at home.

IBM didn't share Gates's vision. Rejecting his proposal, they kept the company's focus on hardware and business services. As a result, IBM is no longer the giant it formerly was, while Bill Gates, who retained his patent rights, became the textbook success story of a generation.

Life Force / **160**

Set realistic goals

Although it's important to keep our eye on the mountain peak, we cannot expect to rise to the heights in a single leap. The journey to success in every field is comprised of many small steps, each of which is critical to the highest achievement. Success is like an infant's progress: we need to sit before we can crawl, and crawl before we can stand, walk, and run.

> So often in life we set ourselves impossible goals.
> Far better would it be to attempt the possible,
> even if we consider it far short of our highest ideals.
> For little successes will strengthen us, and prepare us,
> finally, to win the truly great victories of life. [10]

A step-by-step approach is practical not only for the strength and self-confidence it develops in us but also because each step gives us a broader vision of the terrain. Possible shortcuts, changes, and need for goal adjustment then become apparent.

Adaptability and flexibility

Following a rigidly prescribed direction is unlikely to bring us lasting success. Circumstances change, people change, the market changes, tastes change, the climate changes, and most of all, *we* change. When a couple marry, as the joke goes, the wife believes she will change the husband, while the husband imagines that the wife will never change. They are both destined to be disappointed.

Benjamin Franklin said: "Change is the only constant in life. One's ability to adapt to those changes will determine your success in life."

During the Covid lockdown, when many restaurants closed their doors, others developed home-delivery services and survived. Many businesses allowed their employees to work from home using rapidly evolving technologies for tele-conferencing. My hairdresser swiftly adapted to the physical distancing requirements by creating barriers between the stations and expanding into an adjoining space that was left vacant by a business that couldn't adapt.

Necessity is indeed the mother of invention and the midwife of success.

Patience

Impatience is a sign of the ego's need for control: wanting things to unfold exactly as we wish. But when we enlist the help of others and approach our work as partners, we find our success amplified by contributions beyond the ego's narrow control. When we plant seeds and water and feed them, we can be sure that they will sprout in their own good time, quite apart from any desires or impatient demands we might be harboring. Maximum energy on our part, combined with patient faith in the Law of Magnetism, is the winning formula.

> Patience is the prerequisite.... and the straightest and smoothest highway to every type of success.[11]

Non-attachment

Exercising creative initiative requires a balancing act between wholeheartedly pursuing a clear direction, and remaining calmly unattached to the results.

A defining quality of prosperity is "flow." Prosperity comes by entering the already-existing flow of abundance. When we try to grab the flow tightly in our hands and control the outcome, the result is anxiety, nervousness, and tension – for there is no way to contain its mighty wave. The satisfaction and invigoration we find in doing our best at every moment will be our richest, most satisfying reward.

> Don't work with the thought of what you might get out of it. What comes of itself, let it come. Work to serve God, and for the supreme satisfaction of pleasing Him.[12]

> Don't be attached to success or failure. Successful people work primarily for the joy of doing what they feel inspired to do. They are less concerned with returns on their labor. Nonattachment helps a person to live fully in the present tense – to do his best *right now*.[13]

Contentment

Closely related to non-attachment is contentment, which Patanjali, in his Yoga Sutras, names as *santosha*, calling it the greatest of all virtues.

Contentment means to be grateful and at peace with what we have, yet at the same time not resigned to the *status quo*. Both non-attachment and contentment are attitudes that open the floodgates of prosperity.

In Yogananda's words we recognize again the need for a delicate balance between putting out maximum energy to achieve our desired goals, and not letting ourselves become enslaved by runaway ambition for the results.

> Life will give you more than you ever dreamed, if only you will define prosperity anew: not as worldly gain, but as inner, divine contentment.[14]

Self-confidence

Humility may be the opposite of bravado, but we should not confuse humility with an inferiority complex.

> An inferiority complex is born of contact with weak-minded people and the weak innate subconscious mind. A superiority complex results from false pride and an inflated ego. Both inferiority and superiority complexes are destructive to self-development. Both are fostered by imagination, ignoring facts, while neither belongs to the true, all-powerful nature of the soul. Develop self-confidence by conquering your weaknesses. Found your self-confidence on actual achievements, and you will be free from all inferiority and superiority complexes.[15]

Everything on earth has its unique qualities, but nothing on earth possesses all possible qualities. There are perfumed roses, and roses that are multicolored but without scent. Some trees bear fruit while others give shade. Some people are quick off the mark, and others are slow and steady. Comparing ourselves to others prevents us from discovering and developing our unique talents.

> It is unfair for anyone, in his true self,
> to have to stand comparison to others.
> There is in each of us a special song to be sung.
> None of us is more important, or less so, than
> any other. Our simple duty is to find our unique
> song deep within us, and to sing it to perfection.
> That perfection will come only when we have
> learned to sing our own soul-song to God, offering
> back to Him the inspiration of *His* love.[16]

No matter how great our talents and accomplishments, they all pale in comparison to what we can achieve when we look past egoic self-preoccupation and connect with our Source.

✺ AN ESTEEMED WAY OF BEING ✺

No matter how many accolades and awards I received for my public talks, every time I had to give a presentation or speak in public, I had to do battle with a deep sense of incompetency. It made me so nervous that I would become disoriented and forget my script. I consoled myself that it was humble to feel this way. But then I listened to a talk in which Swami Kriyananda disabused me of this notion. He said, "High or low self-esteem are not different from each other: both of them arise from excessive ego-consciousness."

My self-criticism and my desire for perfection were seemingly only signs of too much egoic self-preoccupation. There was always one more milestone I felt I had to pass in order to prove my worthiness.

These dysfunctional attitudes made it difficult to relax and rejoice in my own and my teammates' successes. Although I was forging ahead quite well in my career, there were times when the nervousness and desire to withdraw impacted my performance. I knew there was an opportunity for growth somewhere in it all, if I could only stay focused in the moment and not in my fears.

Quite unexpectedly, a challenging opportunity suddenly came, accompanied by a surprising solution. I was scheduled to speak at a global conference of young entrepreneurs. When I took the stage, the audience had pretty much lost interest in the speeches and were engaged with their smartphones. Normally, my confidence would have spiraled into nervousness, but this time was different. A fresh thought came into my mind: how could I help these distracted millennials become fulfilled and successful entrepreneurs?

That thought inspired a flood of enthusiasm, and with it a flow of words that were much more relevant than the ones I had planned. Heads came up, synergy returned to the room, and soon everyone was raptly involved in my presentation and the ensuing discussion. The applause at the end was satisfying, but even more so was the joy and relief of having intuitively found a solution that I could use from then on.

Since that victory, I have made a conscious effort to replace thoughts of inadequacy with the genuinely humble thought – "How can I help?" In the process, I forget myself and my inadequacies and expand my heart to embrace others' realities.

This was made possible by regular meditation that naturally filled my inner void and bestowed a feeling of wholeness. To reinforce this esteemed new way of being, I have been using one of Swami Kriyananda's affirmations: *"Mine is the power of the universe, channeled for my own awakening and the awakening of other sleeping souls!"* –**Madhu**, *Mumbai*

In the Bhagavad Gita, Krishna assures his disciple, Arjuna.

> To those who meditate on Me as their Very Own, ever united to Me by incessant worship, I make good their deficiencies, and render permanent their gains. (9:22)

Service

A serviceful attitude is critically important for success: that whatever we want to offer should be genuinely useful, and that we should work not only for personal gain, but also include the welfare of others.

> Your work in the world, in the sphere where your karma, your own action, has placed you, can only be performed by you yourself. And it can only be successful when it serves your fellow man.[17]

The stories we've encountered in these pages – about George Washington Carver, India's President Abdul Kalam, and renowned botanist Luther Burbank – reveal these great souls as remarkable innovators. Their lives demonstrate how success, simplicity, contentment, and service go hand in hand in a successful life. The following story demonstrates how a serviceful attitude led to remarkable success.

❈ The best bellboy in Boston ❈

He was only a humble bellboy, yet the guests who regularly returned to the luxurious Boston hotel unfailingly requested – and even insisted on – his services.

Walter was nine when he left school to help support his impoverished family. Even in those days, when child labor was not regulated, it wasn't easy to find work. Walter was so grateful to the hotel that hired him that he determined to be the best bellboy it had ever employed. His salary was $8 per month, and in the busy summer months he could expect tips of perhaps $100.

He made sure the guests were well settled in their rooms and suites. He would get them ice water or whatever they required, shine the shoes they left outside their doors at night, and when an infant awoke crying and hungry at five in the morning, he would happily go out to buy fresh milk. The guests were wealthy and tried to tip him generously, but Walter wouldn't accept a dime. No – it was his job to be a help to them, and he spared no energy in offering them the best service in Boston.

In his little free time, he began to sketch and paint, and when the hotel guests saw his work, they recognized clear signs of genius. They bought paintings amounting to $850, far more than he could make in tips. Five wealthy families made offers of legal adoption, which he courteously refused. Walter established lasting friendships with the guests, who commissioned many paintings and portraits and referred their friends to him. With these funds, added to what he earned playing the organ at church, he enrolled in art school and soon became a sought-after portrait painter of children, as well as of many notable people, including Mrs. Theodore Roosevelt and her children, and Archbishop Corrigan.

Walter Russell went from success to success. He would receive recognition and awards for his book and magazine illustrations, as a war correspondent, and in architecture, real estate development, writing, philosophy, and sculpture. His busts of Thomas Edison, Joan of Arc, Franklin Delano Roosevelt, George Gershwin, and Charles Goodyear are breathtaking, as is his monument to Mark Twain, portraying the American author with twenty-eight characters from his books.

The magnetism he generated by his loving and selfless service as a bellboy rewarded him not only with abundant riches; it opened many doors for the expression of his prodigious talents.*

---

* "Walter Russell," Wikipedia, https://en.wikipedia.org/wiki/Walter_Russell.

Joy

> Joy is the true lord of this world. People are ruled by what they most desire. And what do all men want, truly? Joy! Even when they think it is money or fame or good health, joy is always their "ulterior motive." [18]

True success is measured not by our bank account or our possessions, but by the satisfaction we feel at the end of a day well lived.

> The best test is to analyze yourself and find out whether you are happier today than you were yesterday. If you feel that you are happier today, then you are progressing, and this feeling of happiness must continue. [19]

These lyrics by Swami Kriyananda describe such happiness.

There's Joy in the Heavens

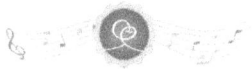

There's joy in the heavens,
A smile on the mountains,
And melody sings everywhere.
The flowers are all laughing
To welcome the morning;
Your soul is as free as the air.
Leave home in the sunshine:
Dance through a meadow —
Or sit by a stream and just BE.
The lilt of the water
Will gather your worries
And carry them down to the sea.
Men hunger for freedom,
But don't see their dungeon
Is only the thought that
  they're bound!
Desires are their shackles:
The hope that tomorrow
The doorway to joy will be
  found.
There's joy all around us!
Why wait till tomorrow?
We've only this moment to live.
A heaven within us
Is ours for the finding,
A freedom no riches can give!

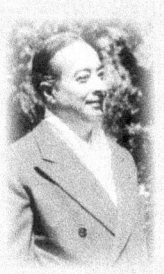

YOGANANDA'S RECIPE FOR PROSPERITY [20]

- Success is for the hardworking man.
- Success is for the man of creative ability.
- Success is for the man who knows how to economize.
- Success is for the man who thinks and asks opinions of financial experts before he invests his money.
- Success is for the man who tries harder to make money after each failure.
- Success is for the man of incessant working ability.
- Success comes to the man of character.
- Success comes to the man of regularity.
- Success comes to the man who seeks for more with dissatisfied satisfaction—who does not rest on his laurels.
- Success comes to the man who does little accomplishments very well.
- Success comes to the undaunted.
- Success comes to the man who advertises his business rightly and sells the best articles.
- Success comes to the man who spends less than his income and not more.
- Success comes to those who make money by making others more prosperous.
- Success comes to those who spend for God's work with as much spontaneity, naturalness, and pleasure as they do for themselves or their own families.

NOTES | PART XI

Title Page
1 Yogananda, Yogananda, *Super Advanced Course No. 1*, Lesson 6.
2 Yogananda, *Scientific Healing Affirmations*, 62-63.

Chapter One
1 Yogananda, "The Surest Way to Prosperity," *East-West*, October 1932.
2 Yogananda, "Divine Abundance," *Inner Culture*, June, 1940.
3 Yogananda, *Praecepta Lessons*, Vol. 2:47-48.
4 Yogananda, "The Surest Way to Prosperity," *East-West*, October 1932.
5 Kriyananda, *Do it NOW!*, July 11.
6 Yogananda, "Spiritualizing Business–Henry Ford's Five-Day Working Week," *East-West*, November-December 1926.
7 Yogananda, "My Divine Birthright," *Attributes of Success*, 1.
8 Yogananda, *New Super Cosmic Science Course*, Lesson 5.
9 "Transcendence: My Spiritual Experiences with Pramukh Swamiji", https://en.wikipedia.org/wiki/

Chapter Two
1 Kriyananda, *Money Magnetism*, 18.
2 Yogananda, "The Ocean of Abundance," *Attributes of Success*, 7.
3 Yogananda, "How to Unleash Your Secret Magnetism," *Praecepta Lessons*, Vol. 2: 47-48.
4 Yogananda, *Super-Advanced Course No. 1*, Lesson 8. See the complete article in the online Appendices.
5 Yogananda, "Recipes," *East-West*, May-June 1927.
6 Yogananda, *Praecepta Lessons*, Vol. 5:116.
7 Yogananda, *Super-Advance Course No. 1*, Lesson 6.
8 Yogananda, Lesson 8.
9 Walters (Swami Kriyananda), *Education for Life*, 158.
10 Yogananda, *Yogoda Course*, Lesson 10.
11 Yogananda, "Failure as a Stimulant," *Attributes of Success*, 4.
12 Kriyananda, Swami, "The Science of the Future," Unity in Yoga Conference, May 27, 1995.
13 Yogananda, "Meditations and Affirmations," *East-West*, August 1932.

Chapter Three
1 Kriyananda, *Hindu Way of Awakening*, 220.
2 Yogananda, "Acquiring Magnetism," *Inner Culture*, July 1941.
3 Kriyananda, *Material Success Through Yoga Principles*, Vol I:134.
4 Yogananda, *The Attributes of Success*, 2.
5 Yogananda, "The Ocean of Abundance," *The Attributes of Success*, 7.
6 Yogananda, *Super-Advanced Course No. 1*, Lesson 6.
7 Yogananda, "The Second Coming of Christ," *Inner Culture*, January 1940.
8 Yogananda, "The Surest Way to Prosperity," *East-West*, October 1932.
9 Kriyananda, *Art and Science of Raja Yoga*, 279, 280.
10 Yogananda, "The Value of Meditation," *The Attributes of Success*, 8.
11 Kriyananda, *Money Magnetism*, Chapter 92-93.
12 Yogananda, "The Dynamic Power of Will," *The Attributes of Success*, 3.

13 Kriyananda, *Money Magnetism*, 101.
14 Kriyananda, *Art as a Hidden Message*, 98.
15 Yogananda, *Yogoda Course*, Lesson 8.
16 Yogananda, "Will Power," *Inner Culture*, November 1938.
17 Kriyananda, *Art and Science of Raja Yoga*, 297.
18 Yogananda, *The Essence of Self-Realization*, 15:5.
19 Kriyananda, *Art as a Hidden Message*, 98.
20 Kriyananda, *The Light of Superconsciousness*, 19.
21 Cohn, Patrick, "How Olympians Use Mental Imagery To Improve Success," *Peak Performance Sports*, https://www.peaksports.com/sports-psychology-blog/how-olympians-use-mental-imagery-to-improve-success/.
22 Yogananda, "The Value of Meditation," *Attributes of Success*, 8.
23 Yogananda, "Recipes," *East-West*, November-December 1927.
24 Yogananda, "Failure as a Stimulant," *Attributes of Success*, 4.
25 Kriyananda, *Art and Science of Raja Yoga*, 296, 297.

Chapter Four

1 Kriyananda, *Money Magnetism*, 12.
2 Yogananda, "Real Prosperity," *Inner Culture*, January 1939.
3 Yogananda, "Four Recipes," *East-West*, July-August 1928.
4 Yogananda, "Spiritualizing Business — Henry Ford's Five-Day Working Week," *East-West*, November-December 1926.
5 Yogananda, "Divine Abundance," *Inner Culture*, June 1940.
6 Kriyananda, "How Much Wealth is Available?" *Money Magnetism*, 54.
7 Yogananda, "Recipes," *East-West*, July-August 1928.
8 Yogananda, "Four Recipes," *East-West*, July-August 1928 and January-February 1929.
9 Yogananda, "Interpretation of the Bhagavad Gita," Verse 2:33, *Inner Culture*, March 1935.
10 Yogananda, "Spiritualizing Business–Henry Ford's Five-Day Working Week," *East-West*, November-December 1926.
11 Yogananda, "Meditation and Affirmations," *East-West*, March 1933.
12 Yogananda, *New Super Cosmic Science Course*, Lesson 5.
13 Kriyananda, *Money Magnetism*, 50.
14 Yogananda, *The Essence of the Bhagavad Gita*, 485, Verse 16:3.
15 Kriyananda, *The New Path*, 253.
16 Yogananda, "Recipes," *East-West*, January-February 1929.
17 Kriyananda, *Material Success Through Yoga Principles*, Vol. I: 298-299.
18 Yogananda, "Recipes: Creating Your Happiness," *East-West*, August 1932.
19 Kriyananda, *Material Success Through Yoga Principles*, Vol. I: 305, 21.
20 Kriyananda, *Money Magnetism*, 79, 58.
21 Yogananda, "Recipes," *East-West*, August 1932.
22 Yogananda, "Spiritualizing Business — Henry Ford's Five-Day Working Week," *East-West*, November-December 1926. You can find this article in the Appendices.
23 Yogananda.
24 "The Man Behind Good Business and Good Chocolate," Hershey, https://www.thehersheycompany.com/en_us/home/about-us/the-company/milton-hershey.html.
25 Kumar, Rusen, "Corporate Social Responsibility (CSR) in India," *Indiacsr*, https://indiacsr.in/corporate-social-responsibility-csr-in-india/
26 Yogananda, *Autobiography of a Yogi*, 121.
27 Yogananda's predictions can be found in these books by Swami Kriyananda: *The Road Ahead*; *Intentional Communities: How to Start Them and Why*, published in

one volume with *Cities of Light: A Plan for This Age;* and *Hope for a Better World: The Small Communities Solution.*
28 https://www.ananda.org/find-ananda/
29 Kriyananda, *Material Success Through Yoga Principles,* Vol. I: 296.
30 Kriyananda, "Gratitude," *Affirmations for Self-Healing,* 114.
31 Yogananda, "Meditation and Affirmations," *East-West,* May 1932.

Chapter Five

1 Kriyananda, *Money Magnetism,* 74.
2 Kriyananda, *Material Success Through Yoga Principles,* Vol. II: 150.
3 Kriyananda, *Money* Magnetism, 73.

Chapter Six

1 Yogananda, *Attributes of Success,* 8.
2 Yogananda, *Yogoda Course,* Lesson 10.
3 Yogananda, "Analyze Yourself," *Attributes of Success.*
4 Yogananda, "Recipes," *East-West,* January-April, and May-June 1927.
5 "Luther Burbank Quotes," *Goodreads,* https://www.goodreads.com/author/quotes/227459.Luther_Burbank.
6 Yogananda, "Luther Burbank: An Appreciation," *East-West,* May-June 1926.
7 Yogananda, "Recipes," *East-West,* May-June 1927.
8 Kriyananda, *Material Success Through Yoga Principles,* Vol. II: 255, 263.
9 Yogananda, *Attributes of Success,* 2.
10 Kriyananda, *Money Magnetism,* 121-122.
11 Kriyananda, *Do It NOW!,* December 5.
12 Kriyananda, *The New Path,* 249.
13 Kriyananda, *26 Keys to Greater Awareness.*
14 Yogananda, *The Rubaiyat of Omar Khayyam Explained,* 52.
15 Yogananda, *Super-Advanced Course No. 1* Lesson 9.
16 Kriyananda, *Art as a Hidden Message,* Chapter Nine.
17 Yogananda, "Analyze Yourself," *Attributes of Success,* 5.
18 Kriyananda, *Eastern Thoughts–Western Thoughts,* 90.
19 Yogananda, *Praecepta Lessons,* Vol. 3:53.
20 Yogananda, "Recipes," East-West, May-June 1929.

PART XII
VIBRATORY HEALING

Different rates of vibration, balanced in the cosmic rhythm, produce before us the majestic cosmos.[1] —Yogananda

Everything in life is vibration. We are slowed down sound and light waves, a walking bundle of frequencies tuned into the cosmos. —Albert Einstein

If you want to find the secrets of the universe, think in terms of energy, frequency, and vibration. —Nikola Tesla

PART XII   CHAPTER ONE

The Vibratory Structure of the Universe

> Consciousness and vibratory matter are the two natures of one undivided, unmanifested Spirit. The difference between consciousness and matter is relative. The former is a deeper and the latter a grosser vibration of the one Transcendental Spirit.[1] –YOGANANDA
>
> In all creation, nothing exists except vibration. Even the rocks are insubstantial: Science has found that matter is only a particular vibration of energy. Were vibration to cease, matter would revert back to its essence, Spirit.[2] –KRIYANANDA

Everything in creation is in motion. Plants reach out with their tendrils to climb walls and fences. Our thoughts travel at supersonic speeds. Our earth orbits the sun at 16,000 miles per hour – as Galileo said: "And yet it moves!" The galaxies revolve at tremendous speed, while moving away from each other as the universe expands.

What we perceive with our physical senses, and everything that exists outside the range of our senses, is essentially the result of consciousness and movement.

> By creation, the hitherto unmanifested Spirit manifests two natures—one consciousness, and the other vibration. Consciousness is the vibration of Its subjective nature, and vibration is the manifestation of Its objective nature.[3]

Every movement in physical creation produces waves. The motions of subatomic particles produce seemingly solid matter, including the infinite variety of life forms that inhabit the physical world. Similarly, waves of thought and energy create the causal and astral worlds, respectively. In the world of physical matter, vibrations create musical sounds and colors that we perceive with our senses.

The musical, mathematical, and geometric foundations of the universe

After its debut performance in 1918, Gustav Holst's haunting musical suite "The Planets" became popular for its musical suggestion of distant worlds. Swami Kriyananda used it as the background for a recording of himself reading a selection of Yogananda's "Metaphysical Meditations."

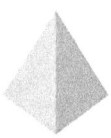
TETRAHEDRON

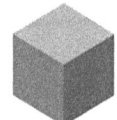
CUBE

The notion that heavenly bodies emit music as they travel through space is attributed to Pythagoras, the Greek philosopher and mathematician of the sixth century B.C. Pythagoras surmised that the universe was created from a single central vibration that manifested sounds particular to each aspect of creation – thus all plants, planets, and human beings had their own unique frequencies. Pythagoras spoke of the "music of the spheres"[4] – melodies that emanate from the planets – and a grand cosmic symphony of the combined sounds of all created things.

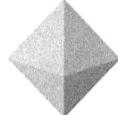
OCTAHEDRON

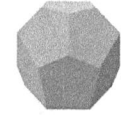
DODECAHEDRON

Vibrations produce sound, and according to Pythagoras, sound produces a form unique to each frequency – mathematically based patterns that are repeated throughout all nature, from the smallest subatomic particles to the largest galaxy. In Pythagoras' view, there are five perfectly symmetrical, archetypical shapes on which the universe is constructed: cube, tetrahedron, octahedron, dodecahedron, and icosahedron. Later known as Platonic solids, these shapes are used by certain healers to amplify healing energies.[5]

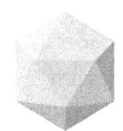
ICOSAHEDRON

> "In the context of healing, Sacred Shapes are elemental shapes that complete the toolkit of Sacred Geometry Healing. Placing or visualising these shapes at the seven chakras or energy centres of the body can help activate the virtues and vibrations related to those meridians."[6]

All sounds, including the human voice, produce forms, which sensitive instrumentation has been able to detect. Here is a fascinating story told by Swami Sivananda of Rishikesh.[7]

✸ SINGING A DAISY ✸

Sounds are vibrations. They give rise to definite forms. This view has recently received corroboration in experiments carried on by Mrs. Watts Hughes, the gifted author of "Voice Figures." She delivered an illustrated lecture before a select audience in Lord Leighton's studio to demonstrate the beautiful scientific discoveries on which she has alighted, as the result of many years of patient labor.

Mrs. Hughes sings into a simple instrument called an "Eidophone," which consists of a tube, a receiver and a flexible membrane, and she finds that each note assumes definite and constant shape, as revealed through a sensitive and mobile medium. At the outset of her lecture, she placed tiny seeds upon the flexible membrane. The air vibrations set up by the notes she sang, danced them into definite geometric patterns....

Once when Mrs. Hughes was singing a note, a daisy appeared and disappeared. "I tried," she said "to sing it back for weeks before at last I succeeded." Now she knows the precise inflections of the particular note that is a daisy, and it is made constant and definite by a strange method of coaxing an alteration of crescendo and diminuendo. She then sang a series of daisies of great beauty, some with succeeding rows of delicate petals.

The flowers were followed by sea-monsters, serpentine forms full of light and shade and detail. After these came other notes that produced trees, trees with fruit falling, trees with a foreground of rocks, trees with the sea behind them.

In France, Madam Finlang's singing of the hymn "Ave Maria" brought out the form of Mary with child Jesus on her lap. The singing of the hymn to the god Bhairava by a Bengali girl studying in France gave rise to the formation of the figure of Bhairava, with his vehicle, the dog.

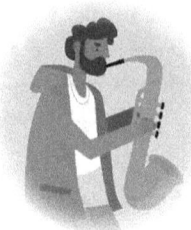

There are sounds that soothe, sounds that excite, sounds that lull us to sleep, and sounds that awaken us. Certain sounds evoke fear, whereas others elicit delight. Each sound contains a power to manifest or dissolve.

In his autobiography, Yogananda speaks of sounds that can extinguish a fire.

> Charles Kellogg, the California naturalist, gave a demonstration of the effect of tonal vibration on fire in 1926 before a group of New York firemen. "Passing a bow, like an enlarged violin bow, swiftly across an aluminum tuning fork, he produced a screech like intense radio static. Instantly the yellow gas flame, two feet high, leaping inside a hollow glass tube, subsided to a height of six inches and became a sputtering blue flare. Another attempt with the bow, and another screech of vibration, extinguished it."[8]

City dwellers today are prey to a cacophony of sounds that enter through our senses and penetrate the central nervous system, affecting our emotions and even the vibratory composition of our body cells. Protective measures such as multiple-pane windows and avoiding noisy locales when possible, are highly advised.

Sound frequencies and health

Frequencies of sound are indicated in hertz (Hz), or cycles per second. Low-frequency sounds, called infrasound, are produced by cars, trucks and rail traffic; air and water craft; by heavy industrial machines; and by household equipment such as washing machines, heating units, and air conditioning units.

Extended exposure to infrasound creates a general sense of disturbance and lowers our immunity to disease. Such exposure can negatively affect blood pressure, balance, and membranes of the inner ear; as well as produce fatigue, hypertension, depression, abdominal distress, headache, depression, sleep disorders, and anxiety attacks.[9]

These low frequencies lower our body's defenses and make us more vulnerable to disease. Higher-frequency sounds, including flowing water, birdsong, and natural sounds such as wind in the trees recharge the brain, slow the heart rate, lower blood pressure, and strengthen the body's immunity.[10]

Dr. Robert Becker, whom we met in Part IV, observed in *The Body Electric*:

> "The human body has an electrical frequency and much about a person's health can be determined by it. Frequency is the measurable rate of electrical energy flow that is constant between any two points. Everything has frequency."[11]

In recent research, Bruce Tainio has measured the frequencies of the human body using an instrument of his creation, the Calibrated Frequency Monitor. Tainio found that the healthy human body vibrates at a frequency between 72 and 90 megahertz Hz. When the body's frequency drops below these levels, diseases can more easily invade.[12]

> HUMAN BODY: 72-90 MHz
> BRAIN: 72-90 MHz
> DISEASE: starts at 58 MHz
> COLDS/FLU: starts at 57-60 MHz
> CANCER: starts at 42 MHz
> DEATH: starts at 25 MHz

The healing methods described in Volume One are intended to be used to maintain the body's vibrational frequency at a healthy level. Particularly effective in this regard are the practice of meditation, the Life Force Energization Exercises, and the Full Body Recharge, especially when these exercises are practiced repeatedly throughout the day.

We will soon explore other salutary frequencies that can help keep the body's vibrational "tone" and defenses strong. But first we will look at the three qualities that pervade the material universe: the *Gunas*.

PART XII   CHAPTER TWO

The Three *Gunas*

> The three *gunas* represent the progressive stages of manifestation outward from the oneness of Spirit.[1] –KRIYANANDA.
>
> The Infinite One vibrated a part of Himself to become two, then many, until the cosmic vibration produced stars and galaxies and planets, flowers and trees and human bodies.[2] –YOGANANDA

Just as numbers play a fundamental role in the Pythagorean concept of the physical universe, so too in metaphysics, numbers can help us understand the invisible vibratory nature of creation.

In the metaphysical lore of ancient India, the number One refers to the unmoving Spirit beyond creation – Satchidananda ("ever-existing, ever-conscious, ever-new joy," as Yogananda defined it).*

The number Two refers to duality: the vibratory force that pure Spirit projected out of itself in order to manifest the universe.

The number Three refers to numerous metaphysical concepts. For our present purpose, it refers to the *gunas*: the three qualities that characterize the created worlds. This is one of the deepest topics of the Vedic teachings. It is explained with exceptional clarity in the Bhagavad Gita, and is mentioned in the writings of many masters through the ages.[3]

> All creation...is a mixture of the three *gunas*, or basic qualities of consciousness. The lowest of them is *tamo guna* (the darkening quality).

---

* See Volume One, Part One for a discussion of the origins of creation.

> Next comes *rajo guna* (the activating quality).
> The highest of the three is *sattwa guna*
> (the spiritually clarifying, or elevating, quality).
> The universe everywhere manifests
> predominantly one or another of these qualities.
> Indeed, the Master told us that entire galaxies
> manifest primarily one or another *guna*.[4]

Everything in creation expresses a mixture of these three qualities: they define the quality of the food we eat, as well as of our thoughts, the places where we live, work, or visit, the people we encounter, and our outward activities – in short, every facet of our lives.

> Every human being manifests these three
> qualities to varying degrees, depending on the
> vibrations of his consciousness and energy.
> If his flow of energy is entirely upward, it gains
> in refinement until at last he passes beyond the
> three gunas into the pure, vibrationless Spirit.
> If the flow is downward, his understanding
> becomes increasingly dull until there is little,
> apart from his human form, to distinguish him
> from the lower animals. And if he lives, as most
> people do, in a state of indecision and inner
> conflict between these two directional flows,
> he remains tossing back and forth,
> forever agitated and restless.[5]

Each of the gunas holds secrets for how to improve our health and prevent illness. As we explore them in this chapter, you will learn how they relate to your diet, your thoughts, the environments and people in your life, and your efforts at self-improvement.

Sattwa Guna
⊛ LET YOUR LIGHT SHINE ⊛

O Sinless One (Arjuna)! Of these gunas, the pure quality of sattwa bestows health and understanding.... When the light of discrimination shines through all of a person's sense gates, it is clear that sattwa predominates in him. (BHAGAVAD GITA 14:6, 11)

The concept of light plays a prominent role in metaphysical teachings. It is one of the first manifestations of Spirit [**Then God said, "Let there be light."** (GENESIS 1:3)] and is a defining quality of sattwa guna. In English, the word "light" has two meanings: physical light, as in the rays of the sun, and the act of reducing physical or psychological weight, as in "lighten your burden." Both of these meanings can help us understand and use sattwa guna to improve our health.

In Volume One, Part IV we learned to use the rays of sunlight to enhance healing. In Volume Two, Part VIII, on the practice of affirmation, we learned powerful methods for enlightening our thoughts.

Also inherent to sattwa are the qualities associated with inner stillness. Sattwa represents that still point between every two movements, the point of rest, of *being* rather than *doing*. It is a state where conflicts become resolved and healing can happen.

QUALITIES OF SATTWA GUNA[6]

Balanced	Calm	Clean	Content
Devoted	Discerning	Dutiful	Faithful
Grateful	Harmonious	Impartial	Intuitive
Loyal	Luminous	Modest	Noble
Patient	Philanthropic	Pure	Simple
Tolerant	Truthful	Virtuous	Wise

Sattwic foods

Sattwic foods have a cooling effect on the brain and nervous system. They help us to be calm and centered. They are easily digested, enhance longevity, and support spiritual development. Among the sattwic foods that Yogananda names are fresh fruit, coconut, raw or lightly cooked vegetables, fruit and vegetable juices, unprocessed grains, peanut and almond pastes, honey, nuts, fresh milk, and coconut milk.

In *The Holy Science*,[7] Swami Sri Yukteswar, Yogananda's guru, asserts that the original diet of human beings is primarily fruit (frugivorous). He adds that "various grains, fruits, roots…milk, and pure water…are decidedly the best natural food for man."*

Mental Diet †

Just as we tend to habitually eat the same foods, we also have a habitual mindset, what Yogananda calls our "mental diet." Each thought directly and immediately influences our health, either opening or closing the channel for the flow of healing life force.

> Have you ever analyzed your magnetic mental diet? It consists usually of the thoughts which you are thinking as well as the thoughts you are receiving from the close thought contact with your friends. Peaceful thoughts and peaceful friends always produce healthy, magnetic minds.[8]

Sattwic thoughts reveal our noble soul qualities: *"I am a child of eternity. I am ageless. I am deathless. I am the changeless Spirit at the heart of all mutation!"* [9]

Sattwic thoughts enable us to see the best in others: *"I see the goodness in everything. I will view the world around me…from the heights of divine aspiration."* [10]

They affirm truth – such as "I am strong! I am well!" – rather than fleeting facts, such as "I have the flu, I am weak."

* Detailed recommendations for a healthy diet can be found in Volume One, Part V, Chapter Three.

† More detailed suggestions for improving your mental diet can be found in Volume Two, Part VI, Chapter Three.

A sattwic mind is better able to perceive deep connections, and to see the components of our relationships and undertakings as a unified whole. Sattwic awareness can help us, above all, to perceive the lives of all beings as unified in Spirit.

I recently had a "mental diet" experience. As I waited in the long line at the post office, I noticed that my thoughts were tending toward impatience and judgment, decidedly unhelpful rajasic thoughts. I couldn't resist, however, thinking of the hilarious scene from the film *Zootopia*, where the animal clerks at the Department of Motor Vehicles are played by sloths. As I inwardly laughed, my frustration diffused, and I could then turn my thoughts to compassion for the over-worked clerks. With awareness, we can redirect judgmental thoughts in a positive, more healthy, sattwic direction.

People

Few outward influences affect our lives as powerfully as other people. Sattwic people are themselves calm, centered and serviceful, inspiring in others these same qualities. Their very presence can exert a healing influence on us.

> **We must be careful with whom we associate, because we are continually exchanging magnetism with other people through our thoughts, through shaking hands and through looking into the eyes of another person. The person who is the stronger gives his vibration to the other person. We become like the people we mingle with, not through their conversation, but through the silent magnetic vibration which goes out of their bodies. When we come in the range of their magnetism, we become like them.**[11]

The presence of sattwic people is healing and uplifting. In Chapter Nine we will consider the powerfully uplifting influence of saintly people. If we are unable to spend time in the physical presence of such advanced souls and saints, we can in any case absorb their influence and consciousness through books, sound recordings, and films.

> Read books and keep company with those silent friends who have the power to comfort and inspire.... Books are your best friends. You can quietly hear Shakespeare, Milton, Emerson, Kalidasa, Krishna, Confucius, Plato, Buddha, Christ, talk to you, solace you, and give you infinite advice. If you have no friends, or if they are a drain on your time uselessly, consort with these wisdom friends by entering through the portals of real study into the eternally charming and interesting thought-land.[12]

Yogananda published a monthly magazine, *East-West* (later renamed *Inner Culture*) with a "Recipes" column where he often recommended inspiring literature, such as the following:

- A few lines daily from the Bhagavad Gita by Sir Edwin Arnold, called *Song Celestial*
- One page daily from Shakespeare
- A history of philosophy
- Ten lines each day from the Gospel of St. John
- The poems of Walt Whitman and Ralph Waldo Emerson
- Scientific books, too. Each new finding of science reveals the glory and wonder of God.
- Books about Indian culture and life, written by Margaret E. Noble (Sister Nivedita)
- *The Imitation of Christ*, by Thomas à Kempis
- Tagore's Nobel Prize-winning book of poetry, *Gitanjali*
- Francis Thompson's poem, "The Hound of Heaven"
- *In Tune with the Infinite*, by Ralph Waldo Trine
- *The Man Nobody Knows*, by Bruce Barton
- *Tao and Wu Wei*, by Henri Borel

Environments

Sattwic environments are calm, harmonious, clean, and uncluttered. They exert a relaxing influence on the body and mind, and encourage us to slow down. Think of how you feel in an airport or bus terminal, compared to how you feel in your favorite natural surroundings. A day spent outdoors in nature or a walk in the park can often set our lives back on course.

There are places that have powerful uplifting vibrations, left by great souls who lived there, or due to their unusually pure natural resonances. We will have more to say later about these special environments, and how we can adjust our own environment to support our physical, mental, and spiritual health. For now, consider the effect that your home, workplace, and the places you regularly visit might have on your wellbeing.

Spiritual practices

Spiritual activities including Hatha Yoga postures, pranayama breathing exercises, meditation, and selfless service calm the nervous system and are greatly beneficial to our health. Their power to heal will depend on the specific practices and how, when, and how regularly we use them.

Yoga. The yoga postures (*asanas*) have a remarkable balancing effect on the body and a deeply calming influence on the mind, especially when we do them with focused awareness, slowly, and accompanied with mental affirmations as taught in Ananda Yoga.[13]

Restorative Yoga is a modern adaptation of the classic yoga postures that focuses primarily on conscious relaxation and release of the physical and mental stress that accompany health challenges and life changes. It is suited to yogis of all paths, as well as to people whose physical condition prevents them from doing the classic positions, but who are able to assume the restorative postures with the aid of supports such as bolsters, cushions, and blankets, under the guidance of trained instructors. Ananda Restorative Yoga enhances the relaxing effects of the poses with affirmations that direct the mind to connect with the higher Self, accompanied by spiritually uplifting music, visualizations, and meditation. It is an ideal modern example of sattwic yoga.[14]

Pranayama. Sattwic breathing exercises cool the nervous system and mind. All of the practices in Volume One, Part III, and particularly the Triangular Breath, are useful in calming the mind and emotions in moments of anxiety and stress. Doing these exercise slowly and gently, with closed eyes, will reliably calm the heart rate and emotions.

Meditation. The purpose of meditation techniques is to calm the breath, still the mind, and reprogram the brain away from emotional reactivity. In meditation, the flow of healing life force is unencumbered by egoic interference, naturally bringing body, mind and soul into harmony, along with intuitive understanding to daily activities.

❈ MEDITATION OASIS ❈

It doesn't snow in Israel. Our country is half covered by desert with lush oases scattered throughout. Thus when I visited the Ananda Meditation Retreat in the Sierra Mountain foothills, I wasn't prepared for the sudden fear I experienced: of the cold, and of actually freezing to death.

With the onset of fall, it was already too cold and I was bundling up more and more with each passing day. I vividly remember a day when as part of the program I was taking we meditated outdoors in the early morning, in the picturesque but 4°C (39.2°F), cold and windy Temple of Leaves.

Wrapped in three blankets but still shivering, I sat to meditate, using all my willpower to hold off thoughts of quitting and rushing inside the chilly but not as freezing temple.

Facing the approaching sunrise, I invoked the presence of my Master and began to meditate. Somewhere along the way, I found a warm inner oasis. I think it was my determined will to stick it out that attracted the deep meditation to me.

I am not aware of how or when it happened, but since that meditation the cold no longer bedeviled me again. I spent the next two months living very serenely in a bungalow was covered in snow, and where at no time did I have hot water. I believe I would never have been able to endure if it were not for the healing during that very cold early morning meditation. *–**Ashtara**, Tel Aviv*

Patanjali's *Yoga Sutras* very clearly describe the steps that lead to *samadhi*, the state of freedom in God, beyond the influence of the gunas. It is not until the second-to-last stage of yoga, called *dhyana*, that we are fully able to enter a sattwic state. In dhyana, the waves of our individual personality are reabsorbed into the cosmic ocean of bliss. Listening inwardly to the Cosmic Sound of Aum is one technique for returning to bliss. Other techniques were discussed in Part II.

Sattwic service. A sattwic approach to service embraces attitudes of respect for the dignity of those we are serving, without a desire for recognition or compensation. The highest reward of such selfless service is the unalloyed joy that we experience when we expand our identity to include others. When we devote our energy and our time, talents, and resources to serve others, the flow of healing life force in us is stimulated and channeled to the recipients of our service.

Rajo Guna
~ CHOOSE WISELY! ~

In its purest, most uplifting form, rajo guna is energizing, activating, and stimulating. Rajasic energy can take us in four directions: upward toward expansion and creativity, outward toward restless involvement in material pursuits, downward toward tamasic inertia or dark activities such as addictions. 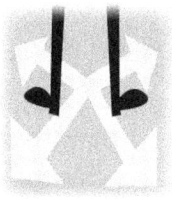 The fourth direction is inward, when we deliberately withdraw energy from the periphery of the body into the spinal highway, and within that channel, direct it upward through the higher chakras to the spiritual eye. There are many spiritual practices that enable us to harness rajasic energy and transform it for healing and Self-realization.

> Rajo guna is the energizing current in Nature,
> and therefore also in man. Rajo guna in the body,
> then, manifests as an upward movement. Indeed,
> we associate any surge of energy— a feeling of
> elation, for example—with an upward flow.

> With developing spiritual sensitivity it becomes clear also that this flow takes place primarily in the spine. Whether or not our awareness is centered there, an upward flow of energy and consciousness in the body produces a tendency to look upward, to stand or sit up straight, and to feel generally "up" about life.[15]

Most of us spend our days operating in spheres of rajo guna – we are outwardly energized and active. When we are in control of our rajasic energies, we can apply them to achieve good health, success, and satisfaction. But when we are victims of rajasic energy, allowing it to overwhelm us, we become restless and overextended, and our health may become compromised.

Burnout syndrome – physical and mental exhaustion, often attended by headaches, fatigue, gastrointestinal symptoms, irritability, and cynicism – is generally the result of excessive, uncontrolled rajasic activity. Burnout usually ends in tamasic exhaustion and inertia.

In the *Bhagavad Gita*, Krishna warns his chief disciple Arjuna about the dangers of uncontrolled rajasic energy.

> Know (the quality of) rajas as imbued with passion, which activates strong desires and attachments and binds one to the body by the intense expectations it develops in him, through his restlessness. (BHAGAVAD GITA 14:6)

Although raja guna can sometimes menace a peaceful meditation, it can save us when we fall into tamasic lethargy.

> Raja guna gives objectifying power to both sattwa and tamas. For tamasic people, it represents the necessary stepping stone to sattwa guna; for sattwic people, it represents the first pull away from spiritual reality, carrying them into worldly involvements.[16]

Life Force / 190

When your life is spinning out of control, and you find yourself moved from your center into a whirlwind of restless activity, a good practice is to take time out to do some slow, deep breathing, a few yoga postures or simple stretches, or go for a walk in the park. Once you have returned to your calm center, you can deliberately take control of your energy and apply it to your work or inwardly in meditation.

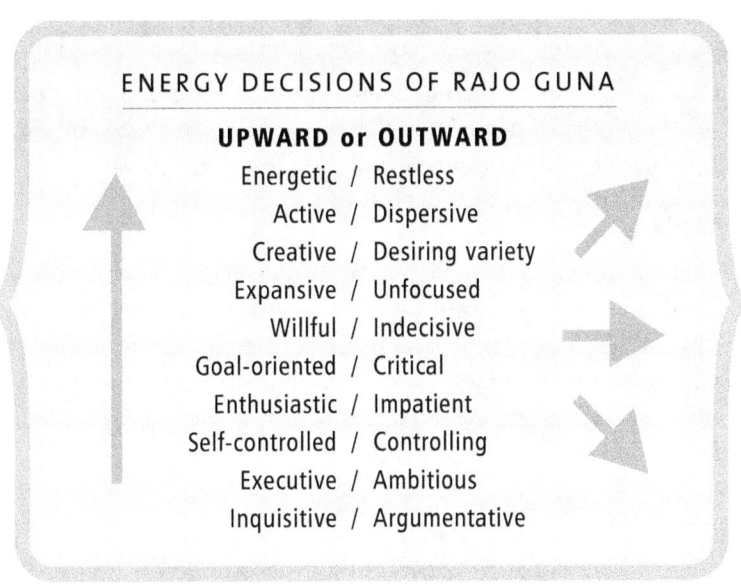

ENERGY DECISIONS OF RAJO GUNA

UPWARD or OUTWARD

Energetic / Restless
Active / Dispersive
Creative / Desiring variety
Expansive / Unfocused
Willful / Indecisive
Goal-oriented / Critical
Enthusiastic / Impatient
Self-controlled / Controlling
Executive / Ambitious
Inquisitive / Argumentative

Rajasic foods

Rajasic foods warm the body, enhance circulation, activate metabolism and digestion, and stimulate the brain. In contrast to sattwic foods, which are quickly absorbed, rajasic foods give energy over a longer period. They are generally cooked, whereas most sattwic foods are uncooked. Rajasic foods include grains and legumes, root vegetables, onions, garlic, eggs, fresh and slightly cured cheeses, chicken, fish, and spices such as salt, peppers, and curries.

Rajasic foods are good friends when we need to do hard physical work, especially in winter or colder climates. They can also help us get our energy flowing in moments of lethargy or discouragement.

Because rajasic foods stimulate the nervous system, they can make us restless. For this reason rajasic foods are best avoided in times of anxiety, fear, or temptation, or if you suffer from gastrointestinal problems or nervous disorders. The strongest rajasic foods, including coffee, black tea, processed sugars, and spicy condiments, excite the nervous system and interfere with proper digestion.

On the other hand, there are rajasic spices that offer valuable healing properties. The ancient Indian healing science of ayurveda includes remedies for specific conditions that take advantage of the healing properties of warming spices to aid digestion and stimulate metabolism – they include turmeric, cumin, black pepper, cayenne pepper, powdered ginger, and curry leaf. Honey is considered rajasic because it warms the body, but without over-exciting the nervous system. It has powerful healing properties when taken in small amounts, and when combined with certain spices.

Mental Diet

Rajasic thoughts are those that motivate us to action. They are useful on a daily basis as we confront our numerous tasks, and especially helpful when we need to ward off demotivating, tamasic thoughts. Training ourselves to meet every duty and every challenge with an energizing mental affirmation opens doorways for a flow of healing life force and for creative solutions.

> "I am awake and ready!"
> "I am positive, energetic, enthusiastic!"[17]

Although rajas can lead us to energetic activity, if we are not attentive it can also lead us to restless, unfocused activity. We want to become more aware of the thought patterns that cause the mind to spin around itself, without moving forward, or which bound indiscriminately from thought to thought, like a jackrabbit caught in the headlights of a car.

When we overextend ourselves, investing rajasic energy past the point where a quiet intelligence is urging us to stop – we soon find our efforts losing focus and momentum, as our body, mind, and soul try to warn us of impending burnout and pull us into rest-and-recovery mode – lest we suffer a complete collapse into health-destroying nervous exhaustion, attended by depthless lethargy, indifference, brainlessness, and despair.

People

Every one of us is constantly emitting a unique vibratory field that will unavoidably affect others. A story in Chapter One tells how a singer was able to "sing a daisy." We may find ourselves in environments where others are silently singing jarring melodies of conflict, spewing toxic negativity into the environment. For our own health, it is better to avoid such environments and people whenever possible. If we have to pass through such places, it will be best to make sure our energy tank is full and our aura shield is intact.*

On the plus side of rajas, there are people who, by their mere presence, can lift us out of discouragement and unwillingness, "infecting" us with a positive outlook and enthusiasm that lifts our spirits and our self-image. The moment our energy flags and becomes less positive, we should reach out to these people.

> **Write down the names** of at least three people whose enthusiasm and positivity uplift you. Connect with at least one of them this week.

Environments

There are places that are filled with invigorating rajasic energy – for instance, the gym. We wouldn't go to the gym to meditate, but when we need to raise our energy, thirty minutes on the treadmill or with weights will do the trick.

There are environments that stimulate the mind and inspire creativity. I happily recall the thrill I felt when I visited the hall where Galileo lectured at the University of Padua — it was the same current of high energy I felt at Tchaikovsky's home in Moscow, at the Nikola Tesla museum in Belgrade, and at the Musée Marmottan Monet in Paris while enjoying Monet's paintings.

During a visit to the United States, I was surprised to see journalists and authors writing for hours at a time in a Starbucks coffee shop. Perhaps their work demanded a public working space. While writing this book, I have been grateful to sit where Swami Kriyananda wrote many of his inspiring books, and to be able to work in silence except for a recording of him chanting Aum that plays softly in the background.

* Ways of protection from negative situations will be discussed in Chapter Eleven.

Spiritual practices

Yoga postures. Some of the asanas of hatha yoga are known to stimulate the brain; these include the inverted postures. Other poses, such as *Bhujangasana*, the Cobra Pose, energize the spine and move energy upward toward the brain. Still others stimulate digestion and metabolism, for example *Uddiyana Bandha*.

Some schools of yoga have a predominantly energizing approach to all the asanas, using them more along the lines of gymnastics, weight loss workouts and body building. However, a well-balanced yoga routine should activate and energize, and then capture the vital energy and bring it inward for meditation.

> Hatha yoga, the yoga of physical postures, is not a separate yoga science in its own right; rather it is the physical discipline of the integral teaching known as raja yoga.[18]

The therapeutic benefits of Hatha Yoga are well known. Medical institutes that include yoga therapy programs, for example, Kaivalyadhama, between Mumbai and Pune,[19] are revered in India and elsewhere for their research on how yoga impacts our biochemical, physiological, and psychological health.

Pranayama Breathing Exercises. Rajasic pranayamas such as Bastrika and Kapalabhati create heat in the body and are known to cleanse and open the *nadis*, the subtle energy channels in the spine through which the life force flows. These exercises improve respiratory capacity and boost metabolism and digestion, as well as activate the parasympathetic nervous system to calm the stress response.

Energization Exercises. Pranayama means control (*yama*) of the flow of life force (*prana*). In Part VI we were introduced to Yogananda's Life Force Energization Exercises,* which are an unparalleled example of a dynamic activity that conserves energy instead of projecting it outward. These exercises combine breathing with contraction and relaxation of various muscle groups to activate a flow of healing prana, and direct it to any body parts in need of healing.

---

* Instruction in these exercises can be found in the online Appendices.

Meditation. Students of Patanjali's *Yoga Sutras* generally associate meditation techniques with the stages of *dharana* (concentration) and *dhyana* (absorption). The Kriya Yoga meditation science includes aspects of pranayama as well.[20]

> The kriya technique as taught by Lahiri Mahasaya is also a form of pranayam. It is the art of switching off the life force from the five senses. Breath control follows life control.[21]

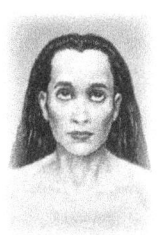

After being lost for centuries, the Kriya Yoga science was revived in the mid-nineteenth century by Mahavatar **Babaji**. In his autobiography, Yogananda writes extensively about Kriya Yoga and the Kriya line of masters. Kriya simultaneously activates a flow of prana while neutralizing past karmic patterns, making it one of the most powerful meditation techniques.

✵ Unwelcome Breathlessness ✵

They say that tortoises, elephants, and yogis breathe only a few times a minute and consequently live long years. When I would go without breath during sleep, no one considered me a great yogi; the doctors announced that I had obstructive sleep apnea, and that it was not a healthy situation.

Due to the frequency of my apnea episodes – up to fifty-seven times in an hour – my sleep was constantly disturbed. As a result, I was so tired that I often fell asleep during the day, which affected my work and my ability to drive safely. The doctors said that the condition, if left untreated, could lead to heart problems and even a stroke.

There are therapies to improve OSA, but none of them cure it. I began to use a cumbersome, uncomfortable machine at night that would force my body to breathe whenever I entered apnea. It helped somewhat, but not exceptionally. To be honest, I found the whole situation rather depressing.

Two years into the apnea therapy, I received Kriya Yoga initiation. The controlled breathing cycles during the technique seemed to stabilize my breathing at night. Little by little, the sleep apnea diminished. Today, the machine is virtually unemployed – it engages only a few times at night, and there are times when it is inactive all night long. As I deepen my Kriya practice, I am convinced that I will soon be able to put the machine in storage.

Kriya has been my salvation. By eliminating the karmic causes of illness, it has given me back a normal life, in addition to the joy it brings me in meditation. If the doctors ask what I have done to improve my former condition, I wonder if I should tell them my secret. –**Piero**, *Pisa, Italy*

Rajasic service. When our service to others is to any degree accompanied by a desire to receive something in return, it is tinged with rajas. There may be an expectation, for example, to have our service recognized and praised. Service to others is also rajasic in nature when we force our attentions on them with little sensitivity for their dignity, and little awareness of their true needs.

Tamo Guna
SHUN THE DARKNESS

Whereas light and lightness are the primary qualities of sattwa guna, darkness and heaviness underlie tamo guna. When rajasic energies flow outward, they can in time lose their focus, dissipate, and by the force of metaphysical gravity be pulled downwards towards tamo guna: to inactivity, laziness, indifference and ultimately to despair.

> O Bharata (Arjuna)! Know the (darkening) quality
> of tamas to produce (spiritual) ignorance, which
> deludes the mind and makes people lazy, heedless,
> and excessively attracted to subconscious sleep....
> When a person's consciousness is dark, lazy,
> neglectful of duty, and inclined to understand
> nothing rightly, tamas is his dominant guna.
> (BHAGAVAD GITA 14:8,13)

Drunkenness is tamasic. Drug addiction is tamasic. Dull-mindedness is tamasic. Stupidity is tamasic. Anything—whether wrong food; habitual inactivity; lack of proper exercise; unwillingness to puzzle anything out or to face any challenging reality; passive acceptance of things as they are, however degrading they may be to one's consciousness, and not caring to see them improved: anything that keeps one from mental clarity may rightly be called tamasic.[22]

Tamasic places and tamasic states of mind are detrimental to our health. In the presence of lethargic energy, the channels of life force close, our energy stagnates, and illness finds a welcome host in a listless body and mind. Whereas an urge to rest may be a warning against impending burnout, if we find ourselves habitually enjoying tamas's indolent ways, we may need to call on rajas to give us a shot of activating energy.

QUALITIES OF TAMO GUNA

Addicted	Apathetic	Confused
Deceitful	Depressed	Dishonest
Dull	Heartless	Ignorant
Inert	Insensitive	Lazy
Negative	Negligent	Obstinate
Passive	Procrastinating	Self-destructive
Stagnant	Treacherous	Unadaptive

Tamasic foods

Tamasic foods burden the digestive system and are unhealthy. They include foods that are old, spoiled, fermented, unpleasantly odorous, over-cooked, processed and preserved, and red meats and alcoholic beverages. Rajasic foods become tamasic when we over-consume them or eat them late at night.

Mental Diet

A low-energy tamasic mindset will tend to produce a pessimistic, negative, complaining disposition. Tamasic thoughts such as "I can't handle this" or "There's nothing I can do about it" can take us on a downward spiral to depression, hopelessness, and despair. As with all forms of tamas, the cure lies in catching them at the outset and injecting them with a healthy dose of stimulating rajasic energy.

People

"Misery loves company" is a saying that Yogananda would likely refute as a "false notion" – what some circles today call an "alternative truth," which is to say, not a truth at all.

The implied idea is that spending time in the company of other sufferers should make us feel at least minimally better, because it is consoling to realize that our situation is not unique and that we are

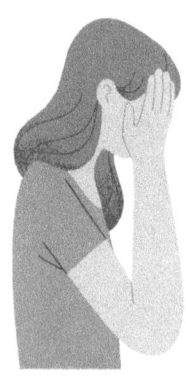

not alone. But the truth is that being with miserable people will only increase our misery, and that our mutual feelings of sadness and misery will amplify each other. Whenever possible, it is the better part of wisdom to avoid or minimize contact with such people at all times, especially when our thoughts and energy are spiraling downward. When we cannot avoid contact with those who are stuck in attitudes of suffering, there are ways to shield ourselves from their downward-pulling influence, as we will discover in Chapter Eleven.

If you find yourself falling into a tamasic state of low energy and hopelessness, the quickest cure is to seek the company of those who are upbeat, positive, and cheerful. A phone call, an online chat, or even a brief visit with such a person – a coffee date, a shopping spree, a walk in the park – can pull us back from the brink of despair.

Environments

Not only are there hellish planets in the astral world where evil reigns, but also here on Earth there are places that have been imbued with vibrations of tamasic, evil thoughts and activities. Just as holy places can heal us, so unholy places can do us immeasurable harm. Stay clear of places that are dark, where you feel heavy and fearful, and where nefarious activities are happening or have happened in the past.

Although the existence of ghosts is another subject entirely, places can be "haunted" by the heavy vibrations of people who live or have lived or died there. If you happen to come into possession of such a place, through ownership or rent, even for a short time, you will want to "cleanse" it with sattwic vibrations. In Chapter Eleven you will find suggestions for purifying an environment and protecting yourself against negative vibrations.

Because clean environments are more likely to support our health, we should take care to keep our home clean, inside and out, including nooks and crannies, storage areas, closets, work spaces, and car. A eminent swami who visited Ananda Village from India many years ago gave the gardeners an important lesson.

❋ The Painted Can ❋

In the early days at Ananda Village, probably 1971, an Indian yogi visited the village garden. Word about our community had spread, and a number of Indian yogis visited us, including Swami Chidananda, the spiritual successor of Swami Sivananda of Rishikesh.

Quietly serene, he didn't say much as we showed him around the community. At one point we were strolling through the tomato garden, and at his suggestion we "circumambulated" the tomato plants — a practice that he said would bring them blessings. In preparation for his visit, we had cleaned and neatly arranged the tools — except for one small rusty can that sat next to a barrel filled with a nutritious organic plant brew.

"What is that used for?" Swami Chidananda asked quietly, nodding at the can.

"To water the young plants," we responded.

"Then paint it, and keep it clean. Lower entities are attracted to *tamas*, and you don't want them taking up residence in these beautiful gardens." –**Shivani** (*the author*)

Spiritual practices

Spiritual practices can lift us into higher levels of peace, love, and joy. But if we do them haphazardly, or go through the motions automatically with wandering thoughts, our practice can take on a tamasic heaviness.

The same goes for letting the mind drift into subconsciousness in meditation. Meditation is a fine art requiring calm, focused attention and relaxed vigilance. There is a fine line between inner states of sattwic peace and tamasic subconsciousness

When we relax, we may fall into a rejuvenating nap. But that is not meditation, which is accompanied by a heightened awareness and a superior wakefulness. The words we use to describe the two states tell the story: we "fall" asleep but we "rise" into bliss. When sleepiness tries to invade our spiritual practice, a good remedy is to open our eyes and do some energetic breathing exercises – for example, the "double breath" mentioned in conjunction with the Energization Exercises.*

The Gunas in ayurveda

The three gunas are a foundational consideration of ayurveda,[23] a science of healing with roots in the Vedic scriptures of ancient India. A person's "dosha" – one's essential physical constitution and psychological makeup – is determined by the proportions of tamasic, rajasic, and sattwic energy that characterize his/her physical, emotional, and spiritual makeup.

The doshas are used as a basis for diagnosing disorders and prescribing the foods, herbs, and other substances that will bring the three doshas into harmony. The doshas are also the basis for determining the composition of herbal medicines to treat specific imbalances. You may be familiar with ayurveda, since it is now widely known and practiced in many countries.

Transcending the Gunas

> O Arjuna, be thou free from the triple qualities,
> liberated from the pairs of opposites, ever balanced,
> and bereft of the thought of receiving and keeping;
> be thou settled in the Self. (BHAGAVAD GITA 2:45)

---

* These exercises are found in Volume One, Part IV.

The spiritual journey of our soul from ego-involvement to ultimate freedom* is colored by the three gunas. In the earliest stages, the quality of tamas prevails, and in the final stage sattwa reigns.

> These four stages have their correspondence in the eternal gunas or qualities of nature, *tamas, rajas,* and *sattva*: obstruction, activity, and expansion; or, mass, energy, and intelligence. The four natural castes are marked by the gunas as (1) *tamas* (ignorance), (2) *tamas-rajas* (mixture of ignorance and activity), (3) *rajas-sattva* (mixture of right activity and enlightenment), (4) *sattva* (enlightenment). Thus has nature marked every man with his caste, by the predominance in himself of one, or the mixture of two, of the *gunas*. Of course every human being has all three *gunas* in varying proportions.[24]

As long as we navigate in the waters of duality, there will be peaks and troughs: cycles when we are progressing in making our lives more sattwic, and other times when we seem to be going backwards. The troughs should not overly concern us, so long as our overall movement is in the right direction.

It is important for our physical, mental, emotional, and spiritual health that we make the best-informed, most sattwic choices possible at each moment. By taking one small step at a time in the direction of happiness and freedom, we will be fulfilling the high purpose of our life, and we will get there in time.

We must all, eventually, pass beyond the cycles of duality, beyond all defining qualities, beyond even sattwa guna, to find complete freedom in cosmic consciousness.

---

* The evolutionary stages of shudra, vaishya, kshatriya and brahmin are discussed in Volume One, Part I, Chapter Four..

> Having transcended the three qualities of Nature, which are the cause of physical embodiment, one is released from the suffering (attendant upon) birth, old age, and death, and attains immortality.(BHAGAVAD GITA 14:20)

> A liberated master, having merged his consciousness in the infinite stillness of Spirit, is spoken of as triguna rahitam: one who has transcended Nature's triune qualities.[25]

On our way to perfect transcendence, there is still a great deal that we can learn about the vibratory influences of our environment – as we will discover in the chapters that follow.

POINTS TO REMEMBER
for developing a sattwic lifestyle

> *Good health requires a sattwic lifestyle, in harmony with nature and with the inner Self.*

- **Silence:** Include a few moments of silence between one daily activity and the next; and for at least a half day once a week.
- **Truthfulness:** Think and speak the truth to the best of your knowing, without imposing your understanding of truth on others.
- **Meditation:** Meditate at about the same times each day.

- **Yoga asanas:** Practice a few asanas before meditation, and have a longer session at least once a week.
- **Nature:** Get outdoors as much as possible and absorb the healing vibrations of Mother Nature.
- **Sleep**: Ensure adequate amounts of deep sleep. Develop a routine for relaxing the body and mind just before falling asleep.
- **Relaxation:** Don't wait for vacations – take time for relaxation during the day and longer periods on the weekends.
- **Diet:** Include more sattwic food, and eat with greater awareness.
- **Compassion:** Keep thoughts of tolerance and understanding uppermost in your mind.
- **Self-awareness:** Observe your thoughts and actions to evaluate their impact on your health.
- **Satsang:** Spend more time with inspiring people, books, and films.
- **Service:** Dedicate your time and resources to helping others.
- **Avoid, reduce, or eliminate:**
    - ~ Overstimulation
    - ~ Mental exhaustion, laziness, sloth
    - ~ Addictions and dependencies
    - ~ Mental resistance
    - ~ Poor hygiene
    - ~ Procrastination
    - ~ Thoughts of judgment, criticism, complaining, and blaming

PART XII CHAPTER THREE

Mantra

OM

A poem by Swami Yogananda

Whence, whence this soundless roar doth come,
When drowseth matter's dreary drum?
On shores of bliss, *Om*, booming, breaks!
All earth, all heaven, all body shakes!
Cords bound to flesh are broken all,
Vibrations burst, meteors fall!
The hustling heart, the boasting breath,
No more shall cause the yogi's death;
All nature lies in darkness soft,
Dimness of starlight seen aloft;
Subconscious dreams have gone to bed...
'Tis then that one doth hear *Om*'s tread;
The bumble-bee now hums along—
Hark! Baby *Om* doth sing His song!
From Krishna's flute the call is sweet:
'Tis time the Watery God to meet!
Now, the God of Fire is singing!
Om! *Om*! *Om*! His harp is ringing.
God of *Prana* now is sounding—
Wondrous, breathing-bells resounding!
O! Upward climb the living tree;
Hark to the cosmic symphony.
From *Om*, the soundless roar! From *Om*
The call for light o'er dark to roam.
From *Om* the music of the spheres!
From *Om* the mist of nature's tears!
All things of earth and heaven declare,
Om! *Om*! Resounding everywhere! [1]

Long before Pythagoras and Plato were contemplating the geometry of the universe, the Indian sages of the Vedic period (circa 1500 B.C.) were teaching mantras – sound frequencies that have healing power.

The word *mantra* has become part of popular usage. People refer to Benjamin Franklin's "mantra": "Early to bed, early to rise, makes a man healthy, wealthy and wise." Popular slogans are often referred to as mantras – Nike's "Just Do It" and "Yes We Can!" – the slogan of former U.S. President Barack Obama's election campaign.

Unlike slogans, true mantras have a very real power to help us change our behavior and improve our well-being. The ancients taught that appropriate mantras can even give us power to manipulate the material and astral worlds.

> The ancient rishis discovered these laws of sound alliance between nature and man. Because nature is an objectification of Aum, the Primal Sound or Vibratory Word, man can obtain control over all natural manifestations through the use of certain mantras or chants.[2]

Certain mantras are meant to help us change our consciousness at the deepest levels. Their power lies in their attunement vibratory potency.

> A mantra is a word or combination of words that exerts a vibratory influence. Mantras can affect events objectively as well as states of consciousness subjectively.[3]

Bija mantras

According to the spiritually illumed Indian rishis in Vedic times, there are universal, pure tones called *bija* mantras, or "seed" sounds.

All of the bijas derive from the primal sound of Aum. Based on these sounds an entire science of mantra has developed, each sound having a specific effect on the mind and often on objective reality.

> Particularly powerful are words that were brought into being purely for their vibrational resonance.[4]
>
> Sanskrit seed sounds, or bij-mantras, when correctly pronounced are capable of effecting great changes in the natural order, or in one's own inner nature.[5]

The Sanskrit alphabet is based on the *bija* sounds, each letter said to have a specific vibratory power.

> Sanskrit...contains in its syllables sounds which the great sages of India have claimed come the closest to the natural sound-vibrations of the astral world. That is why Sanskrit has been known traditionally as Devanagari, the language of the gods.[6]

There is a direct connection between the letters of the Sanskrit alphabet and the chakras in the human astral body. The yoga scriptures claim that each Sanskrit letter resonates with one of the fifty petals of the crown, or sahasrara chakra, this being the sum total of the petals in each of the chakras.

> The Sanskrit alphabet has 50 letters in it. This is exactly the same number of petals or spokes that there are on the flowers or wheels of the total of the first six chakras or esoteric energy centers, located along the spine. This is no accident. The Sanskrit language is a tool for working with the subtle energy potential ... in the etheric body. However, the six major chakras contain the 'map of sounds' written on each of the combined 50 petals on those six chakras.[7]

Chanting Sanskrit mantras harmonizes astral energies in the chakras and resonates as well in the physical brain to alleviate stress.

Neuroscientists from the University of California found that even 10 minutes of mantra chanting blocks the release of the stress hormones adrenaline and cortisol. This soothing effect lasts for up to 48 hours after each mantra session.[8]

Mantric power can be used for good or evil. In Indian mythology, wars were fought using not only the conventional weapons, but also mantras (called *astras*) that were applied to the soldiers' arrows.

The renowned Tibetan yogi, Milarepa, used powerful mantras to destroy the enemies of his family. He later repented and, undergoing severe discipline and penance with the famed guru, Marpa, achieved enlightenment in that lifetime.[9]

Hindu priests chant mantras at the request of people seeking material benefits such as a suitable spouse, a healthy baby, or a success in business. Spiritual gurus traditionally give their disciples a mantra to repeat in meditation: the name of one of God's manifestations or a bija mantra to help slow the breath and calm the emotions and thoughts sufficiently to merge their consciousness with the blissful sound of Aum.

ॐ *The Cosmic Sound* ॐ

The supreme healing mantra is Aum, the primordial sound that sustains all creation, and that is the source of our being.*

> A part of God's consciousness...
> vibrated from its center of absolute peace,
> and produced the appearance of
> a manifested universe.[10]

---

* Yogananda and Kriyananda refer to the Cosmic Sound interchangeably as "Om," and "Aum." Kriyananda explains:
  Aum, which is often written OM in English, with two letters, is more correctly rendered with three letters, *AUM*. The first letter, *A*, represents the creative vibration; the second, *U*, represents the preserving vibration; and the third letter, *M*, represents the vibration of destruction—that which dissolves the created universe back into the Infinite Silence. –*The Essence of Self-Realization* 20:2

St. John refers to Aum in this famous passage from the Bible:

> In the beginning was the Word, and the Word was with God, and the Word was God. The same was in the beginning with God. All things were made by him; and without him was not any thing made that was made. (JOHN 1:1-3)

The "Word" here is the Amen of the Christian Bible, the Aum of the *Vedas,* the *Amin* of Islam, and the *Ahunavar* of Zoroastrianism.

> As words are sounds produced by human thought, so the Biblical "Word" is the mighty Sound Vibration by which God manifested His creative impulse in the form of Cosmic Creation.[11] —YOGANANDA

> I am the Aum chanted in all the Vedas: the Cosmic Sound moving, as if soundlessly, through the ether.
> —SRI KRISHNA (BHAGAVAD GITA, CH. 7:8)

Swami Kriyananda describes the origins of Aum in one of his musical compositions.

The Thunder of Aum

Out of the silence
  came the song of creation,
Out of the darkness came the Light.
Out of the darkness, out of the silence,
Thundered the Cosmic Sound, Amen.
Out of the darkness, out of the silence,
Thundered the Cosmic Sound, Aum.

The power of the Aum mantra lies in the fact that it is the first outward expression of Spirit.

> Aum is, in fact, the highest mantra, attuned as it is to the very essence of all vibrations, the Cosmic Vibration itself.[12]

How to chant Aum

As modern researchers discover the frequencies of the human body and its component parts, resonance therapies are being devised to heal without invasive surgery.

A more all-encompassing form of subtle healing involves bringing the individual parts of the body into harmonic alignment with the vibration of Aum, similar to the way the instruments of an orchestra must be tuned to a tone played by the concert master before they can play together in harmony.

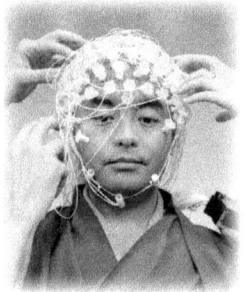

In a study by Bhavna P. Harne, an EEG machine recorded the electrical activity in various parts of the brain while the subjects chanted Aum. The study confirmed that chanting Aum positively affects the brain's prefrontal cortex and the vagus nerve, and that it calms and harmonizes heartbeat and respiration.[13]

Another study using functional MRI found that chanting Aum significantly reduced stress by deactivating the limbic system, the amygdala, the hippocampus, and other stress-involved brain areas.[14]

Chanting Aum, aloud or mentally, brings the body and brain into alignment with its healing frequencies.

> To utter with calm feeling the supreme mantra, Aum, even if it doesn't suggest any particular meaning to the mind, has a transforming effect on every level of one's consciousness.[15]

Aum is written and pronounced differently in various traditions.

> To chant it, pronounce it to rhyme with "home." In English it is usually written *Om*, to keep people from pronouncing the first letter with a long a. Otherwise, it is spiritually more correct to spell Aum with three letters, each letter signifying a different phase of the Cosmic Vibration: creation, preservation, and dissolution.[17]

A common approach to chanting Aum is to intone it on a single note while regulating the breath to create a steady rhythmic repetition. Yogananda introduced another approach that is widely used.

> Aum is traditionally chanted three times, as a reminder of its three aspects. The first time, it is sung high; the second, lower; and the third, lower still. These are the differences in sound between the three vibrations of the cosmic sound. Brahma, the creative vibration, is high-pitched; Vishnu, the preservative vibration, is pitched somewhat lower; and Shiva, the all-dissolving vibration, is a low, deep sound.[18]

We can chant Aum mentally or aloud, alone or in a group, with or without a recording. Try these exercises for drawing harmony and healing to the physical and astral bodies.

Yogananda's *Om* Immersion Exercises

- Concentrate on both feet and imagine a warm electric force trickling all over the soles of your feet. Do the same with calves, thighs, haunches, abdomen, stomach, navel, heart, left and right lungs, each of the fingers, palms, forearms, upper arms, throat, back of head and top of head, in the middle of the head, in the eyes, in the ears, nostrils, and mouth, in the liver, kidneys, intestines, and wherever there is disease or weakness. Concentrate the mind on the weak or diseased part and try to feel that a warm electric force is descending from the mental chanting of "Om," fifteen times in each place or body part.[19]

- Sit on a straight chair, spine straight. Expel the breath quickly, and keep it out, counting mentally 1 to 10. Then inhale slowly, hold the breath counting 1 to 10, exhale quickly and repeat 10 times. Then expel breath and forget it, not caring whether it comes in again or not. Concentrate on the toes of the left foot and say, mentally, "Om" on each toe. Do the same to the right foot.

- Then concentrate on the sole of the left foot. Say, "Om". Do likewise with the right foot. Concentrate on the left and right calves, mentally saying "Om." Do the same with the left and right thighs, left and right haunches, navel, abdomen, liver, spleen, stomach, pancreas, heart, left and right lungs, left and right hands, and arms, left side of neck, right side of neck, front throat and back of neck. Say "Om" mentally, concentrating on the pituitary gland, pineal gland, medulla, point between the eyebrows, mouth, big and little tongues [ovula], on the left and right nostrils, on the left and right eyes, left and right ears, cerebellum, and cerebrum.

- Then go up and down the spine mentally chanting "Om" at each chakra: coccygeal, sacral, lumbar, dorsal, cervical, medulla, and Christ Center at the point between the eyebrow. Try to feel that the whole body is surrounded within and without with the holy vibration of "Om." [20]

Aum at home

The healing effects of Aum can be obtained to some degree by listening to it being chanted, especially by someone of refined and elevated consciousness. A practice that is gaining popularity is to keep a recording of Aum playing very softly, even barely audibly, in your environment day and night. You can find such recordings on the internet. They vary significantly in terms of pronunciation, tonality, rhythm, timber of the chanter's voice, as well as the consciousness of the person chanting.

Personally, I have a recording of Kriyananda's "Aum: The Mantra of Eternity"[21] on my phone, and I keep it playing softly in the background as I go about my daily activities. It has accompanied me during the writing of this book, and I often keep it in my pocket when I work outdoors and in my purse when I travel. Introducing Aum into your environment in this way will bring a sense of harmony to those who inhabit or visit that space. Just being in an environment saturated with Aum can calm our emotions and clarify our thoughts.

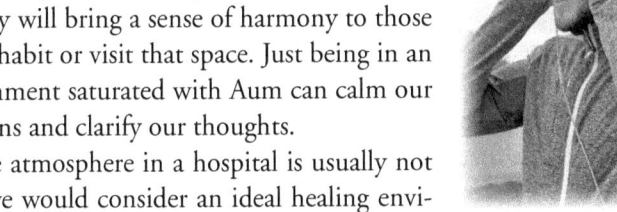

The atmosphere in a hospital is usually not what we would consider an ideal healing environment. When you or someone close to you must be there, consider taking a recording of Aum along in your phone/tablet/computer, and to whatever extent possible, listen to it – best through headphones when others are present. The calming and balancing vibrations of this mantra will nourish you inwardly, create around you a protective shield against the fearful emotions of others, and even if inaudible to others, silently uplift the environment for everyone.

Aum and the Chakras

On a subtle level, the vibrations of Aum harmonize the causal, astral, and physical bodies. Illnesses associated with these bodies,* having a lower frequency, can be neutralized when Aum is properly intoned, or when our consciousness is immersed in Aum through deep meditation.

---

* See Part I in Volume One for a discussion of the diseases associated with our three bodies.

> To experience God as Sound is to commune with the Holy Ghost, or *Aum*, the Cosmic Vibration. When you are immersed in *Aum*, nothing can touch you. *Aum* raises the mind above the delusions of human existence, into the pure skies of divine consciousness. [22]

Chanting Aum at the chakras at the start of a meditation while visualizing the chakras at their locations in the astral spine stimulates these centers of spiritual energy and helps us experience higher states of consciousness.

OPENING THE ASTRAL DOORS OF THE CHAKRAS

Try this practice from Yogananda's Super Advanced Course, which **"will release your soul from the bondage of matter and sense attachment by enabling you to escape through the seven astral doors and become one with the Spirit."** [23]

- Sit upright and straighten the spine to resemble a straight lightning rod. Concentrate the vision between the eyebrows with eyes half open. (Do not frown while doing this; keep the facial expression serene.)
- Now slightly move the spine to the left and right by swaying the body, changing the centre of consciousness from the body and senses to the spine. Feel the astral spine and stop swaying the body.
- Then let your consciousness travel up and down several times, from the coccygeal plexus at the end of the spine to the point between the eyebrows.
- Then concentrate on the coccygeal plexus and mentally chant Om.

- ... slowly travel up the spine, mentally feeling the coccygeal, sacral, lumbar, dorsal, cervical, and medullary plexuses, to the point between the eyebrows, mentally chanting Om in each place.
- When you reach the central point between the eyebrows, return downward, chanting Om at the point between the eyebrows, the medulla, and the five plexuses, and mentally feeling the centers at the same time.
- Continue to chant Om at the seven centers, feeling them while traveling up and down the astral spinal *Sushumna* passage. Practice the above until you distinctly feel that your consciousness is transferred from the body into the spine.

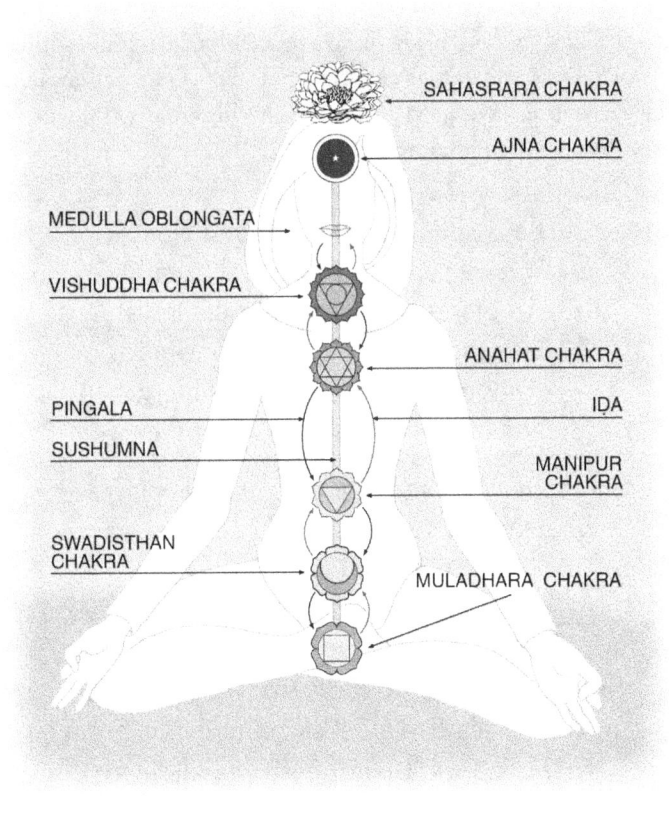

Swami Kriyananda recommends chanting Aum several times in each chakra.

> It is a good practice in meditation to chant "Aum" mentally three times at each of the chakras, moving up and down the spine several times. In this way the energy becomes somewhat withdrawn from the outer body to the centers. Once the energy is felt in the centers, draw it upward by concentrating your attention on the upper centers—especially on the Christ center between the eyebrows.[23]

Meditating on Aum

Although chanting Aum brings us to a peaceful state, it is not sufficient to completely transform our consciousness from egoic self-awareness to Self-realization. We need to hear Aum vibrating within us, and merge ourselves with it completely.

> The Cosmic Vibration is inaudible to the human ear, but can be heard inwardly by the "ear" of intuition." To hear Aum inwardly, we need to be in a quiet place where car horns, construction machinery, and other sounds cannot intrude.
>
> People sometimes get a hint of it in places where there is complete silence. They may hear a soft hum, or a gentle murmur like the whisper of wind in the trees. The sound emerges from no discernible point in space, but seems rather to come from everywhere... What is heard in quiet surroundings is not so much a spiritually uplifting experience

> as simply a whisper—like that of a waterfall from afar—of the mighty thunder of Aum perceived in deep meditation. To attune oneself to that sound, one must commune with it in the inner silence. Deep communion with Aum makes one conscious of the underlying reality of everything in existence, God.[24]

Meditating on Aum is a practice common to many yoga traditions. It is the bridge connecting the unmoving Spirit to vibratory creation, one which we can use through meditation to travel in the opposite direction – backwards from creation to the Source.

> Meditation on Pranava, the divine sound of Aum, is the only way to Brahman (Spirit) salvation.[25]

Listening to the sounds of the chakras

Our journey of meditation begins with the techniques given in Part II of Volume One for calming the mind and emotions by concentrating on the natural flow of the breath. When the mind and emotions are calm, we can explore deeper states of meditation by focusing our attention on the inner sounds of Aum vibrating in our astral body.

Yogananda describes the sound of Aum as "a symphony of all the Astral sounds emanating from the Six Centers."

> The life current in the coccyx is responsible for the solidifying of Life Force and atoms into flesh, and produces the sound of a buzzing bee as it operates.
>
> The sacral center sustains the atoms of all the watery substance in the body and makes the musical sound of a flute as it works.

> The lumbar center keeps up the Astral and electrical heat of the body and oozes out the beautiful sound of a harp.
>
> The dorsal center keeps the oxygen and air elements in the body combining with the flesh and sends forth the sound of a gong bell.
>
> The cervical plexus maintains the etheric background in the body and times it to all spatial vibrations. This cervical center reverberates with the Cosmic Vibration of ocean rumblings.
>
> The Christ Center, in the medulla and in the point between the eyebrows, is the dynamo of consciousness, Life Force, and elemental vibrations, which mainly keep the elements of life, consciousness, flesh, blood, heat, air, and ether of the body continuously recharged.[26]

The symphony of Aum can be perceived at the Christ Center. If you do not hear Aum immediately, you can focus on the sounds of any of the chakras until you become immersed in that sound, which will naturally lead you to the higher sounds, and eventually to Aum.

> Listen intently in the right ear, especially, to any subtle sound you hear. It is not likely that you will hear Aum clearly at first, but concentration on any internal sound will help you gradually to attune your consciousness to the subtle Cosmic Vibration.

The spiritual sounds are usually heard in the right ear, not in the left. If you hear them in the left ear, try to bring that perception gradually to the right ear.[27]

You'll hear this sound first in the right ear. Gradually let it permeate the brain and the entire body, until every cell vibrates with that sound.

After that, try to hear Aum in everything you do, in everything you perceive. This is true japa, when the mind no longer repeats words, merely, but is intoxicated with the bliss of the "music of the spheres."

By attuning one's consciousness to that sound... one enters the stream of vibration that proceeded out of the Spirit, and that merges back into the Spirit at creation's end and at the end of the individual soul's cycle of outward wandering. By merging in Aum, liberation is attained.[28]

When the Yogi's consciousness is able not only to hear this cosmic sound but also to feel its actual presence in every unit of space, in all finite vibrating matter, then the soul of the Yogi becomes one with the Holy Ghost or Holy Vibration.[29]

Success with this technique requires intuitive inward listening, a commitment to practice regularly, and the patience to practice long enough to experience the results. Here is a story of someone who used the Aum technique at a time when other meditation practices were not possible.

✻ Aum Refuge ✻

During the past twelve years, I've had one karmic health situation after another: high, sustained fevers; repeated eye, bladder, and prostate infections; Lyme disease; and burst colon and appendix were just some of the challenges. A doctor said my body was like an army that has been soundly defeated and its forces scattered.

Before this karmic period, I had developed a strong affinity with this practice. During this time, due to compromised breathing and other factors, my usual meditation practices were not possible; but I could listen inwardly to Aum and subtly feel its healing vibrations. By listening to it with love and yearning, I could escape my body to a noticeable degree.

During this period of eight years, I wrote six books in an attempt to escape my body and to be expansive. Hearing Aum wiped clean the slate of suffering, and gave me new revelations and intuitions that made writing a joyous experience. The Lyme disease specialist said I should be in a wheelchair, but due to Aum and through the grace of God, my energy is strong. *—Joseph Bharat Cornell*, California

Using Aum as a vehicle for transmitting healing energy to others

We can offer ourselves as conduits for the healing power of Aum, by immersing ourselves in its current and directing it even over long distances to people, situations, or places that need healing.

> **When you utter "Aum" it travels not only all around the earth but throughout all space and eternity.**[30]

Yogananda's technique for sending healing power to others uses both the hands and the voice as transmitting instruments. A detailed description of this method can be found in Volume Two, Part

IX, Chapter Five. These subtle healing practices are most effective when we can motivate the recipients to awaken their own will to be healed, and when we can help them stimulate their willingness to try self-healing practices while seeking appropriate medical support.

Aum as a transition at death*

Aum is the connecting link between the physical and astral bodies. At death, or in deep breathless states of meditation, the life force withdraws from the physical body, traveling on waves of Aum to find its home in the astral world and reunite with its astral body of energy.

> Yogananda explained also that at physical death the departing soul does in fact hear that mighty sound, manifested as a vibration which corresponds to its own consciousness. That special aspect of the Cosmic Vibration determines the nature of one's state after death, during the interim period between his incarnations on earth or on some other planet.[31]

If you are assisting someone who is making the transition of death, you can help them find their way by playing a recording of Aum softly in the room. You can also, when possible and appropriate, chant Aum aloud in their presence. Yogananda said that the sense of hearing is the last to shut down at the time of death.

Chanting Aum in the dying person's right ear can either help bring them back to the physical body if it is not their destined karmic time to die, or help their soul attune itself to the Aum vibration and proceed on its journey into the Light.

> May this Aum or Amen vibration, conjoined with the music of the spheres, dispel all your darkness and bring joy and understanding in your heart.[32]

---

* You will find a discussion about the transition between life and death in the Epilogue.

CHAPTER 3: *Points to Remember*

- A mantra is a word or phrase that sets up a vibratory force field that influences our consciousness, health, natural surroundings, and objective events.

- *Bija* mantras are pure sounds that have exceptional powers.

- Aum is the highest and most powerful mantra. Listening to it, chanting it, and merging with it in meditation can bring complete healing.

- Playing a recording of Aum softly in the background helps calm the mind and uplift the vibrations of any environment.

- Chanting Aum at the chakras is a good way to begin meditation.

- While transmitting healing energy to to others, chanting Aum can be very powerful.

- When helping a sick friend, if appropriate, playing a recording of the Aum chant softly in the room.

- When helping a dying friend, in addition to playing Aum softly in the room, chanting Aum in the person's right ear will help him or her proceed on the journey into the Light.

PART XII CHAPTER FOUR

The Healing Power of Music

> Music is the language of God.
> –Ludwig van Beethoven

> Our ancestors believed that music has the power to harmonize a person's soul in ways that medicine could not. The Chinese character for medicine actually comes from the character for music.
> –Gao Yuan, Shen Yun Symphony Orchestra[1]

> The future medicine will be the medicine of frequencies. –Albert Einstein

> The medicine of the future will be music and sound. –Edgar Cayce

❋ I Live Without Fear ❋

It was dark night with heavy rain as I drove the steep, winding road to my home. I had driven it countless times, but no there was an ominous feeling of foreboding. Misty tendrils of fog danced in the headlights, and with no other cars on the road late at night I felt a little spooked. The rational mind tried to talk me out of a rising fear. And then I began to sing aloud, with strength and conviction, a song called "I Live Without Fear" by Swami Kriyananda.

"My Lord, in Your presence, I live without fear!" Immediately the fear dissipated, replaced by a deep peace, as I felt a warm glow of comfort fill my body, mind, and soul.

–Elizabeth, *Nevada City, California*

Music has a remarkable ability to penetrate our bodies, hearts, and minds and influence us – it can agitate, energize, and soothe. It can relax whole audiences, or incite them to war. It can inspire or depress.

A song entitled "Gloomy Sunday," also wryly called "The Hungarian Suicide Song," was banned in Hungary because of the rash of suicides that followed its publication. The BBC, along with other stations, also banned it, after its depressing melody and lyrics reputedly incited a number of suicides in the UK.

Martial music has been used as a weapon. The ancient Israelites used trumpets to bring down the walls of Jericho. The Scots went to war while playing bagpipes. Rugby teams in New Zealand perform the Maori *haka* dance to challenge their opponents. Instruments are often used to incite patriotic and militaristic sentiments.

> Sound has been used as an actual weapon of conflict. Music has been used to spur on fighters, antagonize the enemy, and propagandize the public. Military music "stirs the blood," and in order to achieve this, some instruments, some compositions, some sounds are more favoured than others.[2]

Many of the classical composers were sensitive to the emotional impact of their compositions, and the effects of each instrument and various rhythms on the listener. Mozart and Verdi wrote their music to be played at 432 Hz, known as the "Verdi A," which is believed to be the frequency of the electromagnetic field of the Earth. Tibetan healing bowls, Stradivarius violins, and even ancient Egyptian instruments are said to be tuned to it.

> 432 Hz is considered to have the potential to synchronize both hemispheres of our brain: the logical and analytical left brain and the creative and intuitive right brain. This creates what scientists call "whole brain synchronization", maximizing our potential as thinkers, artists, and spiritual beings.[3]

A 2015 study by Professor Peter Sleight at Oxford University found that listening to slow pieces by Verdi and Puccini, and to Beethoven's Ninth symphony significantly lowered blood pressure. In another study, Hans-Joachim Trappe and Gabriele Voit demonstrated that music by Mozart and Strauss markedly lowered not just the subjects' heart rates but also their blood pressure by nearly five systolic points, which is better than some medications. Mozart's Symphony No. 40 in G minor demonstrated the strongest effect.[4]

Effect of sound on plants

Plant health is also affected by sound. When the renowned Indian scientist Sir Jagadish Chandra Bose submitted his research on the sensitivity of plant tissue to sound frequencies, the London Royal Society rejected his findings. Nevertheless, based on his work, modern researchers have used advanced technology and frequencies beyond the audible range to discover that frequencies above 5000 Hz cause plants to grow more vigorously and produce higher yields.

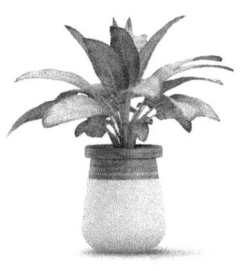

Various genres of music have unique effects on plants. Some classical Indian ragas have increased the yield of rice and wheat by over 50%. Classical Western music by Mozart, Brahms, Beethoven, Vivaldi, and others causes flowering plants to grow toward and even embrace the speakers; their flowers grow bigger, and their seeds are more fertile.

Plants prefer string instruments to percussion, and fewer beats at higher frequencies. Even the rhythmic sound of the bell-clad feet of dancing Bharatanatyam dancers was shown to improve plant growth. Music with heavy bass frequencies causes damage to plants, sometimes causing their death.

Based on the unique frequencies of a wide spectrum of individual plants, researchers have developed music that enhances their growth and controls the proliferation of plant pests. I can recommend this fascinating article, which offers research findings and actual recordings of music for plants.*

> Music... exerts a strong influence on our consciousness. If it can influence plants to grow faster, how much greater is its potential for influencing us.[5]

---

* Sharma, Sanjay, "The Effect of Music on Plant Growth and Pests," *Owlcation*, September 13, 2022, https://owlcation.com/stem/The-Effect-of-Music-on-Plant-Growth-and-Pests.

Divinely inspired music

So much for frequencies and Hertz! Music is more than physical sound. It is a vehicle that communicates consciousness: primarily that of the composer, but also of the performers. This can be said of all art, but it is particularly true of music which more easily and directly enters our inner world than other art forms, and requires no deliberate mental interpretation.

Although art by its nature is inspired by something, not all artistic inspiration is divine: it can derive from subconscious emotions rather than superconscious experience. Much modern art and music is reactive, and in its own way may have social value – I think of the protest songs of John Lennon, Pete Seeger, Joan Baez, Bob Dylan, and others against the Vietnam War.

Musical compositions can be born in the rational mind, and nowadays created by Artificial Intelligence. Music that endures, however, comes from a more refined level of awareness.

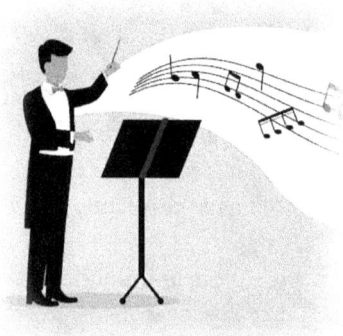

In his book *Talks with Great Composers,* Arthur M. Abell recorded conversations with some of the greatest composers of his day. When asked about the source of their inspiration, they all claimed that it came from a higher source. Brahms quoted Beethoven: "I know that God is nearer to me than to others of my craft; I consort with Him without fear."

When Abell asked Brahms for details of how he himself received omnipotent inspiration, the composer replied:

> "It cannot be done merely by will power working through the conscious mind…It can only be accomplished by the soul-powers within…Those powers are quiescent to the conscious mind unless illumined by Spirit.… I have to be in a semi-trance condition to get such results—a condition when the conscious mind is in temporary abeyance.…To realize that we are one with the Creator…is a wonderful and awe-inspiring experience.…

"I always contemplate all this before commencing to compose....I ask my Maker the three most important questions pertaining to our life here in this world—whence, wherefore, whither. I immediately feel vibrations that thrill my whole being. These are the Spirit illuminating the soul-power within, and in this exalted state, I see clearly what is obscure in my ordinary moods; then I feel capable of drawing inspiration from above....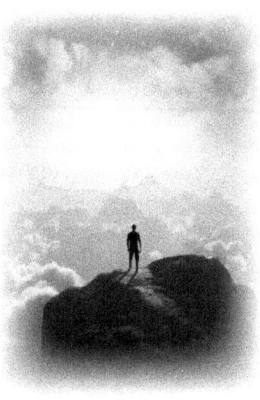

"Those vibrations assume the forms of distinct mental images, after I have formulated my desire and resolve in regard to what I want—namely, to be inspired so that I can compose something that will uplift and benefit humanity—something of permanent value.

"Straightaway the ideas flow in upon me, directly from God... clothed in the right forms, harmonies and orchestration. Measure by measure, the finished product is revealed to me when I am in those rare, inspired moods." [6]

In *Art as a Hidden Message,* Swami Kriyananda gives a similar example.

> *The story is told of George Fredrick Handel, when he was composing the Messiah:*
>
> His meals, which were left outside the room where he was working, went for several days untouched. At last the person who brought his food, concerned for the composer's welfare, opened the door and peeked in. And there he found Handel weeping for sheer joy, so inspired was he by the music he was receiving. In referring to the "Hallelujah" chorus, Handel exclaimed later, ecstatically, "I did think I did see all Heaven before me, and the great God Himself!" [7]

Swami Kriyananda's "Music of Divine Joy"

Swami Kriyananda began to compose music in the 1960s.

> Music has always been a large part of my life. I began...writing songs, hoping through them to touch people's hearts along with their minds. My approach has been superconscious and intuitive... from the perspective of philosophy, trying to understand (music's) deeper meaning.... Many of these songs express a philosophy of joy.[8]

He informally called his music "philosophy in song." In 1979, he introduced a concert with these thoughts.

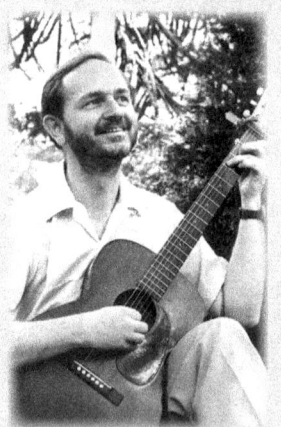

> Some years ago I got the idea to write the philosophy that we teach in song form, so that it could be sung and when listened to more easily absorbed than in a sermon....
>
> It has been interesting to see that music has a language of its own. I had known it abstractly, but in writing music, I have come to know it more definitely... Music's language is different: it carries a certain mood. That mood can be uplifting, it can be depressing; it can be exciting, it can be calming. It definitely speaks. And if it is written from soul consciousness, or from an inner consciousness, it will convey what the composer is intending....

> Whatever we do from an inner
> consciousness—be it music or the other arts,
> be it carpentry or gardening or taking care
> of our children—that consciousness
> expresses itself in the outward form.
> Whatever we do says something about
> our inner consciousness.

Composing music came more easily to Kriyananda than writing books, he once told me in a private conversation.

> "I hear melodies all the time, so many I can
> never write them all down. Before I compose,
> I become crystal clear as to the message
> and feeling I want the music to convey.
> I offer that clarity up to the superconsciousness,
> and almost immediately the melody comes.
> As I write down the notes, I hold each of them
> up to the inner sound of Aum, and feel
> if they are right."

On another occasion he remarked:

> "(Writing music) has been one of the great
> joys in my life. Often, tears of joy have flowed
> down my cheeks as a melody or a sequence
> of beautiful harmonies poured through me
> like a mountain stream, effortlessly." [9]

Having sung and listened to Kriyananda's music for more than fifty years, I can attest to its healing effects. The joy I felt while singing these uplifting pieces was sometimes so intense that I could scarcely continue.

❊ Songs of Joy ❊

On the day of a concert of Kriyananda's music, I was invited to sing with the choir. While I would normally have been delighted, the pain in my hand was so severe that I could only manage a weak smile of consent. I had fallen on the stairs during the night, landing on my hand.

The pain was so intense that I suspected my wrist was broken, but there was no time to go to the hospital – the rehearsal was about to start, and we would perform shortly after.

The songs were heavenly, and even though my English wasn't good enough to pronounce all of the words correctly, I was caught up in the joy of singing. When my roommate asked about the pain in my hand afterward, I wondered for a moment what she was referring to – and then I remembered. A few hours earlier I could barely breathe for the pain, and now it was gone. The hand was completely healed and the pain never returned. –**Natalia**, *Moscow, Russia*

Music is also used to express human tragedy. Can such music have a healing effect? One of the songs in Swami Kriyananda's album *The Mystic Harp* tells the legendary story of Irish noblewoman Deirdre who, loving one man but being forced to marry another, commits suicide.

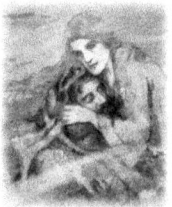

> **The suffering expressed in "Deirdre's Sorrows" is real, and mounts in intensity until it reaches a climax in Deirdre's suicide on the corpse of her beloved. Yet the music manages at the same time to express a healing energy. It is cathartic, for it purifies the listener, lifting him above his own personal tragedies into calm, expansive acceptance of the Eternally Inevitable.** [10]

In a private conversation about this song with friends in Lugano, Switzerland on November 11, 1998, Kriyananda remarked:

> Certainly life has its dark moments, yet we need to realize that even darkness can lift us into recognition of life's impermanence and of eternal verities. Once you reach superconsciousness, or once you get deep into the spine, then you can look back on all these emotions we go through, but they're different, they don't bind you any more, you liberate yourself from them and make even them beautiful.

The power to transform our consciousness was the subject of an interview by Sara Cryer with Swami Kriyananda on February 6, 1996.

> Music opens a window in the mind to a more flowing and unitive perception of reality. What music does words alone can't do is transmit experience. What the composer experiences he can convey—through melody, harmony, and rhythm—states of consciousness, and, if the listener really listens, he finds himself transformed also.
>
> An example of that would be the wonderful choral piece at the end of the St. Matthew Passion. Another example of that would be Handel's Messiah, the Hallelujah Chorus, but all music in one way or another opens the door to states of consciousness.
>
> Music can help us to awaken the hearts longings for higher experiences of life, and music that is really worthy of the term lifts the heart upward toward the superconscious.

Of Kriyananda's four hundred compositions, for me two stand out for their transforming effect on those who sing and hear them. The first one is "Chant of the Angels" (later renamed "Life Mantra").

> I wanted to write a choral piece for an angel choir, not for angels up in heaven, but for people to sing as if they were angels. As I meditated on this, I heard the piece, and it was as though angels were singing it to me.
>
> Suddenly, words and music came pouring over me like a waterfall of sound. The work came effortlessly: I wrote it all out in a single day.... I was thrillingly aware of angelic presences, guiding and blessing my labor.
>
> Something wonderful occurred during an early rehearsal...Only six of our choir members worked on it at first. At one point during a practice session, they were resting. All of a sudden, a sweet voice was heard "out of thin air," repeating the words and melody of one section of the music: "Life is a mission from on high. Life is a quest for inner joy!" Three in the group heard this etheric voice; the rest heard nothing. The angels themselves were indicating their blessings and approval for this work.[11]

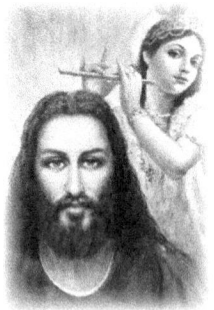

The other defining work that I would name, and perhaps his most important musical composition, is the oratorio, "Christ Lives," which tells the story of Christ's life from the perspective of its meaning for us today.

After a pilgrimage to the Holy Land, Kriyananda shared the inspiration he felt at each place: Bethlehem, Nazareth, the Jordan river, the Sea of Galilee, Canaan, Jacob's well, and Jerusalem. The oratorio's fifty compositions include instrumental pieces, recitatives, solos, duets, trios, quartets, and twelve pieces for full choir.

❄ I KIDNAPPED JESUS ❄

When my parents would put up the Nativity scene before Christmas, I would worry that the baby Jesus might be lonely during the night, so I would kidnap him and bring him to my room. As we both grew older, we remained fast friends.

I became a musician, focusing on violin and guitar. While still living in my native Switzerland I discovered Swami Kriyananda's compositions, and I was especially inspired by his oratorio about the life of Jesus. After moving to California, I joined a choir in time to prepare for a Christmas performance in 2006.

It was for a memorable event in my musical career. I stood in the back row with the tenors, and as the music progressed, "Christ Lives!" became more than a mental concept – it was a tangible experience of Christ's joy-filled loving presence inside me and in everyone in the choir, the audience, and the world.

As we sang the piece for the resurrection, "Christ Is Risen," I felt the clear truth of Christ's victory over death in my heart. He was alive!

But not only Jesus Christ – I knew with a clear inner certainty that every soul is on a path toward the same blissful destination. After the final song, "Thy Light Within Us Shining," I felt his presence so powerfully that I turned around, expecting to see him standing behind us. I was surprised that, even with my Catholic upbringing, I had never experienced the presence of Christ as tangibly as I did during my first performance of the oratorio. Since then, each time we perform "Christ Lives!," I hold Him hostage in my heart. –**Fabio**, *Nevada City, California*

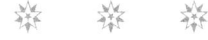

Sing for better health

Numerous studies by the British Academy of Sound Therapy have shown that singing improves our health in specific ways to a greater extent than merely listening to the same music.[12]

1. It reduces the amount of adrenaline, which is linked to heart disease, high blood pressure, and cancer.
2. It reduces cortisol, a hormone related to high stress levels.
3. It increases levels of dopamine, the "feel-good" neurotransmitter.
4. It releases endorphins, hormones that lift our mood.
5. It increases antibodies that fight off disease.
6. It regulates the breath, reducing stress and anxiety, and increasing heart and lung functions.

❋ Singing from Morning till Night ❋

Music came into my life when I needed it most. I had lost two loved ones, and a barrage of karmic bombs seemed to be exploding in my life. I chanced upon a recording of music and mantras sung by the Dalai Lama which began to soothe my inner turmoil, opening something inside me and releasing long-blocked energy. I would listen to the recording at home, and when I went out I would put on headphones and continue to listen.

Not long after I found *Autobiography of a Yogi*, I discovered Kriyananda's music of divine joy. The power in the songs made me long to sing them, and now I sing them every day – while cleaning the house, while working, and when there is a difficult meeting in the offing. I play the recording of Swami Kriyananda chanting Aum so softly that no one else can hear it, but it creates a climate of peaceful acceptance.

I find that I am able to do things calmly now that used to agitate me. I sing when I am tired, when I am sad, and when I am happy. I sing my children to sleep, and they sing with me in the car. When I meditate, music accompanies me like a river that carries me to inner silence. When I sleep, I sing in my dreams. –**Valentina**, *Brescia, Italy*

The benefits of singing are amplified when we sing with others. The Johns Hopkins Center for Music and Medicine formed a choral group for Parkinson's patients. Called the ParkiSonics, the group's participants have demonstrated improvement in both movement and vocal expression, which are often impaired in Parkinson's disease.[13]

Singing or playing music in a group brings a sense of belonging, and of being valued. It keeps the mind active through learning and concentration. Whether singing or playing alone or in a group, the composer's intent and consciousness are experienced much more powerfully than if we only listen to the music.

❈ A Mystical Love Song ❈

When I was seven, I took piano lessons for no more than a year, but I never learned to read music. So it came as a big surprise when an inner urging prompted me to learn to play "Where Has My Love Gone?" – a "mystical love song" by Swami Kriyananda.

This how it came to pass. I was staying at Ananda Assisi, and one day while meditating next to the bed where Swamiji had left his body, I was lamenting that I hadn't known him while he was in the body – and then suddenly I felt his love: it permeated the room, and it was permeating me. It was a communion of our souls.

When I left and got in my car, a CD that I had bought earlier in the day was playing "Where Has My Love Gone?" And as I listened, I couldn't help but feel that Swamiji was singing it to me and for me. In that moment, I understood that the love that I feel for Swamiji and our Masters is an eternal kind of love that knows no limitations of time or space, even though I was never blessed to have the experience of meeting them in the flesh.

When I decided to learn to play the song on the piano, it became an integral part of my sadhana for the next two years. As I played, the meaning expressed through the music penetrated deeper and deeper into my consciousness. "Seek me," she said, "love, out on the sea: boundless the reaches of true love must be."

The music has been a mirror for me, showing me my reactive processes, whether as frustration, impatience, self-deprecation, or any other form of ego involvement. Many wrong attitudes were reflected to me when I played the wrong notes. "Life's made of dreams, friend: dreams that must break, quickly dispersing when we awake."

Much like with the purifying effects of Kriya practice, with faith-filled effort, and with each new attempt, those downward-pulling tendencies were being uprooted.

The power that came from playing the song enabled me to enter into a deep inner attunement with divine love. It helped me deepen my meditations and transcend my attachment to this ephemeral dream. –**Hansa**, *Montreux, Switzerland*

❊ A New Dawn ❊

I remember Swami Kriyananda saying that when you are able to hear the inner sound of Aum in meditation, you will never tire of listening to it. That is how I feel about playing his instrumental compositions for violin – I never tire of playing them.

The melodies are simple. They are not technically difficult, yet their impact is much more than the sum of the notes. They come from a superconscious flow of inspiration that bridges the gap between the Divine and our human experience. When I play them, I cross that bridge, back and forth, throughout each piece.

One piece that I play often is "New Dawn." The first time I performed it, I had a remarkable experience. I felt a power guiding my fingers and the bow to the perfect tone and the right vibrato. I was completely immersed in the flow of the exhilaration of the "new dawn" that had inspired the composer.

Kriyananda wrote a violin solo for me, "Old Men at Sundown." He always valued melody over harmony and other forms of accompaniment, and the violin highlights the melody above all else.

> It was the day of my thirty-sixth birthday, and Kriyananda and I were reviewing a piece that he had just composed. I mentioned that one of the beauties of the violin is that, like the human voice, it can slightly alter the tonality of a note, making it a bit sharper or flatter for the sake of expression and color. As we went through the piece, he indicated where to make these adjustments.
>
> I consider it a rare treasure to have experienced such an intimate contact between composer and performer. I wrote down the adjustments and recall them each time I play the piece.
>
> This music has been one of the great gifts in my life. Performing it is an experience of inner communion with the composer, whose spirit has, in many ways, guided me toward a happier, more fulfilling life. –**Darshan**, *Ananda Assisi*

Playing any musical instruments engages our minds and requires mind-body coordination which strengthens the nervous system. It brings many, surprising physical, mental and emotional benefits.

> Playing music is like doing a workout for every part of your brain. It helps improve your mental performance and memory. There's even evidence that music can help a patient's brain recover from a stroke, as well as slow the onset of dementia and Alzheimer's disease.[14]

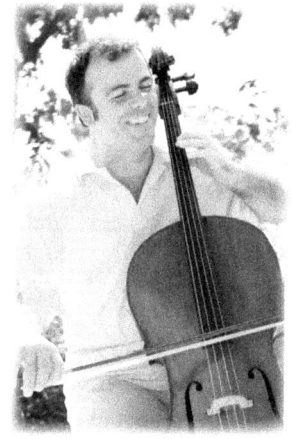

Music can serve us as a convenient and effective mood-changer. When we are feeling down, our thoughts and emotions can feed on each other and trap us in unhealthy moods. When we sing or play music, we experience the world through a new lens, and we become more intuitively perceptive. If the music is inherently uplifting, it can definitely help us break out of negative moods and feel more energized and inspired.

For an enjoyable and effective mood changer, sing along with some of Kriyananda's songs, which you find in the online Appendices for Volume Three.

> **When feeling isolated, sing:**
>
> *All the world is my friend, when I learn how to share my love—*
> *When I stretch out my hand, and smile,*
> *When I live from above.*
> —"All the World is my Friend"
>
>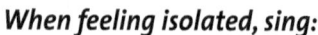
>
> **When feeling burdened, sing:**
>
> *Birds sing of freedom as they soar lightly on the air,*
> *So may our hearts soar high above all curbs and cares.*
> —"Channels"
>
> **When life is difficult, sing like a nightingale:**
>
> *Nightingale, nightingale, sing of joy through the night*
> *Teach my heart to impart everywhere your delight;*
> *Sing of moon rays on the rain; sing that love's not in vain.*
> *Ev'ry grief, ev'ry wrong*
> *Has its ending in song.*
> —"Song of the Nightengale"
>
> **And when all seems dark, sing:**
>
> *I awake in Thy light, I awake in Thy light,*
> *I am joyful, I am free, I awake in Thy light.*
> —"I Awake in Thy Light"

One of Yogananda's close disciples was the famed operatic soprano, Amelita Galli-Curci. She enjoins us:

A final plea: Let music ring throughout your life, and prove to the world what I know well to be the truth, that song shall be the greatest boon for all the world's ills. Banished will be disease, unhappiness, war and strife, till human life will surely become one grand song. SING, OH, SING! [15]

CHAPTER 4: *Points to Remember*

- Music affects us directly and immediately. It can soothe, agitate, excite, or inspire.

- Music that is inspired from a high level of consciousness can lift the listener toward, or even into the same state.

- Choose music that was composed by individuals who are conscious of its effects and intentionally write to uplift the performer and listener.

- Singing and playing spiritual music is more powerfully healing than listening to it.

> Music, more than most human creative endeavors, has the potential to resonate with the higher realities of love and joy. Let us learn to use music and all our creative energies as doorways to the kingdom of heaven, where alone our true home lies.[16] – SWAMI KRIYANANDA

PART XII   CHAPTER FIVE

Songs of the Soul

> Harmonious sound and chants
> impregnated with superconscious
> and soul-force, will-power, and faith,
> awaken the drooping tissues
> of the nervous system by rosing
> vital energy in them.[1]
> —YOGANANDA

> Spiritual chanting is heartfelt prayer,
> deepened by the dimension of music and
> by the building power of repetition....
> The art of chanting correctly is, first,
> to practice it with full awareness of
> its *inner* purpose:... to focus the heart's
> feelings and raise them toward
> superconsciousness.[2] —KRIYANANDA

> He who sings, prays twice. —ST. AUGUSTINE

> Vibratory Healing consists in creating and
> sending vibrations to diseased individuals,
> internally by energy charged by will-power,
> or externally by superconsciously-
> impregnated chants, intonations
> of the human voice, enlivening words,
> phrases, and affirmations.[3]
> —YOGANANDA

✵ Chanting at Carnegie Hall ✵
Paramhansa Yogananda

I was giving a series of lectures at Carnegie Hall in New York City in 1926, and at that time I first suggested to some musical friends the idea of my singing one of these chants, asking the whole audience to join in, without previous rehearsal. My friends thought the chants would be so alien to American understanding that they warned me to expect overripe tomatoes as a possible commentary on my innovation.

I protested that music is the universal language of the soul's devotion to God and that all soulful people, whether familiar or not with Eastern or Western music, would understand the divine yearning of my heart during chanting.

The next evening, while my friends sat behind me on the platform, fearing for my safety, I started to chant "O God Beautiful," and asked the audience, who had never before heard the song, to join me in chanting it. For one hour and twenty-five minutes, the thousands of voices of the entire audience chanted, without discord, "O God Beautiful," in a divine atmosphere of joyous praise. Even when I left the stage, the audience sat on, chanting the song. The next day, many men and women testified to the God-perception and healings of body, mind and soul which had taken place during the sacred chanting, and numerous requests came in to repeat the song at other services.

This experience, which occurred in Carnegie Hall, the musical temple of America and scene of the triumphs of many great singers and artists, was a spontaneous tribute to the universal nature of soul-music.[4]

Music enriches our lives. When we sing, perform, or even listen to music that lifts our consciousness, we feel better and receive healing energy for our bodies and minds. But there is a kind of music that bears even greater and longer-lasting benefits: devotional chanting.

> India has developed a tradition of chanting as an expression of deep, intimate love for God.... Spiritual chanting is different from singing songs or hymns....(they) may inspire, (but they) don't lift the mind into a meditative state.... The highest purpose of chanting is to help awaken us to our own spiritual potential: to bring us closer to Self-realization.... It is to focus the heart's feelings and raise them toward superconsciousness.[5]

In this chapter we look at the tradition of chanting that has been used since ancient times in India, and the distinct form of chanting that was developed from that tradition for the age of Dwapara Yuga by Paramhansa Yogananda.

Bhakti Yoga

The science of Raja Yoga incorporates the methods of the other main paths of yoga as tools for the journey to Self-realization: Bhakti (devotion), Karma (right action), and Gyana (discernment leading to wisdom).

Although devotional practices may not be the preferred tools for everyone's spiritual journey, rightly understood and practiced, they can help us fulfill the two prime prerequisites for experiencing superconscious states: a mind that is still, and a heart that is calm and receptive. Even those who are by nature inclined to devotion may find that past lifetimes of human disappointments have raised protective walls around their hearts. Through chanting, those barriers can begin to fall.

When the young Donald Walters (later Swami Kriyananda) came to Paramhansa Yogananda, he was steeped in intellectual interests. Yogananda valued the new disciple's mental clarity and asked him to write articles for his magazine. But he also urged him to develop devotion.

"Get devotion!" he would tell me. "You must have devotion. Remember what Jesus said"—here he paraphrased the words of the Gospel—"'Thou dost not reveal Thyself unto the prudent and the wise, but unto babes.'"

Swami Sri Yukteswar, a saint of wisdom if ever there was one, and therefore, so one might think, a saint more likely than most to endorse intellectual attitudes, said that love alone determines a person's fitness for the spiritual path. In his book *The Holy Science* he wrote, "This heart's natural love is the principal thing to attain a holy life.... It is impossible for man to advance a step towards [salvation] without it." [6]

I worked hard to develop devotion, chanting and praying daily for the grace of intense love for God. Master one day smiled at me lovingly. "Keep on with your devotion," he said. "See how dry your life is when you depend on intellect." [7]

Indian poetry, scripture and music

Indian scripture, poetry and music are intertwined. The scriptures are written in poetic verse, and are meant to be sung. The word *gita* means song, as we see in the Bhagavad Gita, which is often sung in its entirety at special religious gatherings.

India's great mystic poets sing of the devotee's love for the Cosmic Beloved. Their poems symbolize the story of the individual soul and its relationship with God. The poems of Adi Shankara, Mirabai, Kabir, Sri Ramprasad Sen, Kalidasa, and Rabindranath Tagore are sung to this day.

Such songs are known as *bhajans* – songs of reverence. They are usually lyrical, sung in the native language of the poet, and based on melodic *ragas*. The melody carries the message and mood of the *bhajan*. The singer's voice is accompanied by a principal instrument, which may be a harmonium, a flute, or a stringed instrument: often a simple *tanpura* that provides a tonic background drone.

Yogananda writes: "India has always recognized the human voice as the most perfect instrument of sound."[8] Harmony, beloved in Western music, is not part of the Eastern tradition.

> It is interesting that Indian devotional music, though highly melodic, is devoid of both harmony and sub-melodies. Western religious music, with its intricate counter-melodies and harmonic patterns, is considerably richer....
>
> Richness is something the Indian tradition seeks to avoid, owing no doubt to its stress on personal, inner communion with God. Western religious music is usually associated with communal worship....Indian religious tradition, by contrast, ignores the human personality more or less altogether, and concentrates on the soul's eternal longing for its divine Source in God. Through music, the Indian worshiper is taught to seek attunement, ultimately, with Aum, the Sound-current of the Infinite.[9]

Kirtan chants

The traditional *bhajans* are not the same as the chants that are commonly sung during *kirtans*. A kirtan is a group gathering that is dedicated to singing God's name. The idea is that the vibrations of the Beloved's name will purify our hearts and instill divine qualities in us. They are usually sung in Sanskrit and often include a variety of names for the same deity.[10]

Kirtan is classically sung in the "call and response" manner, with the group responding to phrases sung by the lead singer. The songs may be mantras or compilations of the names of God's manifestations. Often used in kirtans are "*mahamantras*" associated with each of the major India deities – "Om namah Shivaya"; "Sri Ram Jai Ram Jai Jai Ram"; "Hare Ram Hare Krishna"; "Om Namo Bhagavate Vasudevaya" – and many others.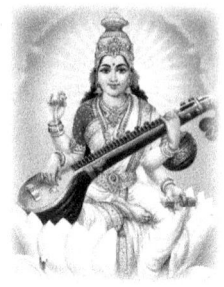

Even though Westerners may not have a personal relationship with or cultural knowledge of the divinities mentioned in kirtan chants, the magnetic vibrations of the Sanskrit mantras and the devotion instilled through the ages in the classic chants can combine to make kirtan gatherings uniquely inspiring and healing.

❈ Vertigo ❈

I had always been athletic – I kept my body in excellent shape with long walks, swimming, and aerobic workouts at the gym. But there came a day when I began to have dizzy spells – recurring episodes of vertigo for which I had to be hospitalized three times.

In the face of the baffling condition, fear crept in, and I stopped exercising. The fear led me to explore Paramhansa Yogananda's teachings, to see if they would suggest something that I could do to overcome the vertigo and the accompanying fears.

While participating in a yoga posture session during a spiritual retreat, I began to feel nauseous and lose my balance. I left the class, and even though I rested for the remainder of the day, the symptoms persisted. That evening, I attended a kirtan, and for an hour I forgot my woes and let myself become absorbed in the music. By the end of the kirtan I was astonished to realize that the nausea, headache and confusion had melted away, replaced by inner calmness.

When I came to the next daily yoga session, the same sequence occurred – nausea, headache, instability, and fear – and in the evening, chanting at the kirtan, followed by the same miraculous relief: all of my symptoms mysteriously disappeared.

Yogananda's chants and Kriyananda's music now accompany me every day, smoothing my path at work and in my spiritual growth. The vertigo is gone, the fear has vanished, and the music gives me the courage to face whatever difficulties my life may bring. An added benefit is that when my husband, who suffers from insomnia, listens to this music in bed with headphones, he easily falls into a refreshing sleep. We are both grateful for this healing musical heritage. –**Marina**, *Bologna, Italy*

❊ KITCHEN KIRTAN ❊

I received an emergency call – the dinner clean-up crew had been double-booked and would be unable to help. Four of us responded, and when we entered the kitchen the mountain of dirty pots, pans, and dishes was discouraging. I'm sure that our shared thought was "We'll be here half the night!" But we rolled up our sleeves and got started.

After little more than a few minutes, someone in the group began chanting: "From joy I came; for joy I live, in sacred joy I melt again." Soon we were all singing.

We got through the dishes, then someone began chanting "Il mio cuore è Tuo" ("You Fill My Heart with Music"), and we got through the silverware.

We switched to mantras for the pots and pans – "Govinda Jai! Jai!" – then "Om Namo Bhagavate Vasudevaya."

We cleaned the counters and the floor to "Door of My Heart."

Instead of working half the night, we finished in record time – I was so full of energy that I continued to chant "Who Is in My Temple?" as I strolled to the temple, where I had a most rewarding meditation. –**Santoshi**, *Ananda Assisi*

Cosmic Chants

Yogananda's mission as an avatar of Dwapara Yuga was to highlight the deeper truths in the Christian and Hindu scriptures, and to revive spiritual practices which, during the dark age of Kali Yuga, had been lost or become perfunctory. His purpose, he would say, was to spiritualize, not 'Indianize' the West.

> He came to do something very unusual: he came to bring about the inwardness of the East and the outwardness of the West,...not to "Indianize" Americans, but to spiritualize America and through America, the West and the world. And he came to bring back to India the practical approach to spirituality that he encountered in this country, because both are now needed as a balance.[11]

> "East and West must establish a golden middle path of activity and spirituality combined," (Babaji) continued. "India has much to learn from the West in material development; in return, India can teach the universal methods by which the West will be able to base its religious beliefs on the unshakable foundations of yogic science."[12]

Yogananda's transforming wisdom penetrated every aspect of the spiritual life, including the practice of chanting.

> Paramhansa Yogananda, as a great yogi whose mission was to disseminate the yoga teachings in the West, introduced a new kind of chanting here. It is based on the repetition of meaningful phrases, rather than of the divine names. Some of the

Life Force / 248

> chants he wrote he translated from Bengali or Hindi songs. Others, he wrote himself. This kind of chanting is more like a repetitive prayer set to music, and is better suited for meditators, who understand the importance of combining the soul's appeal for divine grace with self-effort. For by singing God's names only, what remains in the mind is the thought "God will do it all for me." What Yogananda's method of chanting accomplishes is to awaken in the mind the thought "In these ways I will cooperate with His grace." [13]

He called these songs "Cosmic Chants" and published a compilation of forty of them in 1938.

> I was able to complete at the hermitage a long-projected work, Cosmic Chants. I set to English words and Western musical notation about forty songs, some original, others my adaptations of ancient melodies. Included were the Shankara chant, "No Birth, No Death"; two favorites of Sri Yukteswar's: "Wake, Yet Wake, O my Saint!" and "Desire, my Great Enemy"; the hoary Sanskrit "Hymn to Brahma"; old Bengali songs, "What Lightning Flash!" and "They Have Heard Thy Name"; Tagore's "Who is in my Temple?"; and a number of my compositions: "I Will be Thine Always," "In the Land Beyond my Dreams," "Come Out of the Silent Sky," "Listen to my Soul Call," "In the Temple of Silence," and "Thou Art my Life." [14]

Adopting the style of the *bhajan*, simplifying or composing more singable melodies, and embedding in each chant a prayer and/or an affirmation, Yogananda developed a unique blend of Eastern and Western music.

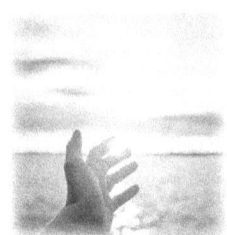

One of the best-known Cosmic Chants is "Door of My Heart." Adapted from a Bengali *bhajan*, it begins with an affirmation: "Door of my heart, open wide I keep for Thee."

And then a prayer: "Wilt Thou come? Wilt Thou come? Just for once, come to me?"

A bhajan-style devotional conversation follows: "Will my days fly away without seeing Thee, My Lord?"

For the finale, a closing affirmation: "Night and day, night and day, I look for Thee night and day."

One of Yogananda's original compositions is this loving declaration to God:

> *Thou art my life, Thou art my love,*
> *Thou art the sweetness which I do seek.*
> *In the thought by my love brought, I taste Thy name –*
> *So sweet, so sweet.*
> *Devotee knows how sweet You are,*
> *He knows whom You let know.*

❊ LIGHT FOR THE MIND ❊

After experiencing a brutal deception and betrayal, I began to lose control of my mind. As my thoughts revolved obsessively around the minute details of my terrible memories, I would cascade into a seemingly irreversible depression that I thought would never end.

When I found Yogananda's Cosmic Chants, I began singing them in an attempt to superimpose their uplifting melodies over my sad thoughts. "Door of My Heart" was a personal favorite, and through its chant-door I began to be healed. In time, I became sufficiently stable to start practicing yoga, energization, and meditation in search of an even more comprehensive healing.

That was three years ago. I continue to chant, pray, and meditate – although no longer for healing, for I am well, but from a heart that is filled with gratitude, and with a longing to know God and share His presence with others.
—**Margherita**, *Brescia*

Spiritualizing the chants

Another unique feature of the Cosmic Chants is that Yogananda "spiritualized" each of them.

> Each of the Cosmic Chants in this book
> has been spiritualized, that is, each song has
> been sung aloud and mentally until
> it has found actual response from God....
> These chants properly repeated will bring God-
> communion and ecstatic joy, and through
> these the healing of body, mind and soul.[15]

Spiritualized chants carry vibrations that can neutralize the vibrational frequencies of disease.

> One who sings these spiritualized songs,
> Cosmic Chants, with true devotion will find
> God-communion and ecstatic joy, and through
> them the healing of body, mind, and soul.[16]

Just as the vibrations of saints linger in holy places for thousands of years, the vibrations of ecstatic joy that are permanently embedded in the Cosmic Chants offer us as a bridge that we can cross to higher states of awakening.

A spiritualized chant has even more power when we ourselves make the effort to then spiritualize it.

> A song which is born out of the depth of true
> devotion to God and which is continuously chanted,
> audibly or mentally, with ever-increasing deep
> devotion until response is consciously received
> from Him in the form of communion, ecstasy and
> boundless joy, is a spiritualized song.[17]

To spiritualize a chant truly, it is best to choose a single chant and sing it over and over until we have unlocked its power.

> Yoganandaji wrote that the greatest benefit comes from spiritualizing a chant oneself, by singing it repeatedly, more and more deeply, day after day until it lifts one into superconsciousness. Thereafter, he said, whenever one sings the same chant it will induce that state of consciousness....
>
> For once, by long practice, a specific practice has been "spiritualized" through some form of divine contact, it will quickly induce a divine state of awareness every time it is undertaken again. In the same way, although a variety of chants may be more interesting, and in that sense more inspiring, than sticking to one chant for a long period of time, the way really to spiritualize a chant is to sing only that one for days, weeks, or months together, taking it deeper and deeper into oneself as you have been taught to do with affirmations, until through it one achieves some definite divine contact.[18]

❋ WHEN THY SONG FLOWS THROUGH ME ❋

Many times, chanting has lifted me out of sad moods, depression, loneliness, and negativity – it has raised me out of my little self into my higher Self, with a minimum of effort.

We will naturally be drawn to chants that resonate with our vibrations, or that magnetize us with the vibrations that we aspire to. In moments of despair, I turn to Yogananda's chant "When Thy Song Flows Through Me."

> *O life is sweet and death a dream*
> *when Thy song flows through me, my Lord*
> *Then joy is sweet, sorrow a dream*
> *when Thy song flows through me, my Lord*
> *Then health is sweet, sickness a dream*
> *when Thy song flows through me, my Lord*
> *Then praise is sweet and blame a dream*
> *when Thy song flows through me, my Lord*

I consider it one of his most beautiful chants – it reassures us that when we attune ourselves to the divine vibrations and offer ourselves as channels for God to others, our life becomes sweet, and all the things that afflict us are seen in their true light, as only a dream.

Many times this chant has helped me open my heart, step out of my ego, and loosen the grip of delusion. It has become so deeply a part of my consciousness that its effects are instantly there whenever I need them. *–Sanjaya, Ananda Assisi*

Japa chanting

> To spiritualize a chant, keep it rotating in the mind –
> for days at a time, if necessary: not only in meditation,
> but as you go about your daily activities.
> This practice is also called japa.[19]

Japa is the practice of continuous mental chanting. It uplifts the mind and strengthens the protective magnetic field around the body.* It can consist of chanting a name of God, a God-reminding thought, an affirmation, or a prayer. Japa focuses the mind and protects it from distractions.

On his first visit to the Indian saint, **Ananda Moyi Ma**, Swami Kriyananda asked her:

---

* See Chapter Eleven for a discussion of the aura, and techniques for strengthening it.

> "Mother, would you give me some personal advice for my spiritual practice?"
>
> "Always practice japa" [she responded]. "Keep your mind busy chanting God's name, and you won't have time to think of anything else."*

Japa is in not unique to Hinduism. Catholics do japa when they recite the Hail Mary consciously and lovingly. The Tibetan Buddhist practice of chanting *Om mani padme hum* is a form of japa, as is the Jesus prayer of Eastern Orthodox Christians: "Lord Jesus Christ, have mercy on me," and the *mahamantra* of the Vaishnava bhaktis – worshipers of Vishnu who chant the "Hare Krishna" mantra.

As part of a slideshow about his recent trip to India, Swami Kriyananda showed us this photo of an exceptionally luminous monk,

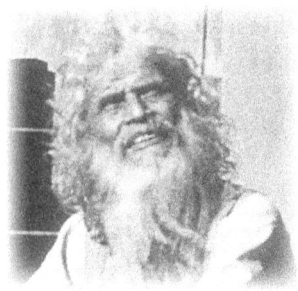

whose face was filled with joy, his eyes as deep as the ocean. Whatever question Kriyananda addressed to this monk, the answer was always, and only: "Aum Guru!" Since that evening, I have taken that as my personal japa mantra.

Yogananda suggested several phrases that we could use as a japa mantra: "Reveal Thyself," "I am Thine, be Thou mine," and "I want only Thee." Swami Kriyananda has written melodies for these mantras, so that they can be sung as well as repeated.

How to chant

Every skill has both technical and artistic dimensions. A complicated dinner menu requires high-quality ingredients, special kitchen equipment, and a detailed recipe – these are the technical elements. Once we have mastered the recipe, we can apply our artistic creativity to embellish its flavor and appearance.

Chanting, too, has technical and devotional aspects. Mastering the technical side will allow us to deepen our practice.

---

*Kriyananda, "My First Meetings with Ananda Moyi Ma," private notes of his visit on 13 February, 1959.

Yogananda emphasizes the scientific principles of chanting in *Cosmic Chants* and *Scientific Healing Affirmations.* To go deep with a chant, we need to sing it in a way that will penetrate the three levels of our consciousness. Although casual chanting may be pleasing, it will not have the power to transform our consciousness. In the prelude to *Cosmic Chants*, Yogananda describes five phases of chanting.

> **The five states in chanting are conscious chanting aloud—whisper chanting—mental chanting—subconscious chanting—superconscious chanting.**[20]

When we proceed through these five stages with faith and devotion, we can tap the power of the chant to heal us.

> In connection with singing, chanting, or intoning away physical disease or worry or or spiritual ignorance, one must know the law of intonation from high to low, low to whisper, whisper to mental, subconscious to superconscious, chanting. This is the method of converting loud meaningful words into realized experiences — assimilating the truth of a word or words by chanting loudly and mentally until they become a part of the soul's realization. In all cases the intonation, whether mental or physical (that is, audible), must be injected with superconscious mentality, faith, and steadiness in the beginning or at the end, to be effective in accomplishing a specific healing.[21]

Loud chanting

When chanting alone or in a group, it is important to begin by chanting loudly to engage the rational mind, which wants to understand the words and learn the melody. Loud chanting also focuses the mind.

> There is...a good reason also for chanting loudly at first. It isn't to get God's attention, but to focus our own thoughts and feelings. It is when we are inwardly focused that we should chant softly, with increasingly inward awareness.[22]
> Loud chanting...commands attention from your thought-soldiers. (It) creates a magnetic flow... (that) can dissolve the eddies of thought and feeling. Once you've got their attention, chant more softly, more inwardly.[23]

> After the notes are learned, one's undivided attention should be given to repeating them with deeper and deeper devotion, striving to fully understand the meaning of the words in the chant, until one is immersed in the joy of singing. This joyous feeling is the first perception of God.[24]

The words to Yogananda's chants are nuanced, with deep spiritual truths to contemplate. Consider his chant, "From This Sleep, Lord."

> *From this sleep, Lord, will You wake, wake me?*
> *From this dream, Lord, will You wake, wake me?*
> *In Thee I dive;*
> *In Thee I rise, in Thy sea, in, in Thee.*
> *From this sleep, Lord, will You wake, wake me?*
> *From this dream, Lord, will You wake, wake me?*
> *In Thee I'm born;*
> *In Thee I die, to live forever in, in Thee.*[25]

While chanting the words loudly, we begin to grasp the truth that we have been sleeping in delusion, and that our soul longs to dive in the sea of bliss and rise into superconsciousness. With continued chanting, we realize that our souls are born of Spirit, and that when the delusion of our egoic separation dies we will be resurrected and able to live in the consciousness of our immortal soul.

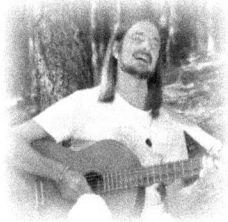

Even when listening to recordings of chants, it is more effective to sing with them. When chanting alone before meditation, we may want to skip the phase of chanting loudly. Nevertheless it is important to take the chant from the conscious level, through the subconscious to the superconscious.

You can use the position of your eyes to help your chanting. Begin with open eyes while looking straight ahead, possibly focusing on an object or image on your altar. Then close your eyes and lower the gaze to instill the vibrations of the chant in the subconscious mind, bringing the high vibrations of the chant to that level and planting the chant in your memory. Then raise your gaze with eyes closed or half-open and focus your attention calmly at the spiritual eye to lift the chant into superconsciousness.

Whisper chanting

As we sing more and more softly, the meaning of the words and the vibrations of the music will filter into the subconscious, where we can begin to experience them directly instead of merely thinking about them.

> Once your conscious mind is wholly engaged in chanting, bring it down into the subconscious by whispering. While chanting in the subconscious, offer the chant there, too, up to superconsciousness at the point between the eyebrows, until you feel your entire being vibrating with the words, the melody, and the rhythm.[26]

Mental chanting

Whisper chanting naturally leads to mental chanting, which reinforces the chant's vibrations in the subconscious.

> All loud affirmations by a group may be started loudly or softly, but must end in chanting them mentally for some time in silence, until the words change into vibratory messengers of thought let loose in the ether to execute their desired errands.[27]

Subconscious chanting

To experience the full healing power of a chant, we must sing it for a long time, not only for a few minutes. At some point, the chant will take on a life of its own, repeating in our subconscious through the day, and even in dreams.

> Subconscious chanting becomes automatic, with internal consciousness only....it will be found that the songs subconsciously repeat themselves in the background of the mind bringing great joy even when one is in the thick of the battle of activity.[28]

As we strive to spiritualize a chant or affirmation, we find it lingering in the background of our awareness, repeating with its own momentum. We can use this ability of the subconscious mind to our spiritual advantage. Instead of being tortured by advertising jingles, we can train the subconscious to feed us only transforming words and melodies of life-changing chants. After listening all day to a softly playing recording of Swami Kriyananda chanting Aum, I continue to hear it, because it has saturated my subconscious.

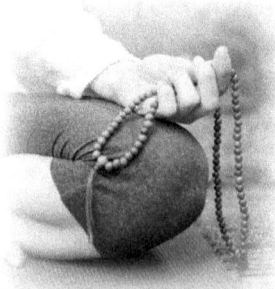

Superconscious chanting

Our chanting journey can bring us now to the superconscious level.

> One must chant deeper and deeper until all chanting changes into subconscious and then superconscious chanting which brings one into the divine Presence....
> Superconscious chanting is when the deep internal chanting vibrations are converted into realization and are established in the superconscious, subconscious, and conscious minds....
> Each of these chants should be sung not once but many times, utilizing the cumulative power of repetition, until the singer feels a great joy break through the radio of his heart. When this joy is felt it is proof that God has answered the devotee, and that his devotion has been properly tuned and the broadcasting of his ardor in chants has been true and deep.[29]

> At last, chant only mentally, at the point between the eyebrows. Let your absorption lift you into superconsciousness. Once it does so, and once you receive a divine response, you will have spiritualized the chant. From then on, any time you sing the chant it will quickly carry you again to superconsciousness as if on a magic carpet.
> To spiritualize a chant, keep it rotating in the mind—for days at a time, if necessary: not only in meditation, but as you go about your daily activities.[30]

This is the stage at which the chant has maximum healing power.

> The moment the phrase reaches super-consciousness..., a volley of energy will shoot down and vibrate and heal the mind, and soul, electrocuting physical bacteria, paralyzing mental fears, and conflagrating ignorance into ashes. Hence, the external method of vibrating the voice according to the aforesaid methods can heal all inharmonious conditions of the body, mind, and soul.[31]

The healing power of chanting [32]

When we sing a chant which we ourselves have spiritualized, it has the power to eliminate physical and psychological ailments because it introduces frequencies which are higher than those of the illness.

✵ THE CHANTING CURE ✵

I didn't want to accept that I was having a nervous breakdown. A serious surgery, and my father's death, were more than I could process. My breathing became erratic to the point of spasm, my heart rhythm was accelerated.

That was my sorry state when I was introduced to Yogananda, meditation, and chanting.

This was years ago, when Ananda had a retreat center near Lake Como, which I often visited. Because I was addicted to psychotropic drugs, I was unable to control my mind in meditation. The one thing that soothed my anxieties and helped calm my thoughts was chanting, which was a common factor in all of the retreat activities.

I sang at the retreat and I sang at home. Several chants were especially meaningful for me: "I want only Thee, Lord, Thee, only Thee," and "From joy I came, for joy I live, in sacred joy I melt again."

As I chanted, I could feel the weight of pain and suffering melting away. It was a remarkable, liberating experience.

Soon I was chanting mentally all the time. Chanting became my refuge. As I sang, anxieties would gradually dissolve; and when I couldn't sleep, I would lie there and chant.

After a few months, I was able to stop the medication completely. I regained my inner balance and rediscovered my inner strength and joy. Despite the trials that my life had brought me, I have never relapsed into depression.

Many years have passed, and I continue to chant. Best of all, I can now meditate deeply. –*Ornella*, *Biela, Italy*

❋ From Joy I Came ❋

We had been together for five years. Yet while I was aware that he had serious difficulties with family members, I had no idea how depressed he had become.

When he called me at work one day, which he had never done, his voice was filled with sadness and despair. I rushed home, barely in time to save his life from a self-inflicted wound in his stomach.

It was a terrible trauma. My entire world was spinning – I could not understand what had happened and why he had not confided in me. I could barely meditate, often not at all, and I couldn't remember the order of the Energization Exercises. But there was one thing I could do: I could chant.

I am by no stretch of the imagination a singer, but one of the chants kept playing in my mind: "From joy I came, for joy I live, in sacred joy I melt again." The words and melody played incessantly and slowly pulled me out of my despair.

Through the chant I felt connected with the masters, and I knew that they were with me. It has been six months since that traumatic day, and the chant has held me and my life together with no need for medication. Each day I become calmer as I sing the chant, and I am now able to meditate once more. My companion is receiving the professional help he needs, and I am continuing to grow stronger through the remarkable healing power of this song of eternal joy. –*Pierangela*, *Pisa, Italy*

When to use Cosmic Chants

In the original edition of *Cosmic Chants*, Yogananda wrote that he had a specific purpose in mind for each of the chants.

> Each of these Cosmic Chants has been composed to satisfy a special need of mind or life. The devotee's various moods and inner desires can be strengthened or changed by the repetition of one particular chant suitable for that purpose.[33]

You will find his suggestions in the online Appendices for Part XII.

Group chanting

When we chant as part of a group kirtan, each chant helps awaken our devotion. Typically, the more rhythmic chants will be sung at the beginning, and the more melodic and slower chants will be sung as the kirtan progresses.

> A group, gathered together in the name of God, can take one of these chants, singing it together loudly, with piano or organ accompaniment, then more slowly, then singing in a whisper without any accompaniment, and finally mentally only. In this way deep God-perception can be reached singly or together.[34]

While chanting privately, we pass through the stages spontaneously; but in group chanting, the leader must guide the process. Each chant should take us through the five stages to superconscious chanting, followed by a brief period of silent meditation. The final chant of the kirtan will lead us into a longer period of meditation.

> After chanting, especially, but also after making affirmations, sit silently as long as you can do so with joy. Meditate. Chanting is, indeed, only a preparation for meditation. Not to use it as a send-off into silence is to leave the airplane after taxiing it onto the runway.[35]

When we chant at the start of a group meditation, the chanting will serve as a prelude rather than the main activity. Depending on the program and the composition of the group, we may choose one or two more inward, less rhythmic chants to awaken our devotion and bring the group more quickly into superconscious chanting, followed by silent meditation.

Chanting is half the battle

One of Yogananda's oft-quoted sayings is, "Chanting is half the battle." There are many battles that we face every day: did he have one in particular in mind? He never specified, so I will surmise, based on many things which he taught.

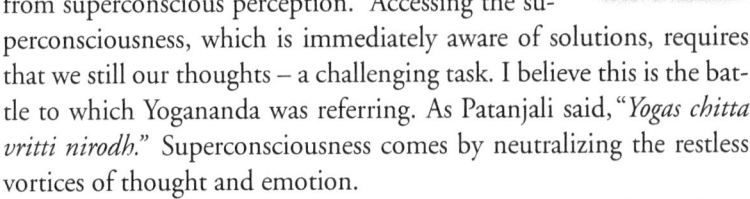

The solutions to all our life's problems come from superconscious perception.* Accessing the superconsciousness, which is immediately aware of solutions, requires that we still our thoughts – a challenging task. I believe this is the battle to which Yogananda was referring. As Patanjali said, "*Yogas chitta vritti nirodh.*" Superconsciousness comes by neutralizing the restless vortices of thought and emotion.

Any activity that absorbs our attention – such as a sport, playing chess, or watching a film – to some degree temporarily takes our minds away from problems. But the effects are not long-lasting or transformative.

Chanting focuses the mind, and through the superconscious vibrations of the words, melody, and music, it calms the emotions and opens the heart to experience divine love, wisdom, and joy. Chanting at the start of a meditation clarifies our vision and opens our heart to perceive the Cosmic Sound of Aum.

* See Volume Two, Part VI, Chapter Five for a discussion of superconsciousness.

> **Vibrations resulting from devotional singing lead to the contact of the Cosmic Vibration or the Word.**[36]

❋ WAR-TIME KIRTAN ❋

To help me open my heart, Swami Kriyananda recommended that I sing in the Ananda Assisi choir. It had the intended effect, and in time I began leading kirtans, playing guitar, and singing.

Many times I have felt the vibrations in the temple tangibly changing as we've chanted, becoming denser, as if the air were filled with an invisible Presence. It would only happen when a group of devotees were chanting sincerely from their hearts to the Divine. I realized that chanting this way can take us deep, just like meditation.

The most powerful experience of chanting that I have ever had occurred in Croatia during the war. Shivani and I traveled to Rijeka to give a series of classes on meditation. When we entered Croatia, we felt the heavy atmosphere of the brutal war that was raging nearby. There was danger in the air, and I admit that I was not free of fear, nor were the people who gathered for the opening program.

We started the evening by inviting the audience to join us in singing one of Yogananda's chants, "I Am the Bubble, Make Me the Sea" – not sure if they would join in. We had learned the chant in Croatian from our hosts, and soon everyone was singing with all their hearts, using the prayerful chant to ask for help from Above.

We sang and sang – it was an unforgettable kirtan, and in that moment I knew that this was the level of intensity that draws God's grace. The heart needs to "churn the ether," as Yogananda urged us, to draw God's response. That is exactly what we did during that dangerous moment – and, yes, we were protected. –*Jayadev*, *Ananda Europa*

❋ ❋ ❋

CHAPTER 5: *Points to Remember*

- One of Yogananda's unique techniques for self-healing is the practice of devotional chanting.
- His *Cosmic Chants* combine the musical style of classic Indian *bhajans* with Western-style melodies of his own composition.
- He spiritualized each of the chants by singing it with such deep devotion that it elicited an actual response from the Divine.
- Spiritualized chants have great healing power.
- You can spiritualize a chant by singing it deeply until you find its power resonating within you.
- To empower a chant to penetrate all of the levels of our consciousness, Yogananda recommends a progression: singing it first loudly, then softly, then in a whisper, and finally with mental chanting alone.
- Chanting in a group kirtan generates a vibration that, when internalized, can lead to healing and the experience of higher states of consciousness.
- Chanting at the start of a meditation focuses the mind, calms the emotions, and prepares the heart to experience divine love.

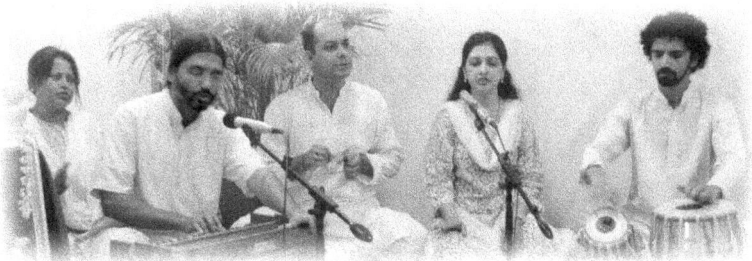

PART XII   CHAPTER SIX

Nature Therapy

❖ NATURE'S GREATEST GIFT ❖

From my earliest years, I have often sensed a loving presence that permeates this world. One day while hiking through a remote valley in Desolation Wilderness, I felt an overwhelming sense of joy—a joy so pervasive that it seemed to animate the flowers, the stones, and the cascading stream. Every blade of grass, every tiny waterfall and mossy rock, seemed to radiate and rejoice in this all-encompassing joy.

I sat beside a small, snow-fed tarn, encircled by huge granite blocks cleaved by a glacier, delighting in the joy around me. Soon, a robust, cheery little bird... came within a few yards of me and began singing.... The bird's vibrant song and its resounding echo greatly amplified the joy I felt that day on the mountain.

Nature's greatest gift, I believe, is in making us aware of the oneness of life. Nature...gives us sustenance, shelter, all our daily needs. Her most precious gift is the experience of her deeper nature: her stillness, harmony, wholeness, and joyful vitality.

–Joseph Bharat Cornell[1]

Nature's Healing Balm

In Indian mythology, each of the three primary gods – Brahma, Vishnu, and Shiva – is considered to be the Creator of the universe. Lord Shiva is depicted as setting creation in motion with his small handheld two-sided drum, the *damaru*, which he shakes back and forth, a small attached bead sounding the Pranava (the Aum) of creation. From these sounds the *ragas* are born – the basic patterns of

Indian music. Shiva Nataraj is considered the progenitor of dance, expressing the rhythm and harmony of life – its *raga* and *taal* (melody and rhythm).

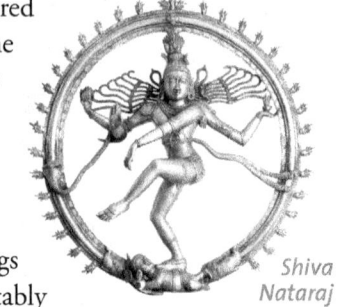

Shiva Nataraj

Everything in life has its inherent song and its perfect rhythm. The planets are dancing, spinning on their axes as they rotate around the sun. We earthlings witness the moon's rhythms as it predictably waxes and wanes. In nature, we observe the seasonal cycles of plants. As the seasons march forward through the year, some locales will experience just one season (Antarctica) or two (lands on the equator), while others may have as many as six (Australia and some others).

Various internal rhythms coordinate the proper functioning of the human body. The twenty-four-hour circadian rhythm that regulates our sleep patterns is coordinated by a master clock in the hypothalamus. The circadian cycle also affects our metabolism, and influences the immune system, as well as our mental health.

All organisms have biological clocks that regulate the timing of their activities. In plants, an internal clock regulates when the flowers open and close. In animals, it regulates when they sleep, hunt, reproduce, and hibernate. In humans, the biological clock regulates hunger, fertility, and much more.

The human body becomes vulnerable to disease when the rhythms of our lives come into conflict with the rhythms of our internal cycles and of nature. A perfectly balanced wheel can spin smoothly at a high rate, but a slight imbalance may cause it to fly off its axis. To maintain our health and sanity, we must align our rhythms to the natural flow of life.

Mother Nature is a powerful healer. Spending time in Her presence can be profoundly therapeutic. Leaving the strictures of our overly busy lives behind for an excursion in nature can reset our physical and mental rhythms and restore an inner sense of harmony.

While listening to the wind, bird songs, the insects, a cheerful brook, or ocean waves, we begin to come back into alignment with our axis. The trees, rivers, fields, and flowers expect nothing – their lives are harmonious and contented; the changes in their existence are imperceptibly gentle and gradual. In nature, vibrations of peace and harmony prevail. No egoic conflicts there, no meetings, no deadlines. Even a short time in nature (without a cell phone) can have a remarkably salutary effect on our mental and physical health.

☼ EARTH WINDOWS ☼

Keiko had endured a troubled childhood. As an adult, she had a remarkable experience during a nature exercise created by naturalist Joseph Bharat Cornell.

I was lying perfectly still under a thick blanket of leaves, gazing upward from the earth to the swaying trees and passing clouds.

I heard an abundance of subtle sounds. I watched leaves dancing gracefully downward, some of them landing softly on me, each leaf making its own light rustle....I heard an insect walking near my ear. I heard sounds nearby and far away. I heard all the sounds *all at once*....The three-dimensional world around me, I realized, was incredibly rich and dynamic, everywhere filled with exquisite detail.

Everything was breathing and sharing the same air. The air in the sky was the same air breathed in and out by the trees, the birds, every animal, and by the people of the earth. I felt myself part of the earth—I had a sense of oneness with everything around me....

Never before had I beheld the earth shining with such radiance and benevolence. Every sound became precious to me and uplifted me. I felt—for the very first time—that my life was a precious gift....

I have been able to access this experience at will since that magical day thirty years ago. The feeling of acceptance and love that came to me in that moment in the forest has never left me. Like a lighthouse, my forest experience has guided my footsteps to this day, helping me to leave behind the sadness of my early years and to embrace the time ahead with joy and gratitude.[2] – from *Flow Learning*, by **Joseph Bharat Cornell**

The healing effects of water

Urban life exposes us to an overload of positive ions – from electronic devices, fluorescent lights, and toxins in paint, carpets, and upholstery. These environmental enemies can affect our mood, exacerbate chronic pain, increase inflammation, and much more. Modern houses, office buildings, and cities are overloaded with disease-inducing positive ions.

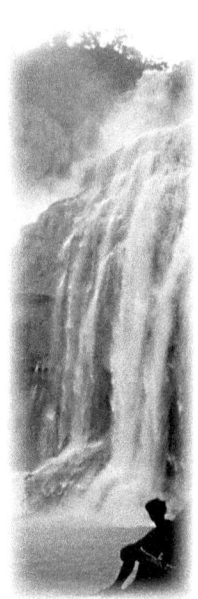

> Sitting by flowing water has a positive healing effect on metabolism, digestion, blood pressure, sleep, the immune system, and emotional state. Among the healthiest places in nature are the ocean, waterfalls, and fast-moving rivers, owing to the release of negative ions.[3]

According to Dr. Elliot Dinetz, of the University of Miami Miller School of Medicine, being near water improves our physical and mental health.

> "Bodies of water, whether freshwater or saltwater, have inherent qualities that offer health benefits.... On the mental health front, being near the ocean, a phenomenon often referred to as the 'blue space effect,' has been linked to reduced stress levels and overall mental well-being.... Activities such as swimming or walking on the beach increase these benefits by improving cardiovascular health and promoting the release of endorphins, the body's natural mood boosters." [4]

The seeker in Herman Hesse's novel *Siddhartha* sits by a river with the wise ferryman Vasudev, who asks him:

> "Have you also learned that secret from the river; that there is no such thing as time? That the river is everywhere at the same time, at the source and at the mouth, at the waterfall, at the ferry, at the current, in the ocean and in the mountains, everywhere and that the present only exists for it, not the shadow of the past nor the shadow of the future." [5]

Nature's wonders can serve to symbolize higher realities.

> Mount Carmel has long been for Christians a symbol of everyone's spiritual climb toward perfection; Mount Meru, for Hindus, is a symbol of the challenge to divine attainment; and the river Jordan, for Jews and Christians alike, is a symbol for baptism not only into their respective faiths, but (for those with deeper understanding) into the stream of energy in the spine.[6]

> The rain, Paramhansa Yogananda said, is a message to us of Divine Compassion; the flowers whisper to us of God's love and joy; the tenderness of Mother Nature reminds us of the consciousness in which She wants us always to live. On the other hand, Her elemental fierceness is also a warning to us not to live proudly, as if we were above divine law.[7]

One of Swami Kriyananda's songs is aptly entitled, "Channels."

Channels

Birds sing of freedom as they soar lightly on the air.
So may our hearts soar high above all curbs and care.
Trees standing firm hold the secret of inner power.
Give us when tested strength to endure.
Stars send a message of light through eternity.
Lord when in darkness your radiance we see.
Mountains remote and still hint of higher worlds unseen.

So may our lives be soaring and serene.
Rivers seek passage unhindered by rock or tree.
So may our lives flow steadfast toward the sea.
Flowers so soft and fragile stay fragrant,
Though pressed to the ground.
May we thus learn forbearance,
for in kindness love is found.

Bringing nature indoors

Call to mind how you feel at the bank or post office. Now remember how you feel in a garden center or flower market. Does one environment make you happier than the other? When winter is almost gone, but before it is warm enough to plant, I enjoy visiting the flower growers just to walk through the greenhouses and drink in the vibrancy of the plants. No matter what my mood was like when I arrived, I leave with a song in my heart.

Bringing as much of nature as possible into our indoor spaces vastly improves our physical and mental health. Exposure to sunlight stimulates healing – thus, we will want to maximize the amount of natural sunlight entering our indoor spaces, by keeping curtains and windows open as much as possible.

In northern countries where the sun hardly shines in winter, there are uncommonly high rates of depression, alcoholism, drug addiction, and suicide. Full-spectrum lights have proved far more effective than fluorescent lights for warding off seasonal affective disorder (SAD), and they also help the growth of indoor plants.

Most indoor plants improve air quality through a healthy exchange of oxygen and carbon dioxide, increasing oxygen levels and cleaning the air of up to 87% of dust pollutants and other toxins. Having live greenery in a room has been shown to hasten recovery after surgery, improve concentration, increase productivity, and stimulate creativity.[8]

Flowers have a language of their own: each variety, color, and fragrance has its own vibratory impact. Cultivating them around your house or on your balconies, and having them inside your home and work space will increase the healing magnetism of that area.

For personal and professional use, essential oils are now widely employed for their healing effects. Flower essences such as the Bach remedies and the Spirit-in-Nature Essences, reinforce the positive qualities of the mind. These intriguing methods of healing are beyond the purview of this book but are well worth investigating if you feel drawn to them.[9]

It is possible to neutralize some of the positive ions in our home environment by adding the element of moving water.

> When water evaporates from an indoor fountain, negative ions are released. These negative ions can help cleanse the air by removing pollutants such as dust, mold, and other allergens.[10]

In addition to the benefits of negative ions generated by moving water, its sound is also therapeutic.

> Many psychological studies have suggested that the sound of running water can have a positive impact on our minds. Water sounds are naturally soothing and many people have used running water in meditation practices for years....The sound of running water can provide multiple benefits, including:

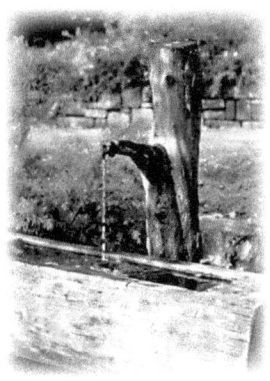

- Anxiety relief
- Stress relief
- Increased concentration
- Better sleep quality
- Natural meditation assistance
- Increased feelings of relaxation
- Noise control.[11]

Reestablish a more natural rhythm in your life. Invigorate your home and work space with nature's vibrant healing gifts of sunlight, plants, flowers, and flowing water. Make time as well to enter Her domain: find the closest place nearby where the asphalt ends and healing nature begins – a small park will do – and go there alone, even for ten minutes. Turn off your phone and be still. Breathe deeply, listen to the sounds of nature rather than your thoughts, and absorb Mother Nature's healing gifts.

PART XII   CHAPTER SEVEN

Colors Communicate

> Colors should resonate with your nature as it is, and with the qualities you would like to develop in yourself.[1] –KRIYANANDA

The ability to see colors enriches our life. Not everyone is endowed with this gift — some people are not able to distinguish certain colors, and, more uncommonly, some people perceive the world only in black, white and shades of grey. The healthy human eye can distinguish, according to some researchers, upwards of ten million colors.[2]

Every color vibrates at a specific frequency, possesses a unique energetic quality (a blend of the gunas), and contributes to the vibratory atmosphere within us and around us. The colors we wear, and the colors we invite into our homes and workspaces impact our energy and our thoughts, moods, and creativity, our human interactions, and ultimately our health. As you read this section, look around you to become aware of the colors in your space, and try to evaluate their influence on you and your activities.

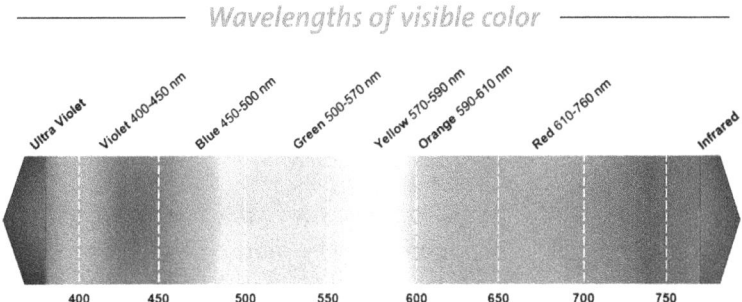

More than we realize, colors have a profound effect on our health.

Research as early as 1932 showed that visible wavelengths of light may have a direct effect on the endocrine system as they are able to reach the pineal and pituitary glands in the brain through neurochemical channels that operate independently of the optic nerve. This means that color may not actually have to be 'seen' to have an effect! [3]

As we become more aware of their influence, we can bring colors into our environments that are in harmony with ourselves and the activities that take place in the spaces we inhabit. Certain colors favor peaceful rest and are suitable for the bedroom. Some colors are helpful in areas where we engage in mental work, and others are favorable in spaces dedicated to physical activity. There are appropriate colors for areas devoted to study, contemplation, and meditation. In recent decades, careful attention has increasingly been given to the color choices for environments dedicated to health – doctors' offices, clinics, massage and physical therapy rooms, and environments dedicated to mental and emotional healing, etc.

The colors we wear and surround ourselves with communicate something about us. When a color vibrates in tune with our unique frequencies, and with the energetic needs of the moment, we are better able to relax, feel centered, and be at the top of our game. Be aware of the colors of the clothes you choose to wear daily, that they vibrate in harmony with what you aspire to accomplish. The wrong color choices can amplify a mental state of irritation, impatience, discouragement, or lethargy – while the right choices can help set the stage for a happy and successful day.

Here are suggestions from Kriyananda,[4] in italics, interspersed with those from the author.

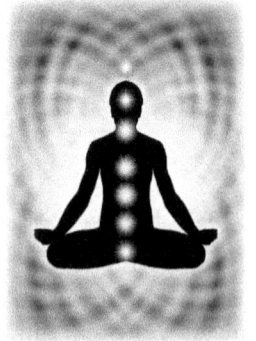

The colors of the rainbow are components of what may be called your "energy body.... [They] have not only a visual impact. They can also affect you vibrationally, when they resonate with the field of energy surrounding you—that is to say, your aura. Surround yourself with pure colors. Muddy hues can obscure mental clarity. Bright hues can induce brighter emotions.

RED

The color red signifies an outwardly directed energy. It can be cheerful, making you brighter, happier.

Red is the warmest of the colors, and as such is rajasic. When your energy is flagging, when you are depressed or discouraged and need a boost, put on something that has red in it. When an activity calls for high energy or when a presentation is meant to persuade, bright red is a good choice. When you want to be strong but not overpowering in a presentation or in a meeting, red mixed with some blue to tone it down would be appropriate, perhaps not wearing red from head to toe. Lighter shades of red, moving toward pink, communicate friendship and affection.

In your home, touches of red can be helpful in areas of activity, e.g., where you exercise, but not where you do yoga. To help stimulate digestion, the kitchen and dining area should have warm colors like red, which can be included in curtains, table settings, serving dishes, aprons, and so forth.

In your work space you might want to include some red from time to time: in flowers, a pen holder, or other items that are not necessarily permanent. Not every work project will require the stimulation of red. Depending on the nature of the work at hand, you need to choose the appropriate supportive colors.

When not to use red. Red is best avoided in hot climates; when we are feeling upset, angry, or somewhat lustful; in the bedroom; and in other rest areas. If you need to be present in an environment, but prefer to stay in the background, don't wear it. If you have a health condition where cells or cysts are proliferating, you should not wear red, a color that stimulates growth.

ORANGE

The color orange suggests fire. It is the classic color worn by swamis in India. *It helps one to generate enthusiasm for burning away all obstacles and destroying all desires and attachments.* As a warming color, orange is good for stimulating digestion and can give a softer energy than red when your body is ill or you are feeling depressed.

Orange is a good color to wear as the weather turns cool in the fall. Softer shades of coral and peach will be helpful as spring approaches. Orange is a color that wants to be noticed. When spending time with people in a primary or secondary role, it is often a better choice than red. Orange is more inviting of the opinions and participation of others, whereas red is more about making a statement. Orange is social, thus a good color to include in advertising and visual presentations.

In the home, orange in its various tonalities will bring warmth to an area and can brighten corners where there is little natural light. It works well in the kitchen, and you can bring it into your work area to

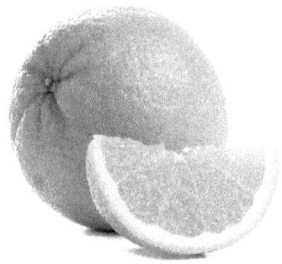

stimulate enthusiasm and creativity, perhaps on a colorful coffee cup, file folders, notebooks, and other accessories.

Healing spaces need both warming and cooling colors. The softer shades of orange, such as peach, apricot, and other pastels would be appropriate.

Orange is also the color of such highly nutritious, immune-strengthening foods as pumpkins, carrots, sweet potatoes, mangoes, papayas, and of course oranges.

When not to use orange. Except for the lightest hues, orange is not suggested for rest areas. It is best not to paint the walls of a meditation space orange. If you tend to fall asleep in meditation, you might try wearing soft orange colors or using an orange shawl as needed.

YELLOW

Yellow suggests the sunlight of wisdom; insight; creativity; and impartial acceptance of things as they are...As the sun's rays shine outwardly upon the earth, so yellow suggests wisdom applied outwardly.... It is symbolic of the joy of our own being....If what you seek in life is progress, yellow may help you to become more creative.

Whereas red and orange can be warming to the point of burning, yellow is more softly warming and more mildly rajasic. It invigorates without agitating the mind and enhances concentrated thinking and creativity. It can be used in most rooms of the home, and in healing studios. Including yellow in your choice of clothes, perhaps as an accessory, can brighten your mood and bring the sun into your environment on a cloudy day. It is an ideal color to include in the kitchen, and it is especially good for consultation rooms.

A golden yellow is one of the colors of the spiritual eye, the outermost color around the border. It represents the Aum vibration, and it invites us inward, into the dark-blue field of higher consciousness.

When not to use yellow. Too weak a shade of yellow can be debilitating. *This color can also be disturbing for those who shrink from meeting challenges. An impure yellow can have a somewhat sickening effect on the mind.*

GREEN

Green is the color of health and harmony; it is most visible among growing things. Green gives a heightened sense of physical and mental well-being.

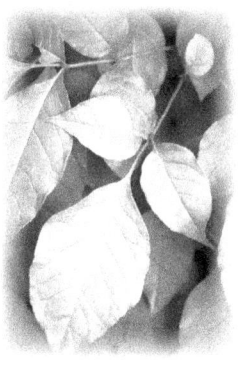

It denotes the vitality of spring, of life bursting forth from the dormancy of winter. It is the color that combines the warming hues of rajas with the uplifting tonalities of sattwa. It is the color that is most restful for the eyes.

When you are unwell, green is both nourishing and vitalizing. Surround yourself with vibrant shades of green, in your clothing and accessories, in plants, and in green foods. To enhance healing, spend time outdoors, gazing at and absorbing the variegated shades of green in the trees, bushes, and fields. Breathe in green vitality. In healing spaces, include an abundance of green plants, and as a counselor, include green in your workday wardrobe.

As a choice for clothing, green can go most anywhere, anytime. It is especially useful when vibrations of harmony or conciliation are needed. During meetings where differing perspectives are being voiced, it is a good color to have in the room. Green plants help create a healthy, harmonious environment at home and at work. Make sure every room in the house contains touches of green.

When not to use green. There are shades of green, especially when mixed with yellow, that can be debilitating and discouraging.

BLUE

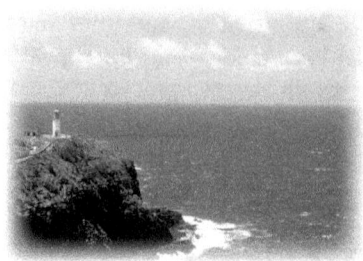

Blue is the color of...calmness, space, infinity, kindness, and an expansive consciousness.

Blue is a cool color, calming the mind and nervous system, and thus is suitable for meditation and other quiet and contemplative activities. It has a predominance of calming sattwic vibrations, while being a dynamic color.

Some illnesses, especially those with fever, will benefit from the cooling and calming effects of blue. In meetings, when the coordinator wears blue, it helps the group stay calm and centered. Because of its expansiveness, it is a good color to wear while making presentations that deal with philosophical and spiritual themes. Wearing blue or using a blue shawl for meditation helps still the mind and emotions. The lighter shades and blue pastels are good for psychological and psychiatric consultation rooms, less so in areas dedicated to physical therapy and bodywork.

A dark vibrant blue is the primary color of the spiritual eye, symbolic of infinite space and expanded consciousness. The three colors of the spiritual eye – gold, deep blue, and silvery white – are the colors adopted by Yogananda and Kriyananda to represent the path of Self-realization.

When not to use blue.
If it lacks warmth, however, its effect on the feelings can be chilling. It is not an ideal color for advertising and promotions, although a rich cobalt blue makes an excellent background instead of black. As an impersonal color, it is not best suited for gatherings where warmth and personal exchange are encouraged.

INDIGO

Indigo implies pure feelings, devotion, and the love of beauty in all its manifestations. Choose this color to deepen your love for others, and for God, as well as your appreciation for everything good in life. Indigo has its negative aspects, however, especially for those whose emotions take them downward. Don't let indigo generate in you attitudes of rejection or withdrawal.

VIOLET

Violet, together with indigo...are actually the most spiritual colors. Violet is the color of high thoughts, high principles, noble aspirations. This color will help you to rise out of the lower emotions into the realization that you, in your true Self, are pure Spirit.
Violet in its negative aspects can erect a psychic wall between yourself and the earthly realities around you, making your ideals unrealistic and impractical.

WHITE

White is the most sattwic color. It is *a blend of all the colors of the rainbow. Its vibration is of all-forgiving innocence, mental clarity, a heart kept open to the needs of others.*

It is the color favored for the practice of yoga, initiation ceremonies, and is well suited for meditation and other inward activities. *Choose white to develop non-attachment to worldliness. If the energy moves up the spine toward the brain, white can inspire a consciousness of purity.*

White is commonly used for the walls of kitchens and bathrooms. Both areas need warmth, so adding a touch of a warm color to the white paint will help. In healing and consultation rooms, starkly white walls and furnishings create a cold atmosphere. If you are able to paint the walls, add a warm color to the mixture. If you are stuck with white walls, add warm but not exciting colors to the room in the other ways mentioned.

When not to use white. White is a cool and impersonal color, not well suited to public or business presentations, and is not recommended when being televised. *White may suggest a bland lack of interest. Don't choose it if your nature is too passive.*

BLACK

Whereas colors are expressions of the light spectrum, black is the absence of light, and as such is tamasic. Although popular in the fashion world, it does not contribute to health. Instead of stimulating the flow of life force, black is enervating.

Black is the absence of color and as such, lowers energy. A long road trip in a car with black upholstery virtually guarantees that the people inside the car will feel exhausted after an hour or more of driving. Wearing black clothing reduces body energy and metabolism and hence is not the slimming effect that overweight individuals desire.[5]

You might consider eliminating black from your wardrobe, at the very least for clothes worn on the upper part of the body, as well as from your living space, substituting deep shades of blue – like "midnight" blue – and green, as in "forest green."

BROWN

Earth tones, and varieties of brown, give a sense of stability, of solidness. They can be worn to good effect on the lower part of the body: pants, socks, and shoes. Earth tones also, however, vibrate with the force of gravity, drawing energy downward. It is best not to wear them in the areas of the higher chakras. A touch of brown in white paint, creating a beige or ivory color, can warm up starkly white walls. Usually, when brown is mixed with other colors, it gives them a sense of heaviness and unclarity.

In the home or office, dark brown furnishings, including tables, chairs, and bookcases, can communicate a message of seriousness and authority – appropriate for law offices, though such furnishings are best avoided in spaces dedicated to health and healing.

In the next chapter we will consider how the vibrational qualities of colors, together with the colors of the three gunas, can help us create healing environments in the home and workplace.

PART XII   CHAPTER EIGHT

Healing Habitats

> Everything one does reflects one's philosophy of life. Buildings, too, ought to be expressions of a conscious philosophy.[1]
> —KRIYANANDA

Long before the Covid pandemic of 2020, people were wearing face masks outdoors to protect themselves against toxins in the air. Every year, nearly seven million people worldwide die prematurely due to air pollution. Add another one and a half million deaths from polluted drinking water and the story is grim. Living in densely – and tensely – populated urban areas does not promote health.

> Of supreme importance is environment, both natural and human. The subtle influences of the city act harmfully on the nervous system, deranging it. The impurities in the air, the speed of the traffic, the threat to one's privacy that is felt from the crowds, the heterogeneous vibrations of countless human beings with diverse and conflicting desires and interests—all of these conspire to produce tension, the supreme disease of our times.[2]

This chapter brings happier news! We will consider how the vibrations of certain places are healing, and how, even amid polluted environments, it is possible to create healing spaces.

For example, a new skyscraper in densely populated Singapore, the Capita-Spring, incorporates 80,000 trees and plants across 90,000 square feet of landscaped area, with a "Green Oasis" a third of the way up its 51 stories, where a spiral garden path winds past exercise equipment, benches, and tables on its journey through four stories of tropical flora. On the roof, a 4,500-square-foot "farm" supplies fruits, vegetables and herbs, to three on-site restaurants.[3]

We return now to one of Yogananda's most incisive teachings: **"*Environment is stronger than willpower.*"** The extent to which our environment influences us is far greater than we might imagine.

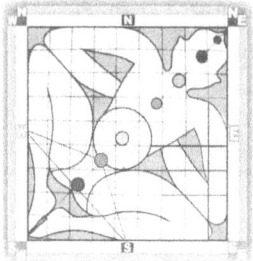

Rather than being helpless victims of unhealthy influences, we can learn to avail ourselves of positive influences that are close at hand, and we can learn to modify the environments where we spend most of our time – our home and work spaces – and transform them into sources of well-being.

The geographical placement of buildings has real consequences. Situating them correctly will align them with the healing vibrations of the earth. *Vaastu* is the science of harmonizing human habitations with the vibratory forces of nature to provide protection, well-being, happiness, and prosperity.

The oldest known treatise on the science of architecture, the Vaastu Shastra, is from the Yajur Veda, dating back roughly to 6000 B.C. Originally applied to the geographical placement, design, and construction of royal palaces and temples, *vaastu* principles are used today in the design of schools, businesses, condominiums, and private homes. At the Ananda World Brotherhood Village in California, and at the Ananda Europa community near Assisi, Italy, there are private homes that were built entirely on the basis of the *vaastu* science. When visiting these homes, I feel a vibrant atmosphere, and a sense of harmony and deep inner stillness.

> Vastu's purpose is to align our architectural spaces with the beneficial effects of subtle laws of nature, earth, and cosmic energies. Vastu works with prana…to enhance the freshness, vitality, and life-supporting qualities of our environment..[4]

As we have seen, Pythagoras and Plato conjectured that certain geometric shapes have healing properties. The shape of a building emanates vibrations that are favorable or harmful to the flow of life force.

A building's shape exerts a subtle influence on people's minds. Square or rectangular buildings... box in thought and inspiration....Walls, corners, ceilings...exert a definite, if subtle, influence on the mind. Flat ceilings...press down on the head and oppose expansion of the spirit....Rounded ceilings, which correspond to the shape of the head... reflect energy back harmoniously.....[5]

(In) planetariums I had visited, I'd felt a peace in them that was palpable, long before the stars came out and images of the galaxies flashed upon the inner surface of the dome....

The Sioux Indians believe that roundedness in a building helps one to feel in tune with the earth and the universe....(They) built tepees to correspond with the round horizon. The steep height of their tepees had something of the soaring quality of the Egyptian pyramids. And the openings faced east whence, they claimed, "all good things come."

A home I'd once visited in Arizona had its corners rounded off on the inside. The room walls were conventionally straight, but I found, to my surprise, that there was a certain feeling of peace in those rooms that seemed to result from those rounded corners, rather than from the furnishings or from the consciousness of the people living there.[6]

Although you cannot easily change the shape of the corners of the walls, there are ways to soften them, such as by installing a corner shelf with a curved front.

If you are planning to build any kind of structure, you are well-advised to consult an architect who is knowledgeable in *vaastu* principles, so that the placement of the building on the lot, the position of its doors and windows, and the location of the rooms will take advantage of the natural flow of healing life force.

> Architecture is, I think, in one respect the most important of all the arts. For a painting in someone's living room, a sculpture in his secluded courtyard, can be enjoyed by only a few, but the building in which one lives can inspire and delight every passerby.[7]

Remodel for improved health

Looking now at the structures we currently inhabit, there is much that we can do to render them more beneficial to our health.

You don't need to consult a psychic to tell you where the energy in your home is low or blocked. You can analyze the vibrational qualities of each space by considering the gunas and the colors as points of reference, while relying on your feelings to help you understand whether a space is sufficiently harmonious.

Ideally, we want to ensure the most nourishing and calming atmosphere possible in each space by increasing its sattwic qualities and eliminating or attenuating tamasic influences. Even the most highly charged work environments can be attenuated to improve their health and productivity.

The place to start is "tamas patrol." Areas that are dirty need to be cleaned. Objects that are old, stale, or unused need to be discarded. Places where things are left unattended, waiting for a tomorrow that may never arrive, need to be sorted and prioritized. A yearly spring cleaning will not be enough to keep your space sattwic. If you aren't enamored of deep cleaning, you can hire someone to help you. A daily dusting, a weekly refresh, and a monthly deep clean will help ensure that your living spaces stay sattwic.

Next on tamas patrol is to look for areas that are dark: places where natural light doesn't reach, areas with inadequate lighting, and places where furnishings or heavy curtains are blocking windows. Light is a sattwic quality; it brings vital energy to a room. Unless the sun is too bright or hot, keep the curtains open during the day to energize the house. Look out for shadows that are created as the sun moves past the windows, and add extra lighting there. Dark rooms harbor low vibrations and diminish the flow of life force. People who are often ill or depressed tend to keep their rooms dark. Was not God's first commandment: "Let there be light"?

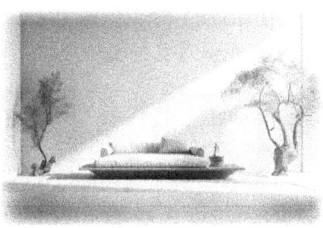

Dark areas can be uplifted with full-spectrum light fixtures and by adding warm colors. Consider adding touches of yellow, orange, and even red to those places, using curtains, paintings, photographs, or murals. A Himalayan salt lamp will create a warm, inviting atmosphere, as will plants with yellow and green foliage. Furniture that is heavy and dark can be brightened with covers, pillows, and other colorful accessories.

Another tamasic quality is stagnation. Fresh air brings prana into the living space – if the air outdoors is indeed fresh. All of the rooms should be aired every day, even in winter, remembering especially the bedroom and bedclothes – keeping the bedroom well-aired each morning and cool for sound sleep. Airing out the closets will keep the energy of your wardrobe fresh, as will putting the clothes you wear each day in fresh air to cleanse them of unpleasant odors and negative vibrations absorbed in other environments. If the outside air is polluted, you will of course not want to invite those toxins inside. Air filters and purifiers in each room then become a necessity.

A rajasic-tamasic quality that interferes with the harmonious flow of life force is confusion. Areas that are cluttered leave little space for the mind to relax. A family with young children will be hard-pressed to keep the house clutter-free. Even so, areas such as the master bedroom, kitchen, and work spaces can be considered with an eye to keeping them tidy.

Let's look further into the use of colors to create healthy environments.

> Colors, for example, are vitally important as expressions of states of mind. Whatever the shape of a house, its colors can be changed at any time. Light colors express expanding awareness. Dark colors, especially if they are dull, absorb energy; they have a dimming effect on one's awareness.[8]

Depending on the main activity in each room, choose the appropriate colors for the walls, wallpaper, curtains, carpets and rugs, art works, and other objects.

> The pictures a person hangs in his home should be thought of as members of the family—loved, cherished, and enjoyed anew every time he looks at them. The pictures that people select for their homes are usually chosen without much thought for the fact that, every time a painting is hung on a wall, the artist's vibrations are being invited into the home....If what he depicts doesn't harmonize with your real feelings about life, why invite him into your home as an unpaying—indeed, well paid!—permanent guest? [9]

Your bedroom

Special attention should be given to the vibrations of the bedroom, since we spend nearly a third of our lives there. Sound sleep is extremely important for good health.

The entire bedroom environment needs to be conducive to restfulness. When visiting the Uffizi gallery in Florence, I was surprised to see the over-sized painting of the Battle of San Romano which Lorenzo de'Medici had hung in his bedroom. The spilled blood, slain soldiers and dying horses might have been appropriate for his war counsel room, but I wondered how much this painting contributed to his slumbers.

The bedroom furnishings, including the bedclothes, should be a restful, cool color. Items that we tend to store under the bed have their own vibrations, usually a cacophony that can interfere with restful sleep. It is best not to have anything under the bed – admittedly a difficult temptation to resist.

A touch of nature

Bringing the healing vibrations of nature indoors in the form of plants, flowers, and fountains with gently running water will greatly improve the atmosphere in your living and work spaces. Even a wall mural of a natural scene can relax and expand the mind.

There are ways to reduce noise pollution at home, where many imperceptible but harmful (infra sounds) abound indoors. Water fountains create a restful vibration and produce healthy negative ions. A recording of Aum chanting, even if barely audible, will override many harmful frequencies. Friends of mine had a small garden area outside their New Delhi home. To cancel the traffic noise, they placed a loudspeaker in a tree where a recording of Aum chanting played day and night.

One of the best home improvements I've made was adding wind chimes to my porch. I carefully selected harmonic tonalities, a combination of medium and higher frequencies, which at the moment I write this are creating a soothing atmosphere.

Your work space

If you work at home, you can consider adjusting your space per the suggestions above. Keep in mind adequate lighting and good ventilation. Keep your work tools conveniently at hand, and keep other things stored nearby to avoid clutter and distraction. Include colors appropriate to the quality of your work, bearing in mind that warm colors are stimulating and cool colors are calming.

If you do consultations or bodywork, the right combination of warm and cool colors will be helpful: soft, warm colors and pastel cool colors. It is important to include green in healing areas. A small fountain can be soothing, and a few carefully selected wall hangings can help create an appropriate atmosphere.

If you work in a shared space with other people and you are unable to transform the entire space, you can include some healing touches at your desk; a lively patterned coffee or tea cup; colored paper clips, stapler, file folders, clipboards, etc. Eliminate clutter where possible: on your work surface keep only what is truly essential. Empty the waste basket every evening, and trim your to-do list to a minimum.

CHAPTER 8: *Points to Remember*

- Bring light and air into your living and work areas.

- Clean these areas often to enhance physical and mental health.

- Eliminate or attenuate dark areas with good lighting and uplifting colors.

- Use colors in each area that harmonize with the activities that happen there.

- Give special attention to the bedroom – keep it well-aired and uncluttered, and include calming colors.

- Adjust the vibrations of your work space to be more stimulating or calming, as required.

As we have seen, there is much we can do to improve the healthful atmosphere of our living spaces. We can also take advantage of those places on earth that are naturally endowed with healing vibrations. Our pilgrimage begins in the next chapter.

PART XII   CHAPTER NINE

Pilgrimage: Sacred Shrines and Saintly Souls

> All places of pilgrimage wherein many people gather and concentrate on divine thoughts possess divine healing vibrations and also help to create faith in persons desirous of divine healing.[1]
> —YOGANANDA

Every year, tens of millions of pilgrims make their way to holy shrines, many of them with the hope of being healed—to Mecca and Medina; to Jerusalem and Rome; to Amritsar and Badrinath. Although the places of pilgrimage mentioned in this chapter may not be readily accessible to all, you may be surprised to find that places of healing power exist in your own part of the world.

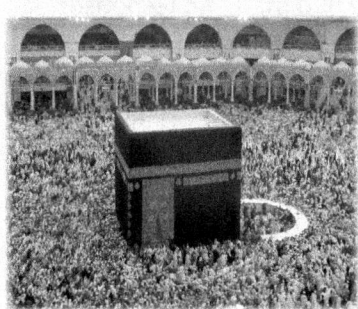

The benefit of going on pilgrimage to holy places... is not because of their rich history, but for the fact that divine blessings can be experienced when visiting them. Their very soil is impregnated with a higher consciousness.[2]

Not every pilgrim is healed, of course. Pilgrimage itself is an act of devotion and an effort of will; yet something more is needed.

> When visiting holy places, we should tune in
> sensitively to their vibrations, with a deeply
> prayerful attitude. If our hearts' feelings are
> uplifted calmly to receive the divine blessings, the
> benefits we gain will be enduring.[3]

I have received blessings from many holy sites, in Europe and in India, and I have felt there the devotion of those who over the centuries have stood on the same spot. Yet often I have observed pilgrims who arrive at their destination, say a standardized prayer – or have the pujari say it for them – and quickly leave.

To receive the transforming vibrations of places of pilgrimage we must know how to attune ourselves to their high vibrations. In *Autobiography of a Yogi,* Yogananda recalls a day when he visited the revered Kali shrine at Dakshineswar together with his sister and brother-in-law. Before they set out, his sister had begged him with desperate urgency to pray for her husband, that he be healed of his cynicism about spiritual matters.

> My mind was concentrated on Goddess Kali....
> My aspiring zeal increased boundlessly,
> accompanied by a divine peace. Yet, five hours
> had passed, and the Goddess whom I was
> inwardly visualizing had made no response....
> "Divine Mother," I silently remonstrated,
> "Thou didst not come to me in vision, and now
> Thou art hidden in the temple behind closed doors.
> I wanted to offer a special prayer to Thee today
> on behalf of my brother-in-law".... My inward
> petition was instantly acknowledged....
> the stone figure of Goddess Kali...gradually
> changed into a living form, smilingly nodding in
> greeting, thrilling me with joy indescribable.[4]

The grace that Yogananda received in that moment soon thereafter penetrated the heart of his brother-in-law, who experienced a profound spiritual conversion and became devoted to meditation for the remainder of his life.

There are many healing places on earth that emanate exceptional spiritual power, some world-famous, others known only to the few who have been blessed there.

> Every religion teaches that in certain places on earth there are holy vibrations. God is equally present everywhere, but His *manifestations* are not all equal. A rock is different from a plant. God's blissful consciousness, too, is manifested *variously* everywhere. In some places, the divine vibrations are particularly potent, owing to the fact that divine miracles have been performed there, or that spiritual masters have lived there.[5]

In the places where "avatars"* of God have lived, the blessings of their presence linger for centuries, even millennia—in Jerusalem and at the Sea of Galilee; at Bodh Gaya and Sarnanth; in Brindaban and Ayodhya.

Especially charged with healing vibrations are places where there have been apparitions. On the mountain top of La Verna is the retreat where **St. Francis** would go for long periods of prayer and inner communion. He lived in a cave where every day Jesus appeared in the flesh and conversed with him. Once, when meditating there, I personally received a very special spiritual grace.

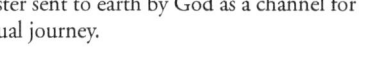

---

* An avatar is a fully-liberated spiritual master sent to earth by God as a channel for His will and to guide others on their spiritual journey.

Close to this cave is the rock on which Francis spent all night to be worthy to experience the Passion of Christ. When morning came, the signs of the stigmata, the five wounds of the crucifixion, were visible on his body. St. Francis was the first in recorded history to receive the stigmata, and the chapel that was later built on that spot is charged with supernatural blessings.

The Virgin Mary has appeared to the faithful at Lourdes, Fatima, Medjugorje, and other sites where countless healings have since occurred, including people who were blind from birth and received the gift of sight, and those who were paralyzed and were suddenly able to throw away their crutches and walk.

❈ Basilica of the Annunciation ❈
Jerusalem

The last eighteen months have been excruciatingly difficult. In May last year, I lost my beloved husband, and then I had to do battle with pancreatic cancer. Fortunately, I was able to win the victory, but it has been a painful, tiring, and very saddening time.

When I departed on pilgrimage to the Holy Land, I thought that I had overcome my grief. But at the very holy pilgrimage site of the Basilica of the Annunciation in Jerusalem I began to feel a devastating physical pain in my heart, just as we were singing the "Angelus." It was the deep pain for the loss of my husband.

And then, the moment I began to pray to the Divine Mother, I felt that She was enveloping me in a warm, tangible divine energy that was bigger than my suffering. As She enveloped me in Her loving embrace, the unbearable pain melted away and was replaced by Light and Peace. No effort of mine could bring such peace – only the Divine Energy could transform such pain. –**Carlotta**, *Locarno, Switzerland*

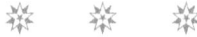

The lore of pilgrimage is replete with stories of miracles that have occurred even in small village churches that are dedicated to Mary.

✳ Our Lady of Grace ✳

Nearly twenty years ago, I brought our daughter to be baptized at the shrine of Our Lady of Grace near Foligno. Later in the day, as I set out for a long hike up a mountain near the shrine, I stopped at the church to meditate. For years, I had been troubled by chest pain whenever I exerted myself, and I hoped that it would not prevent me from reaching the mountain top.

As I meditated, suddenly I felt that the Divine Mother was saying: "What can I do for you?" I was overwhelmed with joy. As tears of gratitude streamed down my face, I placed my attention on my chest, and in that moment I felt the karma of the problem being removed.

I drank the holy water outside the shine and walked all day without pain. I thank our Lady of Grace not only for the physical healing, but for her blessings of joy. –**Massimo**, *Assisi, Italy*

Places where saints have lived, even centuries ago, are still charged with healing vibrations, perceptible to those whose hearts are open.

> **God works through channels. His grace comes to man primarily through those great souls in whom its presence is already revealed.**[6]

Having completely attuned themselves to God's will, these saints, and many others, continue to serve as conduits for His grace.

- Saint Teresa and St. John of the Cross in Avila, Spain
- Saint Catherine in Siena, Italy
- Sri Ramakrishna at Dakshineswar and Cossipur in Bengal, India
- Shirdi Sai Baba at the Shirdi Sai Temple at Sainagar, India
- Saint Seraphim in Sarov, Russia
- Paramhansa Yogananda in Mt. Washington and Encinitas, California
- Swami Sri Yukteswar in Puri, India

The places where the physical remains of the saints are preserved continue to emit a very real power of blessing—the crypt of Saint Francis in Assisi, Italy; the mausoleum of Rumi in Konya, Turkey; the Katapur Sahib of Guru Nanak in Pakistan; the Trinity Lavra of St. Sergius in Russia.

Yogananda considered Saint Francis his patron saint. Francis appeared to Yogananda many times at his hermitage in Encinitas, California. On his way to India in 1935, travelling by car through Europe, Yogananda came to Assisi to visit the saint's tomb. He wrote to a disciple about his experience there: when he put his head on the shrine step, St. Francis appeared, and Yogananda then saw him enter and disappear in a tunnel of blazing light.

In ways that science is at a loss to explain, some saints' bodies remain incorruptible even centuries after their passing. The almost perfectly preserved body of Santa Rita, who died in 1457, can still be seen in the Basilica dedicated to her in Cascia, Italy. Padre Pio's incorrupt body is preserved in a glass casket in the new church at San Giovanni Rotondo, Italy. The preserved body of Saint Joseph of Cupertino, the "levitating saint," is preserved in a basilica dedicated to him in the town of Osimo, Italy. Yogananda's incorrupt body is in a crypt at the Forest Lawn Cemetery near Los Angeles, California. It has been my personal experience that each of these places is charged with vibrations of divine healing.

There are shrines where objects associated with a saint emit spiritually charged vibrations.

- In the Golden Temple at Amritsar, where the Sri Guru Granth Sahib, the holy scripture of the Sikhs, is kept.
- At the Cathedral of Turin, Italy, where the Holy Shroud is preserved—the linen cloth that is believed to hold an image of Jesus at his burial.
- In many mosques where relics of the prophet Muhammad are revered.
- In churches and monasteries throughout the Eastern Orthodox world, where relics of saints and the presence of holy icons possess miraculous healing powers.

❋ The Chalice ❋

Life in Moscow was wild in the 1990s, after the collapse of the Soviet Union. I was a law student, studying hard and partying, and drinking day and night. In time, I became addicted to alcohol.

When I was twenty-three, I lost my younger brother and was devastated by unbearable grief. In my sadness I lost interest in everything – I felt as though I was dead, and stayed home all day and drank.

I had not been baptized in the Orthodox Church and had never attended the ceremonies. But now I found myself praying, "Please save me."

Not everything was bleak. I had met my future husband, and I had secured a coveted position as the deputy general legal director of a corporation that manufactured devices for the Russian space agency. It was a good job, but it was challenging and stressful. I continued to drink, coming to work with a hangover and even drinking on the job. I had no self-control, and I was deeply afraid that I would lose everything – my job, my partner, and my dignity.

While holding tightly to my coffee cup one morning, I shared my fears with a coworker. She told me about a holy icon, known as the "non-intoxicating chalice," that was supposed to have power to heal alcoholics and drug addicts. It would be in Moscow for only a few days.

There were few people in the church when I entered, and I my eyes immediately went to the icon. The baby Jesus was portrayed standing inside a chalice, his arms raised in blessing, with Mother Mary behind him, her arms also outstretched in benediction.

As I waited in line to come face to face with the icon, I prayed silently and continuously to Mary and Jesus, "Please save me!"

I arrived at the icon and read the prayer dedicated to it, then I knelt and kissed it, and with all my heart and will I asked the Mother and Jesus to save me from alcohol.

I suddenly felt a complete inner stillness such as I had never experienced before. I felt as safe as a child held in her mother's arms against her bosom. For a moment of eternity, I was in another dimension without space or time.

Since then I have not touched a drop of alcohol – not at parties or on New Year's Eve. I have now been completely sober for twenty years. I thank God, Divine Mother, and Jesus for using the icon to heal me and save my life.
—**Guelena**, *Moscow, Russia*

In the first chapter of *Autobiography of a Yogi*, we learn how Yogananda was healed as a young boy by a photograph.

> I was stricken with Asiatic cholera. My life was despaired of; the doctors could do nothing. At my bedside, Mother frantically motioned me to look at Lahiri Mahasaya's picture on the wall above my head. "If you really show your devotion and inwardly kneel before him, your life will be spared!"
>
> I gazed at his photograph and saw there a blinding light, enveloping my body and the entire room. My nausea and other uncontrollable symptoms disappeared; I was well. At once I felt strong enough to bend over and touch Mother's feet in appreciation of her immeasurable faith in her guru.[7]

What is the power that endows such places with healing blessings?

> The uplifting vibrations of certain places are due also to the fact that devout pilgrims for centuries have worshiped in them.[8]

❋ Devotion of All Religions ❋

In my travels as a leader of group pilgrimages, I have visited many sacred places that are dedicated to religions that I do not profess, yet there is no question that I have felt powerful vibrations there.

In Abu Dhabi I visited the Sheikh Zayed Grand Mosque, an architectural marvel and one of the largest mosques in the world. Written on the walls in golden script are excerpts from Islamic scriptures. As I sat to mediate, I felt the power of those truths resonating in the space, and within me I felt the power of the devotion of the people who had prayed there. It was an uplifting meditation.

In Kochi, in south India, I led our group into a sixteenth-century Jewish synagogue. The scrolls of the Torah are covered in gold and silver, and housed in an intricately carved teak ark. As our group sat to meditate, I could feel the peaceful, transforming vibrations of centuries of devotion.

Whenever we go to India on our tours, an essential stop is at the cave of the sage Vasishta on the banks of the Ganges near Rishikesh. Not only have generations of Hindu saints meditated there, but it is also said that rishis of Vedic times are still meditating behind a stone wall that prevents visitors from penetrating any farther into the cave.

The overwhelming sensation inside the cave is of a deep, profound silence – far deeper than anything I had experienced elsewhere. On the day of our visit, as I was repeating a meditation mantra mentally, I heard a clear voice from behind the wall – *"Quiet! You are disturbing us!"* I immediately ceased my repetition of the mantra and bathed in the silence. –***Arjuna***, *Ananda Assisi*

Jesus said, "Wherever there are two or more gathered in my name, there I am in the midst of them." (Matthew 18:20) In holy shrines, it is the faith and devotion of the people who visit them that call down the divine presence – especially in places that the faithful have visited continuously for centuries.

An interesting case is the Basilica of the Holy House in Loreto, Italy. No saints are buried here, there have been no apparitions, and there are no relics. Yet it is one of the most visited pilgrimage sites in the Christian world, well known for miraculous healings.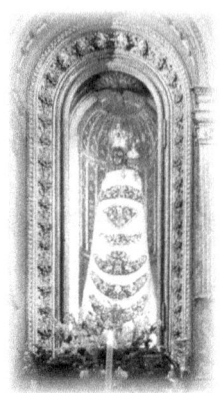

The legend of the shrine dates back to the end of the Crusades, around 1263, when the Holy Land came under Islamic control. It is believed that the three stone walls of the house where the Holy Family lived in Nazareth were carried by "angels" for safekeeping to various locations, one of which was a site near Trsat in Croatia, from where it was brought to its current location in Loreto in 1295. Historical records indicate that members of the noble "Angeli" family who participated in the last Crusade transported the walls by ship.

Since that time, pilgrims have come in an unbroken stream, some hobbling on their knees as penitents, many too ill to walk. Whether history, legend, or myth accounts for the blessings, what is undeniably true is that healing miracles happen at this holy site almost daily.

Ashrams and meditation retreats

Peaceful environments where people have gathered for spiritual activities, especially daily meditation, prayer, and worship, become permeated with healing vibrations. People who arrive bearing the weight of troubles are often able to put their burdens behind them after visiting such places.

✳ JOY DISCOVERED ANEW ✳

I had been unable to feel at peace within myself for months. My heart was closed, and I was filled with fears and ill will, even toward close friends. My spiritual practices were not helping, and my life held no joy.

Not far outside of Moscow, the monastery of Optina Pustyn offers retreat programs. The weekend I came there happened to be the celebration of the birthday of the Blessed Virgin Mary. I went to confession and liturgy, and at the suggestion of a priest, I read Psalm 50 many times every day:

"The Mighty One, God, the LORD, speaks and summons the earth from the rising of the sun to the place where it sets. From Zion, perfect in beauty, God shines forth. Our God comes and will not be silent..."

In exchange for my stay, I was assigned to serve in the vegetable barn, where I washed the jars in which food would be stored for the winter. I discovered that with each clean jar, a little joy was returning to my heart, and when I left three days later, I realized that I was completely healed.

–*Tatiana*, *Nigniy Novgorod, Russia*

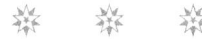

Living Saints [9]

A saint is a person whose consciousness is completely harmonized with the living presence of God within. The vibrations of oneness can be so powerful that those who are receptive may be drawn into the same state. The saints usually profess no special powers, but are simply who they are. Physical, mental, and spiritual healings can happen spontaneously through their touch, or by simply being in their presence. As Swami Adi Shankaracharya said, "Even a moment in the company of a saint can be your raft over the ocean of delusion."

❊ A HEALING EMBRACE ❊

The doctor decreed, "You absolutely cannot travel! We *must* operate on both conditions immediately!"

The MRI had revealed a splintered meniscus, the cartilage between the shin bone and the thigh, which was quite painful and posed a major obstacle to my teaching yoga. To make matters worse, I suffered from endometriosis that had now worsened with the growth of new cysts, which the doctor wanted to remove – also right away.

But I had purchased a ticket and felt that a three-week stay at the ayurvedic ashram in Kerala might heal or at least improve these conditions. So, against the doctor's advice, I left for India.

Along with the ayurvedic therapies, I spent long periods introspecting to try to identify the underlying causes of the illnesses. I also used Yogananda's technique for removing karmic grooves in the brain.

It was a difficult, emotionally painful process. In meditation one day, I felt a guidance to take a day off from my rigorous routine.

When I arrived in the capital city of Trivandrum (now called Tiruvanathapuram), I ran into such a huge crowd that it was impossible to walk down the street. The popular woman saint, Mata Amritanandamayi (Ammachi), was in town, and thousands of devotees were waiting to see her and receive her embrace.

I didn't feel well enough to wait for hours in line, yet I found myself at the table where they were giving out cue numbers – and the one they gave me was the very next number to be called!

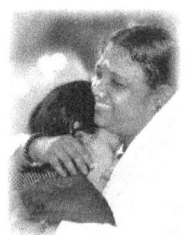

The embrace I received from this saintly woman was saturated with maternal love. I was able to surrender in the moment and let go of all resistance, and when I returned to the ashram to continue the healing process, I realized that something had changed. Gone were the tension and heaviness. I felt supported and able to enter into the natural flow of healing.

When I returned to Milan and saw the doctor, he was stunned. The results of the gynecological exam showed no sign of endometriosis, and an MRI showed that the meniscus no longer needed surgery.

I am back to teaching yoga, able to assume the lotus and other postures without pain, and deeply grateful for the healing embrace from a saintly woman. –**Shraddha**, *Assisi, Italy*

※ THE AGELESS SWAMI ※

When our Ananda Himalayan Pilgrimages group visited Swami Paramananda for the first time, he was 120 years old. As a boy, he had seen Lahiri Mahasaya. He met Yogananda at university and knew most of the saints mentioned in *Autobiography of a Yogi*.

We weren't sure if he would be well enough to receive us this time, but when we arrived we discovered a vibrant, robust and joyful 133-year-old saint.

As was our custom, at the end of the satsang we asked for individual blessings. Not only did he bless us, he also hugged each of us, women included – me included! Swamis in India do not touch women, but in this Swamiji's elevated consciousness we were Spirit, not men or women.

When he hugged me, it felt as if I was embraced by the Divine Mother Herself. I started to weep as I felt a heavy weight lifted from my chest. It was not a specific burden that I could give a name to, but a purification of something deep inside me. —**Santoshi**, *Ananda Assisi*

There are individuals who lay no claim to saintliness or healing power, yet whose presence is naturally and spontaneously uplifting. Perhaps you have been fortunate to meet them. When our energy is spiraling downward, the company of such a person, or merely speaking with them on the phone, can lift our spirits out of the pool of suffering into a place where the sun is shining, the birds are singing, and the skies are blue.

❋ Front row seat ❋

When I became attracted to the teachings of Paramhansa Yogananda, I moved to the Ananda community in Italy. I knew little about Yogananda's direct disciple Swami Kriyananda, who was in residence at the time. While I appreciated his work in founding the Ananda communities, I felt no particular connection with him.

I suffered from frequent severe headaches that could last for days, and I was in the midst of an outbreak when I came to the Temple of Light to listen to Swami talk. I sat in the front row, more out of respect than with any desire to listen closely.

After a few moments, I noticed that the headache had vanished completely. "Strange," I thought, feeling deeply relieved, but not giving it any particular importance.

The next time I went to hear him speak, I again had severe head and neck pain, and I again sat in the front row. When, after a few minutes in his presence the pain disappeared, I realized that, just as the sun radiates its energy to all, a person who is able to serve as a channel for the Light can emanate healing vibrations even to those who, like me, are not particularly attuned.

On another occasion, I brought a document to his house that urgently needed to be signed by one of his personal staff. Swamiji was present when I arrived, and he greeted me courteously, with a radiant smile, and asked my name. When the document was signed I left immediately. I had spent only a few minutes in his presence, yet that night I was so filled with energy that I could barely sleep. The next morning I wasn't tired at all, and the headaches disappeared for a long time. It was an important lesson, to learn to meet advanced souls with openness and gratitude.

—**Manu**, *Ananda Assisi*

The following story relates one of the many healings that have occurred at the site where Kriyananda lived and where he left his body on April 21, 2013. The Moksha Kutir near the Ananda center in Assisi is open for meditation at scheduled times during the week, year-round.

❈ Moksha Kutir ❈

The operation to repair my husband's aorta was followed by a long and arduous healing, with many setbacks. We were both feeling exhausted and discouraged, unable to see an end to the long tunnel of suffering.

I went alone to meditate at the Moksha Kutir. No sooner had I entered the room than I was enveloped by a great wave of love that instantly removed all the layers of tiredness, heaviness, suffering, and pain that had accumulated over months. It was deeply healing every fiber of my being –

I felt as if I had been lifted into a dimension of peace, joy, and divine love.

I remained in the meditative state for a long time, and when I rose I had a clear feeling that something had changed. I was no longer the exhausted and unmotivated soul who had entered the room – I was once again energetic, serene, and full of faith, as if I had been cleansed and baptized by a divine hand. It was a true healing.

When I called the hospital and spoke with my husband, he told me that at exactly the time when I had the healing experience, he had been lifted by a wave of love that had warmed his heart and soothed his physical and emotional pain, infusing him with courage, hope, and renewed will to struggle.

I realized that *this* is the power that is imprinted in places where the saints have lived, and that knows no limits of space or time. I know now that the saints are omnipresent channels of God's love, and for His healing power.
–**Nandini**, *Ananda Assisi*

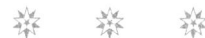

Create your own healing shrine

In Italy and India, there is a saint for every day, and a shrine in every village. In all cultures there are sacred places – they may be churches, temples, mosques, mandirs, special places in nature, or places where people gather to rejoice in God's creation.

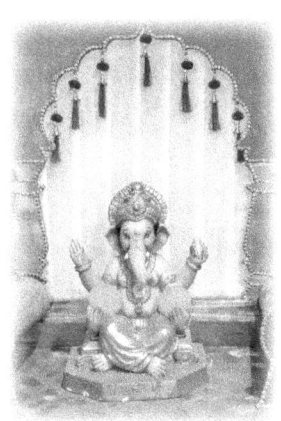

"Seek and ye shall find," Jesus assures us. Spending time in such places, and absorbing their vibrations of peace even briefly, can help us keep our lives on an even keel.

Yet it might be only once in a lifetime, or never, that we can make such a pilgrimage.

Don't despair! We can create a spiritually uplifting and healing atmosphere right where we live.

HOW TO MAKE A PERSONAL SHRINE

- Look around your home and garden for a secluded spot where you can be alone and get in touch with your higher Self.
- It could be a closet or a corner of a basement or attic where you won't be disturbed.
- Fill the space with objects that remind you of your higher Self.
- Visit your shrine daily and meditate deeply there.
- Every day use one of Yogananda's techniques for drawing healing energy to yourself.
- Practice his technique for transmitting healing life force to others.*
- Let this be your refuge, your oasis of peace, and the destination of many inner pilgrimages.

> Whatever places of pilgrimage you visit outwardly, and whatever outward rituals you perform, the ultimate "pilgrimage" must be within. And the ultimate religious rite must be the offering of your life-force on the altar of inner God-communion.[10]

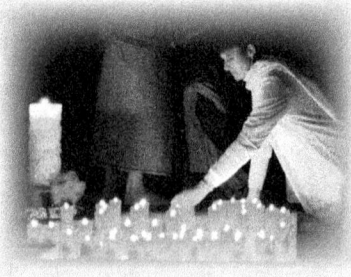

---

* You will find this technique in Chapter Five of Part IX, Volume Two.

PART XII   CHAPTER TEN

The Power of Ceremonies and Rituals

❉ The Sacred Dog ❉

He was just a lad of six when his grandfather passed. All of the adult family members were busily preparing for the funeral which would be held in the temple. There wasn't much that he remembered about the ceremony, but one thing still stood out in his mind: the dog!

The flowers and the offerings of food, ghee, and fire – everything was in perfect order. The pujari had arrived, but just as the ceremony was about to begin, a stray dog wandered into the temple. Chaos ensued! Everything was removed from the temple, which was scrubbed and cleansed from top to bottom. To avoid a repetition of the unwelcome intrusion, the dog was tied to a post in the courtyard.

Our little boy missed the frenzy inside the temple – he was sitting with the dog, the only one who had noticed him.

Time passed, and the boy grew to manhood, in time becoming a householder with his own family. When his father died he was entrusted, as the eldest son, with arranging the funeral rites. Trying to recall his grandfather's last rites, his memories were vague. He did, however, remember the dog, which seemed to have been a main focus of attention. Not owning a dog, he combed the village until he found one to borrow. Before the rites began, he ceremoniously tied the dog to a post in the courtyard.

Time passed, and his son grew up and became a prosperous young businessman. When the time arrived

> for him to arrange the rites for his father, he purchased a dog but had the ordinary stake replaced with a beautiful hand-carved, elaborately decorated small pillar – he even insisted that the pujari bless the dog before the rites began. To this day, funeral rites in that village are known as "the sacred ceremony of the dog."

Rituals and ceremonies are an integral part of every religious tradition – lighting the candles at the start of the Jewish sabbath; receiving the host at the Catholic mass; the morning and evening *aratis* performed in Hindu households; purification and fire ceremonies; initiations and coming-of-age rituals, the prayer of gratitude before eating; baptizing newborn souls, and bidding them farewell.

Ceremonies and rituals are the outer shell of spirituality, the exoteric aspects that are meant to lead us to the inner fruits of direct spiritual experience. Rituals that are performed with little understanding of their symbolic meaning cannot bring us to the inner sanctum. The above Sacred Dog story portrays the emptiness of ritualistic observances that have long lost their initial meaning.

Ceremonies and rituals are symbolic outward observances that are meant to remind us of the inner experience of communion with the Divine.

> Religious ceremonies are symbols of wisdom. To idolize the symbol by the mechanical performance of ceremonies without understanding their significance is of little use. Mechanical ceremonies, worship of forms without understanding their spiritual essence, is idol worship and creates ignorance. That is why the worship of symbols and the performance of religious ceremonies must be done with perfect spiritual understanding and devotion.[1]

Are there rituals that can truly help us raise our consciousness and improve our health?

The answer is both "yes" and "it depends." A true ritual creates a vibratory space where human faith and divine grace can interact, and where true healing is possible. The following story describes a healing that acquaintances of mine experienced during a sacred ceremony.

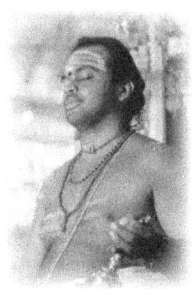

☸ A Touch of Light ☸

The ophthalmologist was optimistic but frank in his assessment of my husband's condition: the hole in the center of the retina of his right eye could be repaired, but the operation – a vitrectomy – was a delicate procedure. Flavio could expect a long post-operative recovery, during which he would have to lie in bed with his head held very still.

Before the operation, we visited the Ananda Assisi community, which we consider our spiritual home. We prayed and meditated long and deeply, asking God and our Master for their protection.

We concluded our visit by attending the Ceremony of Light on Sunday morning. As part of the ceremony, the congregation are invited to come forward and receive the "touch of light" from a minister. Placing his forefinger at the center of the participant's forehead, the site of the spiritual eye, the minister asks God to transmit a blessing.

When I came forward, I felt the light penetrating deep inside me. Returning to my seat, I closed my eyes to absorb the experience. When I opened them for a moment, I saw Flavio standing before the minister, who was positioned in front of a photo of Yogananda. I suddenly saw a beam of light flashing from the photo and enveloping the minister, and traveling through her hand to Flavio's third eye. I thought, "It is healing him."

Later, on the train home, Flavio exclaimed, "There's no spot in my vision anymore! I can see perfectly." I then told him what I had seen during the ceremony, but we could say no more in the presence of the overwhelming feeling of joy.

When we saw the doctor several days later, he had to repeat the full examination a second time. He said, "You must tell me which saint you have in heaven, because you are healed. We can cancel the operation, and I will see you after a year for a checkup. I want to ask a favor, though – may I have your permission to show your records to my colleagues? In the medical books we read that spontaneous healings of this condition are extremely rare. It has never happened to any of my patients."

When we returned home, we picked flowers from our balcony and placed them before a painting of Yogananda, saying, "Thank you, thank you," over and over. –***Paola and Flavio***, *Turin, Italy*

> ### *Rituals as channels for grace*
>
> The transformative power of a ceremony will depend on the following elements:
>
> - **Truth:** The power inherent in the ritual
> - **Attunement:** The celebrant's ability to serve as a channel for grace and healing
> - **Receptivity:** The participant's openness to receive grace
> - **Satsang:** The enthusiastic participation of those present
> - **A sacred place:** The spiritual vibrations of the location

1) Endowed with the power of truth

The power of a ceremony is rooted not in its ritualistic aspects but rather the truths on which it is based: The ceremony is merely a container for the power that it is meant to confer.

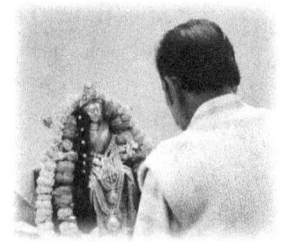

> The real purpose of religion is not to
> mask reality: It is to show the way to personal,
> inner spiritual awakening. It is to inspire people
> to seek the deeper truths for which symbols
> are simply a focus, but never a substitute....
> Certain symbols... have universal relevance,
> especially if they derive from superconsciousness.
> In this case, they may have deep power,
> resonating with fundamental realities of existence,
> and thereby amplifying our awareness.
> Such symbols stir our hearts and uplift our
> consciousness; they may even awaken us
> to some degree of soul-recognition.[2]

Once we get beyond the outward symbols used in ceremonies, we often find hidden secrets for healing ourselves of the fundamental disease of ignorance. "Disease," Yogananda says, "is anything that keeps us from God-realization."[3]

The healing power within the rite of Holy Communion, observed variously by different Christian denominations, lies in what Yogananda refers to as "inner communion: worshipping God not outwardly in form, but deeply within the silence of our soul. Through inner Holy Communion with God we may experience the highest state of healing, that of uniting our souls with the infinite Spirit. As Jesus taught us to affirm: "I and my Father are One."

The weekly Judeo-Christian observance of the Sabbath (meaning "to cease") can be deeply healing for body, mind and soul. Yogananda offers this healing recipe for the Sabbath.

> Observance of the Sabbath Day....
> signifies the willing cessation of all activities
> which scatter and divert the mind.....
> spending it in seclusion, fasting,
> and meditation.[4]

Ceremonies, rituals and spiritual observances provide a channel by which we can open our hearts to the source of healing Light and welcome it into our lives. Whether the ceremony involves lighting Sabbath candles or arati lamps, it is a channel by which we can satisfy the universal longing for understanding, higher guidance, help in times of need, and the heart's yearning for peace and joy.

In India, the "festival of lights," called Diwali, is celebrated by Hindus, Jains, Sikhs, and Buddhists, to honor the triumph of good over evil, of light over darkness.

In creating the Festival of Light, Kriyananda's intent was to remind us that it is God's Light that sustains us and unites us as one. He writes that through this ceremony "God's light is invoked to flow down to earth, and into the hearts of worshipers both present and afar."[5] Here's one of the songs sung by the congregation during the ceremony.

Thy Light Within Us Shining

Thy Light within us shining
Has shone where freedom lies:
From earthly walls confining,
To soar in Spirit's skies!
How oft like sheep we've strayed apart!
Now, guided by Thy ray,
In inner freedom of the heart
Our night has turned to day.

In the story about Flavio's experience, *it was the Light referred to here that healed his eye.*

2) The attunement of the celebrant

That the power of a ceremony be ignited is the responsibility of those entrusted with leading it. Before each celebration of the ritual they need to align themselves with its inherent power, and offer themselves as instruments to channel that power to the participants.

Eye witnesses reported that St. Joseph of Cupertino (1603-1663) would routinely levitate while saying the Mass, remaining airborne for as long as half an hour. Many of those present were able to experience a state of grace.

When Padre Pio celebrated the Mass, it was no mere ritual, but a direct experience of Christ's living presence that transmitted powerful blessings to those present and receptive.

"He found himself in a state of spiritual ecstasy and joy. Seeing him in this state, his followers could see that God was with him at that moment. He not only experienced the Passion, but also prayed for and saw in God all those who had recommended themselves to him." [6]

«On one occasion, when offering the Host to a supplicant, he caused her to rise up off the ground in levitation." [7]

Sri Ramakrishna Paramahansa, a nineteenth-century saint in Bengal, served for a time as a *pujari* (a Hindu temple priest) at the Kali temple in Dakshineswar. While performing the *arati* ceremony he would see the statute of the Goddess Kali come alive, and in a state of ecstasy he would dance with Her. Many of those present at these moments would be drawn into an elevated state of consciousness.

The power of a ritual lies dormant, and needs to be activated by a qualified person. Who is qualified and capable of doing so? Being invested with the authority to conduct a ritual is no guarantee.

Religious institutions ordain ministers who have completed a course of training. Depending on their inner attunement, they may or may not be able to awaken the full power of the ceremonies they have been charged to perform.

Significantly different is the case when someone is empowered to serve as a channel for grace. Jesus empowered his disciples to preach and heal in his name – meaning that he endowed them with the spiritual power to serve as his channels. When Ramakrishna lay dying, he appointed his chief disciple, Swami Vivekananda, as his successor by transferring to him his full spiritual powers.

In India there is the tradition that recognizes the possibility that someone can be directly empowered by God. Although this is possible since all power comes from God, those who claim to be so endowed often are not, while others who lay no claim to divine illumination might be. God's ways are, indeed, mysterious to behold.

Paramhansa Yogananda was empowered to spread the message of Kriya Yoga.

> My heart was set to go to America, but even more strongly was it resolved to hear the solace of divine permission....There came a knock outside the vestibule adjoining the Gurpar Road room in which I was sitting. Opening the door, I saw a young man in the scanty garb of a renunciate. He came in, closed the door behind him and, refusing my request to sit down, indicated with a gesture that he wished to talk to me while standing.
>
> "He must be Babaji!" I thought, dazed, because the man before me had the features of a younger Lahiri Mahasaya.
>
> He answered my thought. "Yes, I am Babaji....
> "Our Heavenly Father has heard your prayer. He commands me to tell you: Follow the behests of your guru and go to America. Fear not; you will be protected....You are the one I have chosen to spread the message of *Kriya Yoga* in the West. Long ago I met your guru Yukteswar at a *Kumbha Mela;* I told him then I would send you to him for training."[8]

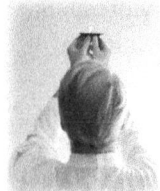

Later, Yogananda would empower many of his disciples to serve as instruments of God's blessings through Kriya. One of these was Swami Kriyananda, who, on his guru's behalf, has empowered others.

Yet even this "empowerment" is not eternal: it needs to be reestablished by the celebrant's inner attunement each time he or she conducts a ceremony. Even the most powerfully-endowed rituals, when performed perfunctorily, will have little if any transformative effect. On the other hand, a person of deep faith will be able to draw grace through a ritual despite the celebrant's imperfect attunement.

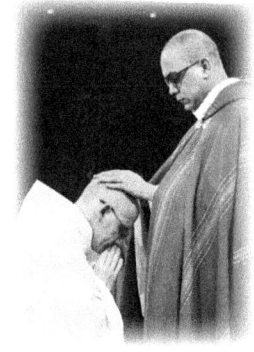

In Flavio's story, *the ministers who blessed both Paola and Flavio are well known for their deep attunement and inner preparation before each ceremony.*

3) Receptivity

Not everyone present at a miraculous healing event is aware of it, or affected by it. It was only the woman who touched the hem of the cloak of Jesus with absolute faith who was healed.

> This woman, by her will-power,
> through her hands contacting the hem
> of his garment, had taken out some
> life force from his body into her body
> which like an x-ray had burned out the
> disease afflicting her.... When he said,
> "Thy faith hath made thee whole,"
> he emphasized the soil of healing.[9]

Flavio and Paola came to the temple *in the hope of gaining inner strength to face a risky operation and long recovery. During the week preceding the Ceremony, they opened their hearts through prayer and meditation. They came to the altar that Sunday to receive the "touch of light" with full faith and devotion.*

Sincerity and receptivity are essential if we hope to experience the healing power of a ceremony or ritual. During the Purification Ceremony offered weekly at Ananda Assisi, participants are required to first affirm their desire and willingness to be healed.

✻ I SEEK PURIFICATION ✻

I would visit the Ananda retreat near Assisi as often as possible, and when I returned home I would always try my best to meditate regularly and find inner peace. Yet the tendency to become upset and angry persisted.

I had long realized that anger doesn't solve anything, and that it was interfering with my health and relationships. And so I determined to eliminate it forever.

On Thursday mornings at the Temple of Light there is a long meditation, followed by a Purification Ceremony. Eventually, a day came when I felt that I was truly ready to be relieved of anger.

The participants in the Purification Ceremony are invited to write on a piece of paper a quality that they want to get rid of, or that they would like to increase in themselves. I wrote a single word: "anger." After praying deeply for the grace to be free of this troublesome quality, I knelt before one of the ministers, and with as much intention, sincerity, and faith as I could muster, I said, "I seek purification by the grace of God."

Placing a finger over my heart, the minister intoned the words of the ceremony: "The Master says: 'Open your heart to me, and I will enter and take charge of your life.'"

It is hard to explain it rationally, but I felt that something was being lifted from me.

I then went to the altar and lit my scrap of paper with the word "Anger" in the candle. I placed it in the urn and watched it burn, and with it my anger, feeling a great sense of relief. When I returned to my seat, I wept for a long time, and for an entire year after I did not get angry. Since then, even if I have sometimes lost my temper, it was never again to the same degree. –**Clarita**, *Rome, Italy*

4) The healing power of satsang

Another important factor that contributes to the power of ceremonies is *satsang* — gatherings where people come together to create a spiritual force field that will magnetically attract blessings to all.

> In the Indian scriptures you find one
> thing stressed: satsanga, good company.
> Master used to say that company and
> environment are stronger than will power....
> You need to be in the right kind of
> environment to be able to soar.[10]

Prayer groups that meet regularly, whether in person or online, develop a magnetic power that charges their prayers with a power that is greater than the sum of their individual prayers. The same is true of people who gather in groups to meditate together.

> Meditating together increases the
> degree of Self-realization of each member of
> the group by the law of invisible vibratory
> exchange of spiritual magnetism.[11]

Of course, not every group will have a unified intention – some people will be willfully and consciously present with joyful expectations, while others will be reluctant, skeptical, or uninvolved. As any experienced teacher or lecturer knows, the inspiration flows more strongly if a group is interested and eager to learn.

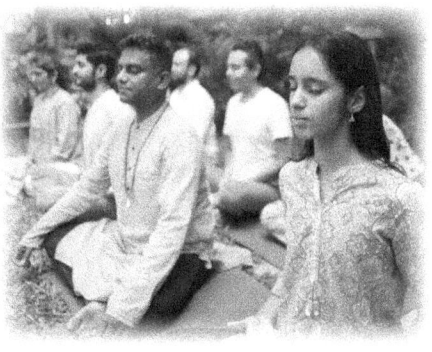

When a congregation is familiar with the ceremony, and especially when many have experienced blessings from it, their enthusiasm and expectation create a magnetic atmosphere

The atmosphere *on the day of Flavio's healing was especially charged due to the presence of Ananda's worldwide spiritual guides, and the many people who had often experienced the blessings of the ceremony.*

5) Spiritually-charged places

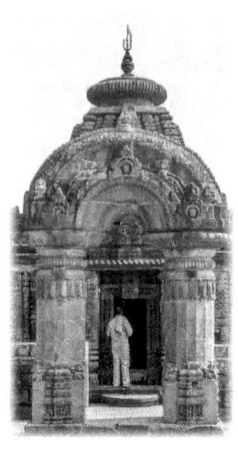

Over years, decades, and centuries, places that are dedicated to spiritual aspiration become charged with sacred vibrations. Wherever spiritual ceremonies are regularly performed, vibrations will be built up that enhance the power of the ceremony. There is a remarkable difference in magnetism between holy places which are used daily for individual worship and ceremonial celebrations, and those which are active only occasionally or which have become historic monuments and museums.

The Temple of Light *where Flavio experienced his healing, although active only since 1996, is the site of daily meditations, weekly ceremonies and frequent initiations, weddings, baptisms and spiritual celebrations. Aside from ceremonial times, it is open day and night for silent meditation, which has created an atmosphere of deep peace and inner awakening.*

Initiation Ceremonies

Our lives are blessed by many new beginnings. Perhaps you can rejoice even now in the long-ago memory of your first day at school, when vast horizons seemed to open before you. Or your first summer camp, and the thrill of being independent of your parents for a time. Or perhaps your first long bicycle ride, and the sense of freedom and adventure it brought you. Or your early experiences of the exhilaration of sports.

Each new beginning stands out in our memory for allowing us to experience the joy of exchanging a limited reality for a more expanded and happier one.

Similarly, spiritual initiations can mark the beginning of inner awakening, of a healing at the innermost level of our being.

In many religious and spiritual traditions, special moments of passage are marked by initiation ceremonies that signal our entry into a life of deeper spiritual study and practice—for example, the *bar mitzvah* of Jewish tradition, the sacraments of Catholicism, the *upanayana* sacred thread ceremony of the Hindu Brahmins, and similar rituals of ancient mystical and new religious movements.

An initiation ceremony marks a fresh beginning in our lives, and if we understand its meaning and participate with open and devoted hearts, it can open channels for a flow of healing grace.

The tradition with which I am most intimately familiar is Kriya Yoga, a spiritual science with roots in ancient times that is designed to help us achieve Self-realization.

In describing the life-transforming power of Kriya, my hope is that if you are already practicing it, you will come to a deeper appreciation of its spiritual riches. Or if you are curious about Kriya, I would like to help you learn more.[12]

If you have been initiated in another tradition, I believe you will be helped to understand its healing powers more deeply. And if you are preparing for a spiritual initiation, I believe you will be encouraged in your chosen path.

When the Kriya technique is practiced with understanding and devotion, it brings us two types of healing. During the initiation ceremony, and in our daily practice, Kriya helps us neutralize and burn up the seeds of our negative past karma — that is, the results of our past physical, mental, or spiritual mistakes that may be blocking our progress now. A *Kriyaban* (one who is initiated in and practices Kriya) gradually becomes free of these past karmic burdens and tendencies. As the following story suggests, initiates may even experience healing from past karmic influences during the ceremony itself.

✹ Healed during the ✹ initiation ceremony

I received my first Kriya initiation at Ananda Assisi in September 2017. In my memory, the ceremony shines as one of the most blessed events of my life.

I understood that I was committing myself to a vast undertaking, and I worried that I might not be able to live up to the promise.

During the ceremony, there was a point when I suddenly felt an amazing power flowing from the photograph of Swami Sri Yukteswar and entering and permeating my being. It felt as if an invisible ray of spiritual healing had passed through the air and been absorbed in my brain and consciousness.

I now realize that in that moment my guru burned from my brain a former habit of slipping from promises. In all these years, I have been faithful in my practice, and the healing power has remained with me, helping me to win out over every spiritual obstacle. –**Cristina Shambhavi**, *Milan*

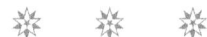

The second type of healing that Kriya initiation and practice can bring us is freedom from spiritual disease.

> Spiritual disease manifests in lack of soul peace,
> want of poise, restlessness, discontentment,
> unbalance, inharmony, unwillingness to meditate,
> habit of putting off meditation, unkindness,
> unforgiveness, melancholia, bigotry,
> lack of introspection, lack of self-analysis.
> These are caused by ignorance.[13]

The blessings imparted during Kriya initiation continue to operate during our subsequent Kriya practice –liberating us from the ego's hypnotic efforts to distract us, arming us against the temptations of Maya, and curing us of ignorance. As we gradually become healed of ignorance and free from the burdens of our past karma, we enter a new phase of life in which we are able to live more constantly in joy.

> Joy and God are One.
> Joy is the healing that you want first,
> the healing of the ignorance of the soul.[14]

PART XII   CHAPTER ELEVEN

Spritual Protection

> A strong, positive magnetic aura around your body will prevent not only people's negative thoughts from affecting you, but also negative or harmful circumstances and happenings, even disease, from coming to you.... No negative energy will be able to penetrate a powerful positive force field.[1] —Kriyananda

I first encountered Kirlian photography at a spiritual fair in Milan in the 1990s.[2] An exhibitor offered to take color images of the fair-goers' auras; and several of us, thinking that it might be fun, volunteered. Looking at the images, we were fascinated by how each person's image was unique in its shape and gradations of color.

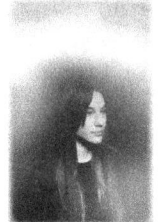

The electric energy moving through a wire creates a magnetic field. Similarly, the life force flowing through the human body creates a protective shield, which in metaphysics is called the person's "aura," the power of which will depend on the strength of the current of energy. Psychically sensitive people can see the aura, and the inventors of Kirlian photography claimed that it could be photographed by their instrument.

> Energy flowing through the nerves of the body... produces a kind of electromagnetic field. This field is much subtler than any with which science is familiar, but it has much greater power to affect people and events. The will determines

> the strength of the energy-flow ("the greater the will, the greater the flow of energy"). If the will power is strong, the body will be filled with energy. As a consequence, the body's magnetic field will be extensive and powerful. ...
>
> If our consciousness is strongly positive, our magnetism will be positive also, and will attract good things to us. It will, in addition, create a "buffer zone" around us, protecting us from harm; like an umbrella in the rain, it will fend off much of the suffering we might otherwise attract by negative karmic vortices (*vrittis*) of energy in the spine. Sri Krishna referred to this protection in the *Bhagavad Gita:* "Even a little practice of this spiritual discipline will free you from dire fears and colossal sufferings." [3]

We are always surrounded by our electromagnetic shield, even as the earth is protected from cosmic radiation and solar winds by its atmosphere. A strong aura serves as a shield to protect us from negative people, environments, and illness – and depending on the aura's strength, even our negative past karma.

The strength of the protection depends on the quantity, quality, and consistency of the flow of prana within us, which in turn depends on the nature and energetic force of our thoughts, as they vary from day to day, and even hour to hour. Whenever our energy is low, our thoughts will tend to turn toward negativity, weakening the magnetic field and making it vulnerable to disease.

It is difficult to avoid the energy that is being generated by dark thoughts – especially now, when ideas can travel around the world at the speed of light, carried by social media, 24-hour news, and the emotions and thoughts of negative and fearful people. Few now believe that the future is bright with promise. Many, if not most, are discouraged, worried, and afraid.

How can we protect ourselves from these external forces, and from our own self-sabotaging negativity?

> Magnetic self-protection may be accomplished by refusing, on the one hand, to respond on a negative level (for example, with fear, anger, or hatred), and by surrounding oneself, on the other hand, with strong positive magnetism.[4]

How to strengthen your aura

The first and most important way to protect ourselves is by keeping our energy reserves high. It is good to have an internal energy gauge and check it throughout the day. If we allow our energy level to dip, due to exhaustion, inadequate sleep, sadness, or disease, or when we overindulge any of the senses or fall prey to behavioral or substance addictions, our aura becomes weak and porous. The moment it first begins to dip is the very best time for a recharge.

The Life Force Energization Exercises* are the most powerful and effective way to keep the aura strong and intact. Doing the entire set at least once a day, and the Full Body Recharge repeatedly during the day, will strengthen our aura and provide excellent insurance against illness and negativity.† The more often we do the exercises, the stronger our aura becomes, and the greater the protection we will enjoy in all situations.

❊ MY ENERGY SHIELD ❊

My husband was in the hospital, fighting for his life against a super bacterium. A few days became a month, then many months – long hours and entire days spent in the waiting room, hoping for good news, or any news. I was exhausted physically and emotionally. Yet I had to stay strong to help my husband keep up his courage

---
* These important exercises are discussed in Volume One, Part IV.
† You will find instruction and guided practice of the Energization Exercises and the Life Force Full Body Recharge in the online Appendices.

and energy, and not be discouraged by the doctors' disappointing reports. And then I had to keep going, day after day after day.

During this period I relied heavily on the Energization Exercises, and especially the Full Body Recharging as my emergency medicine and energy shield. I used them to strengthen my aura when I awoke in the morning, to overcome tiredness during the long hours in the emergency room, to give me strength and calmness before speaking with the doctors, and while visiting my husband to help us stay positive and hopeful.

We were able to emerge from this very trying period, thanks to the invaluable gift of Yogananda's healing exercises, which continue to sustain us as we face our challenges with renewed inner strength and faith. –**Valeria**, *Parma, Italy*

❈ ❈ ❈

It is more effective to fill our energy tank whenever the level falls slightly below full than to wait until our reserves are completely depleted. The more often we let our energy drop, the more vulnerable we become. When the gauge drops past half-full and gets stuck there, drastic remedies may be required, such as a full weekend of rest, disconnected from the internet. A vacation, even a short one, perhaps to a spa or a thermal bath resort. Or, even better, a spiritual retreat.

If you have regular contact with people who are ill, as a healthcare provider or caretaker, monitoring your energy reserves throughout the day is vital. Ill people will draw on your energy, and if you are unable to keep refilling the tank, you will run dry. If you see patients throughout the day, try to schedule time between visits to recharge.* If you are a nurse, take time while walking from room to room to do a mini-recharge: double inhalation through the nose, hold and tense all body parts, double exhalation through the mouth. Recharge your mind as well – generate a positive thought about the next patient, and offer a prayer that you will be able to serve them as a channel for their healing.

* See the Appendices for some one- and two-minute rapid recharging exercises.

When caring for someone day-in and day-out, take energy-recharging "snacks" throughout the day, going outside as often as possible to do them – even for a few minutes. Keep fresh air circulating in the room. Play a recording of Aum softly in the background. Try not to 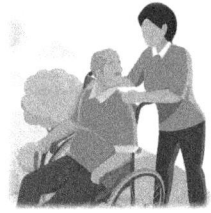 shoulder all of the responsibility; seek the support of professionals and friends. Try to get away for a complete recharge one day a week.

Radiate positive thoughts

We have a choice in every situation to be a passive victim, or to respond positively. As Swami Kriyananda often said: "Learn to be a cause, not an effect."

> Harmonize the vibrations of your heart…
> *Consciously* emanate peaceful vibrations outward
> from your heart center to your environment.
> For human energy has two modes of expression;
> one of them is giving, the other, receiving or
> absorbing. If you can consciously enter the giving
> mode, you will find yourself much less affected
> by outside influences, whether good or bad….
> Send the heart's energy upward to the point
> between the eyebrows. Feel yourself surrounded
> and embraced by the divine light.[5]

Be prepared

If you know that you will be exposed to *tamasic* low-energy vibrations, or to negative people, take time to meditate beforehand. When you are feeling inwardly calm, visualize the situation and the people, and mentally surround them with peaceful vibrations, and with a warm light of impersonal love. Mentally fill the space with thoughts and vibrations of harmony. If you are so inclined, pray that a spirit of peace, harmony, and respect will fill the space and the minds of those present. Prepare your mind with positive thoughts about each person.

Emotion it is especially that creates weakness in one's magnetic "armor." Harmonize your emotions, therefore, by deep meditation. Then, with a conscious effort of will, radiate harmonious feelings outward from your heart center in all directions to the world around you.[6]

Mantra protection

Each mantra has a power to attract a specific result. Some mantras attract prosperity, while others can help us draw a suitable marriage partner, while others can help ward off evil. In Chapter Two, we considered the highest of all mantras: the Cosmic Sound of Aum. Paramhansa Yogananda said, "When you are in tune with [the Aum] vibration, no matter what devastating events occur around you, you will be protected.[7]

Here are some of Swami Kriyananda's suggestions for creating an Aum shield around yourself before entering a negative situation.

YOUR AUM SHIELD

In the privacy of your meditation room, place your arms down at your side. Then, mentally chanting *AUM*, bring them upward, straight out to the side, with your palms up, until you join the palms high above the head. Mentally create an aura of upward-moving light around your body.[8]

[*Author's note:* Repeat several times. If you need to protect yourself while in a business or social situation, you can excuse yourself to the bathroom and practice it there.]

※

Extend your arms before you, your palms touching. Then move them out and around your body in a broad circle until the palms or fingers touch once again behind your back. Mentally, while repeating this process, chant, "AUM-TAT-SAT." (The *a*'s in TAT-SAT are pronounced short, with an "uh" sound: "TUT-SUT.") Repeat this process at least three times.

A *mantra* to repeat in such circumstances is *"AUM hreeng kleeng Krishnaya namaha."* (The first *a* in Krishnaya is pronounced as in our "ah." The other *a*'s are pronounced as in "uh.") [9]

※

The Mahamrityunjaya mantra, from the Rig Veda, is said to eliminate illness and grant health, to ward off calamities and accidents, to offer protection from evil forces, to overcome the fear of death and illness, to avoid untimely death, and to achieve liberation from the cycles of birth, death and rebirth.[10]

Om Tryambakam Yajamahe
Sugandhim Pushtivardhanam
Urvarukamiva Bandhanan
Mrityor Mukshiya Maamritat

If you are beset by negative energies and bad dreams at night, Yogananda suggests this practice.

SAFE SLEEP

Before going to sleep, write an imaginary "Om" or "Amen" word on your pillow with your fingers. Mentally visualize light around your body and look into the spiritual eye and say several times, mentally or loudly: "I am Light. Darkness, fly away." Also touch both of your palms in front of your body, and then swing them behind your back in rapid succession, chanting "Om," and you will be protected.[11]

Spiritual Bodyguard

It is best not to go into negative or conflictual situations alone. Whatever inner strength you may have in the moment could be overwhelmed by the negativity or disharmony of others. When Jesus sent his disciples to preach and heal in his name, he had them go out in pairs. St. Francis also sent his brothers to preach in pairs.

Swami Kriyananda gives the following advice for protecting ourselves in unfavorable situations and environments.

> When you find that you must enter a disharmonious environment, keep a spiritual "bodyguard" with you: someone who is on the same spiritual wavelength as you, to help keep your magnetism strong.[12]
>
> My Master [Sri Yukteswar] used to say, therefore, "Keep a spiritual bodyguard with you when mixing with others." I have always obeyed his advice. I've made it a point to surround myself with a few spiritual souls.[13]

Avoid negative environments.

To keep our protective aura strong, it's important to be very careful in choosing the places we decide to visit, avoiding those that might infect us with low energy and create holes in our aura. Just as the odor of tobacco in a room remains in our hair and clothing, the unwholesome vibrations of negative places can affect us long after.

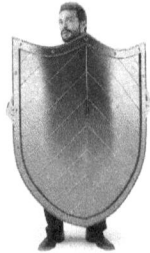

Extra precautions are needed when we are unable to avoid environments that are permeated with the negative thoughts of many people, or with tamasic vibrations of a sensual, violent, criminal, or adharmic nature. Do your utmost to strengthen your aura beforehand, and whenever possible take along a companion who has strong positive magnetism.

Cross of blue light

> If you feel yourself under psychic attack from anyone, use your thumb to place a cross of blue light mentally on the attacker. Do it with sufficient will power, and harmful energy will be unable to reach you, but will return to its sender. Direct good energy along with the blocking energy, that your attacker be cured of his anger.[14]
>
> Imagine that you are using your thumb for this purpose. (Of all the fingers the thumb is the most related to will power.) If you practice this technique with great will and strong faith, any evil coming toward you from others will be arrested at its source, and only good vibrations will be able to reach you. In this way also, while protecting yourself you will not in any way be harming your opponent, though his own negative thoughts may indeed rebound upon him since they cannot reach their intended goal in you.[15]

Good Company

Something over which we have no control is the thoughts and actions of others. When we are unable to avoid being exposed to negative people, we need to be extremely cautious. Yogananda and Kriyananda offer this advice.

> We must be careful with whom we associate, because we are continually exchanging magnetism with other people through our thoughts, through shaking hands and through

> looking into the eyes of another person. As soon as we shake hands with someone, a magnet is formed. The person who is the stronger gives his vibration to the other person. We become like the people we mingle with, not through their conversation, but through the silent magnetic vibration which goes out of their bodies. When we come in the range of their magnetism, we become like them.[16]

> Avoid like the plague anyone whose magnetism has the power to pull you down. Such a person is worse for you than any disease. For physical disease affects only the body, but spiritual disease can devastate you spiritually....

> Try not to look into the eyes of, or shake hands with, people whose vibrations are negative. This avoidance may prove a little socially awkward at times so I don't insist on it, but I should state that these are two of the strongest ways by which magnetism is exchanged between people. (This is one little-known reason for the palms-folded greeting, the *namaskar*, which Indians customarily use in place of the handshake.)[17]

Although we can choose our friends, we have less latitude when it comes to co-workers, and none at all regarding our family. The negative influence of a close family member on our physical and mental health can become a major life issue. In addition to seeking professional support, there are some highly effective spiritual techniques that you can use to protect yourself.

First, there are ways to minimize contact with negative people whom you cannot entirely avoid, even though it may seem impossible. Creating physical and psychic distance will be important. You will want to have "safe zones" – physical spaces where you can retreat and remove yourself from spiraling negative influences. It could be as simple as stepping out on a balcony, or going to a nearby coffee shop. At home, you can retreat to your meditation space. If all else fails, you can make a strategic retreat to the bathroom.

When overwhelmed by phone calls and messages, try to establish "off-line" times during the day, perhaps during the hour or two after waking, then at lunch, and after dinner. The callers will adjust.

When contact cannot be avoided, use the suggestions in this chapter to strengthen yourself. Also, use the techniques of meditation and prayer from the previous chapters to allow God's unconditional, transformative love to flow through you to others. It is not our responsibility to change them, but we can serve as channels for God's love. Realize also that if you are suffering, they undoubtedly are as well.

Associating with positive, inspiring people creates a magnetic environment in which we are more powerfully protected from negative influences than we could protect ourselves. The Latin proverb *Defendit numerus* ("There is safety in numbers") has a solid metaphysical foundation.

> Good company...is extremely important on the spiritual path. Seek out the company of others of like mind. Mix with them lovingly. If you know someone whose spiritual magnetism is particularly strong, spend time with that person. If outward good company is not available, keep good company mentally....
>
> Most important of all, try to keep the company of saints. They will help you, even from a distance, by their subtle magnetic influence. If you know no such people, read their lives; visit places where they have lived; mix with those who knew them. If possible, listen to recordings of their voices.[18]

✺ The Laughing Swami ✺

It was our last day in Badrinath, and we had visited a number of holy people who live there. I had bought some malas (prayer beads) and was lamenting that I had not done so sooner, so that I could get them blessed along the way.

There would be a final satsang at our hotel that evening with Swami Swarupananda. When I saw him for the first time, he reminded me of Hotei, the Chinese god of happiness. He was short, round, with sparkling eyes and a big smile always on his face. From time to time he would unexpectedly erupt in brief bouts of laughter – while speaking, chanting, meditating – for no apparent reason, other than his irrepressible inner joy.

I felt deeply attracted to the swami, and I suddenly remembered my malas. I was seated near him and asked him to bless the malas. As he was holding and turning them in his hand, I had a strange experience: I perceived his voice and his consciousness inside me, in my spine, at my very center. At the same time, I felt as though I was inside him, completely one with him. His laughter was rumbling inside me. The words he was speaking were somehow resounding with great power in my spine, as if their origin was in my soul. Their sound was so pure and beautiful that their meaning seemed secondary to their vibrations.

My identification with my body and ego began to melt and my consciousness began to expand. This was a completely new way of being, full of quiet joy and the feeling of deep oneness with everything. I was at home in my inner soul. –**Andrey**, *Baku, Azerbaijan*

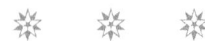

Astrological bangles and gems

The law of karma is mathematically precise. The results of past actions, both good and bad, return to the sender at a predetermined time. While we are responsible for our actions, we have no say as to the timing of their return. How, then, can we protect ourselves from the unavoidable impact?

Yogananda's guru, Swami Sri Yukteswar, explained that the planets in our solar system serve as vehicles for our karma. One of the ways to deflect the karmic influences is by the use of astrological bangles.

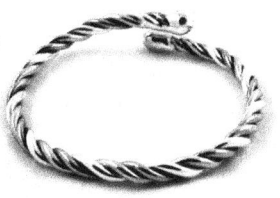

> The relation of the stars to the human body and mind is very subtle. There is a relation of the spinal plexuses to the signs of the zodiac. No matter what environment you may live in, all the surrounding rays of the earth and universe react upon your body. You respond to those rays. There is a reaction between the stars and the rays around your body.[19]

In his *Autobiography*, Yogananda tells how he was struck by a severe liver illness that the doctors said would take six months to heal. His guru, Swami Sri Yukteswar, recommended that he wear an astrological arm bangle of silver and lead,* which he said would reduce the period of illness to one month. The young Mukunda (Yogananda's name at the time) claimed not to believe in astrology, but only in God's power to heal. A portion of the discussion that followed can help us understand the vibratory power of metals and gems to protect us from the bombs of our karma.

> It is only when a traveler has reached his goal that he is justified in discarding his maps. During the journey, he takes advantage of any convenient short cut. The ancient rishis discovered many ways to curtail the period of man's exile in delusion. There are certain mechanical features in the law of karma which can be skillfully adjusted by the fingers of wisdom.

---

* The classic bangle, however, is made from 99.9% pure gold, silver and copper, crafted in precise proportions.

All human ills arise from some transgression of universal law. The scriptures point out that man must satisfy the laws of nature, while not discrediting the divine omnipotence....By a number of means — by prayer, by will power, by yoga meditation, by consultation with saints, by use of astrological bangles — the adverse effects of past wrongs can be minimized or nullified.

Just as a house can be fitted with a copper rod to absorb the shock of lightning, so the bodily temple can be benefited by various protective measures. Ages ago our yogis discovered that pure metals emit an astral light which is powerfully counteractive to negative pulls of the planets. Subtle electrical and magnetic radiations are constantly circulating in the universe; when a man's body is being aided, he does not know it; when it is being disintegrated, he is still in ignorance. Can he do anything about it?

This problem received attention from our rishis; they found helpful not only a combination of metals, but also of plants and — most effective of all–faultless jewels of not less than two carats.... One little-known fact is that the proper jewels, metals, or plant preparations are valueless unless the required weight is secured, and unless these remedial agents are worn next to the skin.[20]

Mukunda duly had a bangle made, and just as his guru predicted, the painful illness lasted only a month. In his later years Yogananda would tell his disciples the story, and add the following advice: **"Never forget that devotion to God is the greatest 'bangle.'"** [21]

✻ Sri Yukteswar to the rescue ✻

Incapacitating migraine headaches have been my constant companions since I was sixteen. They come two or three times a week, and several times a month they are so strong that I have to stay in bed, in the dark, suffering in silence.

I have seen so many doctors! Each has offered a different treatment, but none has worked. The ophthalmologist diagnosed nearsightedness and prescribed corrective lenses. The otolaryngologist found evidence of sinusitis and prescribed aerosol therapies. The orthopedist said the cause was inflamed nerves in my neck and prescribed anti-inflammatories. The neurologist prescribed relaxants and anxiolytics. I was taking all of these medications, as well as painkillers, but none of them brought relief.

I tried changing my diet, taking flower essences, and receiving chiropractic and acupuncture treatments and deep massage – all to no avail.

The headaches interfere with my work and all aspects of my life, as I live in constant fear of becoming paralyzed with pain. Since I have been on the spiritual path, they have interfered with my ability to meditate and to make progress in my practices.

One night, I had a curious dream. I was seated in meditation on a hillside, and an astrological bracelet of the kind that Swami Sri Yukteswar talks about in the *Autobiography* materialized in front of me. I felt a strong energetic shift within me. I did not connect the bangle to my condition, but following the powerful inspiration of the dream, I purchased a bangle. This was in May of 2021, and I have not taken it off since.

Right away, I began to notice an improvement in the frequency and intensity of the headaches. They come now just a couple of times a month, never disabling me to the point where I need to stay in bed. Is it the bangle, or my faith in the bangle? I think it is both, just as Mukunda discovered when Sri Yukteswar urged him to get a bangle at a time when he was gravely ill. –**Giovanni**, *Milan, Italy*

Protective gems

Another way to protect ourselves against planetary influences is by wearing specific gems that are related to each planet. An intuitive and knowledgeable Vedic astrologer can recommend the gems that will offer you the greatest protection, based on your birth horoscope and the current planetary transits.

The gems may be worn as a ring, necklace, bangle, or bracelet, so long as each gem is at least two carats and is mounted so that it touches the skin. A bangle that includes all nine planets (including the north and south poles of the moon, but excluding Pluto and Neptune) is called a *navaratna*, meaning "nine gems."

The nine gems are:

- **Ruby** for the Sun
- **Pearl** for the Moon
- **Red coral** for Mars
- **Emerald** for Mercury
- **Yellow sapphire** for Jupiter
- **Diamond** for Venus
- **Blue sapphire** for Saturn
- **Hessonite** for Rahu (*the ascending lunar node*)
- **Cat's eye** for Ketu (*the descending lunar node*)

Purifying a negative environment

If you are constrained to live in a place that has disharmonious vibrations, you should clean the space both physically and vibrationally before moving in. You might ask friends to help you, and make it uplifting for everyone by chanting as you clean. Some ideas:

- Thoroughly air out the entire space.
- Deep clean everywhere, including outside areas.
- Replace old furnishings, carpets, and curtains if possible, or have them professionally cleaned.
- Paint the walls with appropriate colors (see Chapter Four).
- Install adequate lighting.
- Play a recording of Aum chanting throughout the process, and play it often thereafter.

- Alternate the Aum recording with other devotional music.
- Burn incense, or place essential oil diffusers in each room with purifying fragrances. Lavender is universally popular.
- Place sacred objects around the space: photographs, icons, statues of holy figures, yantras, or relics.
- When the space and objects have been prepared, arrange an ad-hoc or official blessing ceremony.

We are not alone

When we are children, God's love protects us through our parents, and He continues to watch over us through our "guardian angels" as we grow into adulthood. Ever the ideal "manager," God delegates the responsibility for our protection to others whom we meet along the way, and to those who are helping us from higher planes. One of these angels is our spiritual guide, who may or may not be presently known to us. The guru assumes this responsibility with utmost dedication and is always "on call." In a letter to a disciple, Yogananda wrote:*

> You must never lose courage. Divine Mother sent me to pilot you out of the clouds of your mind. Everybody's difficulty is different, and he or she has to win that test of karma.... Your troubles I do not mind. I will never give up my job about you....Have no fear even though I am gone from your visible eyes. You will never be alone...I shall ever be with you and through Divine Mother guard you from all harm....
>
> A smooth life is not a victorious life — and I will give you lots of my good karma, so you will get through. I will...ever lift you up, no matter how many times you fall...Not only will I invisibly help you but visibly, through many here.

Whenever we need protection, the guru should be our first call.

* This letter had been quoted earlier, and is pertinent here as well.

❋ Drowning in the Ganges ❋

We had received many blessings during our pilgrimage to India, but meditating in the cave of Sage Vasishta was exceptional. Such deep silence is hard to imagine, much less to find. The road back to the hotel in Rishikesh took us along the Ganges, and when our guide said that it was possible to arrange a rafting excursion, I joined the group.

I am a good swimmer, having grown up at the seaside, and had rafted. But the river was uncharacteristically turbulent that day, and when our raft capsized I was thrown far into the rapids. I struggled with all my might, but the current was beyond my strength and skill. Fear gripped my mind and froze my muscles – I was helpless. All I could do was call on my Master: "If this is what you want, Thy will be done."

Within seconds the current carried me into calmer waters, and I was able to reach the shore with ease, thanks to my Guru's protecting hand. Apparently I needed a full immersion in the holy waters as well as the chance to surrender myself to God's will. Knowing that I am loved and protected is a special blessing from the pilgrimage that remains with me to this day. **–Giovanni**, *Milano, Italy*

❋ The Guru's promise ❋

When I took vows of discipleship to Yogananda, I was focused on what I was promising to do, not realizing that at the same time he was promising to guide and protect me. I have experienced his protection on numerous occasions, including when my car rolled over.

As I turned my car around in the driveway, a wheel went off a steep embankment. The momentum of the car's weight took hold as it tipped and rolled over on the driver's side, then onto the roof.

"Aum Guru!" I chanted many times, as I found myself upside down against the ceiling of the car. The window was shattered, but I was able to crawl out. I checked myself for broken bones and found only a deep cut on a finger. How my arthritic sixty-two-year-old body managed to get out of the window with only a scratch was remarkable to me. I continued to chant to keep myself calm and able to deal with the wound, then make arrangements for the car. No matter where I am or what I am doing, I feel his protective shield around me always. –**Dhuti**, *Ananda Assisi*

❈ Demons beware! ❈

I experience severe anxiety attacks from time to time, during which I either can hardly breathe or I hyperventilate. If I could meditate at those times, perhaps I could remain calm – but I can't, which is deeply frustrating, since I love meditation and usually sit for a long time.

One day I found a solution: I would chant my meditation mantra inwardly along with the rapid breathing that accompanies the anxiety attacks. It began to calm me during the attack, and I could then consider meditating.

I started with a short meditation and only a few Kriyas. Soon, I was able to practice a complete cycle of twelve rotations; then two cycles became possible. The day I was feeling very comfortable with my Kriya practice and was about to start on the third cycle, I had an extraordinary vision. I saw Yogananda transform into my body: from my head down through my torso. I was filled with and surrounded by an aura of golden light. In that moment I saw legions of demons flying at me from all sides, trying to get inside me. They were coming unbelievably fast, and Yogananda was swatting them down, just as fast. Swat, swat, swat, swat, swat! It seemed that he had a multitude of arms. He was eliminating each of them before they could get to me. Finally they had all been eliminated, and I was safe.

I ended my meditation at that point with an appreciation for the protective power of Kriya, and the realization that no matter where I am or in what mental condition, my Guru's presence is within me. –**Ashtara**, *Tel Aviv, Israel*

We close this chapter with these sage words from Swami Kriyananda.

> Remember also that it is wise always to remain open and receptive to *good* magnetic influences. Do not, therefore, seek to protect yourself against the harmful thoughts of others by assuming an attitude of coldness or indifference to them. Indifference, though it may indeed protect you, will also deaden you to the finer vibrations in the world around you; it will make you less *divinely* receptive. It is better always to respond with a consciousness of light and of impersonal, divine love. Remember, the good thoughts that others send you must also find an opening in you, to influence you.[22]

CHAPTER 11: *Points to Remember*

- There is a magnetic field around the body, an aura that protects us.
- When it is strong, it repels negativity and disease.
- To strengthen the aura, we need to keep our thoughts positive and our energy high.
- Meditation and Life Force Energization Exercises keep the aura strong.
- Other methods that strengthen the aura include protective mantras, devotional chants, astrological bangles, precious gems, good company, faith in God, and reliance on His channels.
- Whenever possible, avoid negative people and dark places. When not possible, charge your aura before engaging.

PART XII CHAPTER TWELVE

Points to Remember about Vibratory Healing

> Spiritual development creates a positive protective aura, which insulates body and mind against the impact of negative karma.[1]
> –YOGANANDA

- Everything in the manifested universe vibrates at a specific frequency. A healthy body vibrates at or above 72 MHz; if its vibratory rate falls below 58 MHz, it will be more vulnerable to disease.

- The vibratory frequencies of sounds, music, nature, colors, environments, holy places, saints, ceremonies, and rituals can contribute to our health.

- Spending time in nature is an investment in our health.

- Everything in creation is a mixture of the three vibrational qualities of sattwa, rajo, and tamo guna. The more our thoughts and lifestyle reflect pure sattwic qualities, the healthier we will be.

- Certain mantras have healing effects. The most powerful mantra is the Cosmic Vibration of Aum. Hearing it chanted, chanting it ourselves, and listening to it in meditation strengthens us, protects us, and leads us, in time, to the highest state of Cosmic Consciousness.

- The music we listen to has a powerful effect on our health for good or ill. If we aspire to manifest sattwic qualities of harmony, peace, and joy in our lives, we should choose music that vibrates with those qualities.

- Listening to divinely inspired music – and especially singing and playing it – opens our hearts to divine grace.

- Devotional songs, particularly the Cosmic Chants of Paramhansa Yogananda, have been infused with a power to transform our consciousness and heal mental and emotional disharmonies.

- We are powerfully influenced by our environment. Pay attention to the quality of the vibrations in your home and workspace. Make necessary adjustments to ensure that they are vibrating with harmony and light.

- Choose appropriate colors for your wardrobe, home, and workspace that support and enhance your health, happiness, and creativity.

- In places of spiritual power, and in the presence of saintly people, spontaneous healings can occur.

- Create a healing space in your home where you can meditate and recharge physically, mentally, emotionally, and spiritually.

- Ceremonies and rituals can serve as powerful channels for uplifting vibrations and spontaneous healing.

- One of the best protections against negativity and disease is a strong magnetic aura. When you cannot avoid confronting negative people or situations, prepare by practicing techniques that will strengthen your magnetic energy field.

- Strengthen your aura with positive, loving thoughts, Life Force Energization Exercises, mantras, prayers for protection, and astrological bangles and gemstones.

- Devotion is the best protection.

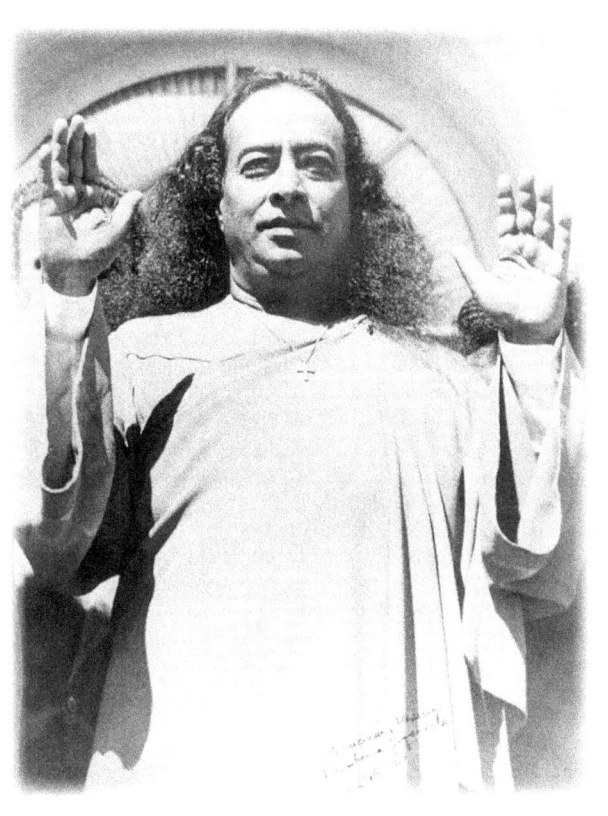

With blessings
Paramhansa Yogananda

NOTES | PART XII

Title Page
1 Yogananda, "Vibration," *Inner Culture*, July 1936.

Chapter One
1 Yogananda, "Consciousness and Vibration," *Scientific Healing Affirmations*.
2 Kriyananda, *The Promise of Immortality*, 29.
3 Yogananda, "Consciousness and Vibration," *Scientific Healing Affirmations*, 31.
4 "Musica Universalis," Wikipedia, https://en.wikipedia.org/wiki/Musica_universalis.
5 "Pythagoras," Wikipendia, https://en.wikipedia.org/wiki/Pythagoras.
    The concept of the Platonic solids was ridiculed for centuries until Professor Emeritus Robert Moon at the University of Chicago demonstrated in the 1980s that the entire Periodic Table of Elements – literally everything in the physical world – is based on these five forms: "Periodic Table of Elements and Dr. Robert Moon," *Cosmic Core*, https://www.cosmic-core.org/free/article-131-atomic-chemistry-part-2-periodic-table-of-elements-dr-robert-moon/.

    "Apart from their natural beauty, many interesting uses of Platonic solids exist in technology. For instance, tetrahedrons are frequently applied in electronics, icosahedrons have proven useful in geophysical modeling, and speakers with polyhedral faces are used to radiate sound energy in all directions."
6 Rajan, Sheetal, "Platonic Solids and Sacred Shapes for Healing," *The Sacred Being*, October 16, 2020, *https://thesacredbeing.com/platonic-solids-and-sacred-shapes-for-healing/*.
7 Sivananda, *Japa* Yoga, The Sivananda Publication League, 1942. Available in a current edition from the bookstore in his ashram in Rishikesh, and also online at https://archive.org/details/in.ernet.dli.2015.128391/mode/2up.
8 Yogananda, *Autobiography of a Yogi*, 158.
9 "Negative Effects of High Level Infrasound," *Noise and Health*, Vol. 23 (109), April-June 2021, National Library of Medicine, https://www.ncbi.nlm.nih.gov/pmc/articles/PMC8411947/#.
10 "The Happiness Revival Guide," Time, https://time.com/6244162/how-sound-can-improve-happiness/.
11 Becker, Robert, *The Body Electric, Electromagnetism and The Foundation of Life*, available at https://www.amazon.com/Body-Electric-Electromagnetism-Foundation-Life/dp/0688069711.
12 Young, D. Gary, "Human Electrical Frequencies and Fields," Quantum Health Consulting, https://quantumhealthconsulting.com/human-electrical-frequencies-and-fields/.
13 Walker, Betsy, "Frequency and the Human Body," Betsy Walker, https://betsywalkerwellness.com/frequency-human-body/.

Chapter Two
1 Kriyananda, *The New Path*, 370.
2 Yogananda, *The Essence of Self-Realization*, 3:10.
3 Chapters 14 and 18 of the Bhagavad Gita include detailed descriptions of the gunas; extensive commentaries by Paramhansa Yogananda on the gunas can be found in his book *God Speaks to Arjuna;* and Swami Kriyananda addresses the gunas in *The Essence of the Bhagavad Gita*.
4 Kriyananda, *Conversations with Yogananda* No. 39.
    "There are entire galaxies where *tamas* predominates. The inhabitants of

the planets in those galaxies are for the most part brutish and incapable of aspiring to spiritual heights. Fierce animals abound there, and cannibalism. The inhabitants are constantly in a state of conflict and warfare. Lust and every animal pleasure are considered the best that life has to offer. Again, there are galaxies where *rajo guna* predominates. The planets in them are peopled by more self-aware beings, whose primary concern is with self-advancement, self-aggrandizement, and self-importance. Our own 'Milky Way' galaxy is such a system....
There are...entire galaxies where *sattwa guna* predominates. The planets there resemble legends of the Garden of Eden. The people there can communicate easily with beings in the astral world. Harmony and beauty are prevalent everywhere."

5 Kriyananda, *Awaken to Superconsciousness,* 170.
6 Yogananda, *Psychological Chart.*
7 Yukteswar, *The Holy Science.* Widely available on the internet from various sources.
8 Yogananda, "The Divine Magnetic Diet," Super Advanced Course No. 1, Lesson 5.
9 Kriyananda, "Immortality," *Affirmations for Self-Healing,* 117.
10 Kriyananda, "High-Mindedness," 123.
11 Yogananda, "Acquiring Magnetism," *Inner Culture,* July 1941.
12 Yogananda, "Recipes," *East-West,* July-August 1926 and 1928.
13 *Ananda Yoga for Higher Awareness* is notable for the transforming effects it achieves by combining traditional yoga postures with mental and vocal affirmations that match the consciousness of each pose. You will find books on Ananda Yoga in the bibliography, as well programs offered through the Ananda teaching centers.
14 Ananda Restorative Yoga is discussed at: https://www.expandinglight.org/yoga/everyone/restorative-yoga-.php.
15 Kriyananda, *The Hindu Way of Awakening,* 105-106.
16 Kriyananda, *The Art and Science of Raja Yoga,* 429.
17 Kriyananda, *Awaken to Superconsciousness,* 26.
18 Kriyananda, 52.
19 Kaivalyadhama, https://kdham.com/about-kaivalyadhama/.
20 Information about Kriya Yoga can be found at www.ananda.org; www.anandaindia.org; and www.anandaeurope.org.
21 Yogananda, "Spiritual Interpretation of the Bhagavad Gita," 2:58, *Inner Culture,* March 1940.
22 Yogananda, *The Essence of the Bhagavad Gita,* Verse 14:8, 453-454.
23 On Amazon excellent books on yoga, Ayurveda, and healing by Dr. Vasant Lad and Dr. David Frawley can be found.
24 Yogananda, *Autobiography of a Yogi,* 379.
25 Kriyananda, *The Hindu Way of Awakening,* 104.

Chapter Three

1 Yogananda, *Whispers from Eternity,* No. 176.
2 Yogananda, *Autobiography of a Yogi,* 158.
3 Kriyananda, *The Hindu Way of Awakening,* 157.
4 Kriyananda, 157.
5 Kriyananda, *The Art and Science of Raja Yoga,* 248.
6 Kriyananda, 248.
7 Ashley-Farrand, Thomas, Kohlapur, India, Saraswati Publications, *The Ancient Power of Sanskrit Mantra and Ceremony,* Volume I, 2002, 12-13. https://www.amazon.com/Ancient-Power-Sanskrit-Mantra-Ceremony/dp/B005MJX19Q.

8 Mank, Natalia, "The Power of Mantra and the Science Behind It," Integral Yoga Magazine, https://integralyogamagazine.org/the-power-of-mantra-and-the-science-behind-it/#.
9 https://en.wikipedia.org/wiki/Milarepa.
10 Kriyananda, *Rays of the Same Light*, 25.
11 Yogananda, *The Rubaiyat of Omar Khayyam Explained*, Quatrain 66, 312.
12 Kriyananda, *Art and Science of Raja Yoga*, 250.
13 Harne Bhavna, "EEG Spectral Analysis on OM Mantra Meditation: A Pilot Study," Research Gate, https://www.researchgate.net/publication/325084616_EEG_Spectral_Analysis_on_OM_Mantra_Meditation_A_Pilot_Study..
14 Wan, Lalita and others, "Review of Scientific Analysis of Sacred Sound Om (Aum)," https://www.researchgate.net/publication/347557728_review_of_scientific_analysis_of_sacred_sound_om_aum.
15 Kriyananda, *Hindu Way of Awakening*, 157.
16 Kriyananda, *The Art and Science of Raja Yoga*, 250.
17 Yogananda, *The Essence of Self-Realization*, 20:2.
18 Yogananda, *New Super Cosmic Science Course*, Lesson 2.
19 Yogananda, Lesson 1.
20 Ananda Sangha Publications, https://anandapublications.com/products/aum-mantra-of-eternity.
21 Yogananda, *The Essence of Self-Realization*, 16:12.
22 Yogananda, *Super Advanced Course No. 1*, Lesson 1.
23 Kriyananda, *Art and Science of Raja Yoga*, 389.
24 Kriyananda, *The Promise of Immortality*, 29.
25 Yukteswar, *The Holy Science*, 55.
26 Yogananda, Bhagavad Gita Interpretations: 1:15-18/2.
27 Kriyananda, *Meditation for Starters*, 71.
28 Kriyananda, *Awaken to Superconsciousness*, 181-182.
29 Yogananda, "Second Coming of Christ," *East-West*, June 1932.
30 Yogananda, *East-West*, June 1932.
31 Kriyananda, *Revelations of Christ*, 332.
32 Yogananda, "Vibration," *Inner Culture*, July 1936.

Chapter Four

1 "Interview with Gao Yuan," Shen Yun Performing Arts, https://www.shenyunperformingarts.org/news/view/article/e/QrYhYohmjxM/composer-interview-gao-yuan.html.
2 "How music is used as a weapon of war," CBC Radio, July 17, 2019, https://www.cbc.ca/radio/ideas/the-nerve-pt-3-how-music-is-used-as-a-weapon-in-war-1.5215235#.
3 "About 432 Hz Music: Theory, Science & Benefits," *Mind Vibrations*, https://www.mindvibrations.com/432-hz/. You can listen to nine classical pieces which are known to have calming effects on the brain and nervous system: https://www.cmuse.org/calm-classical-music/.
4 Beethoven and Verdi lower blood pressure," Boon, Maxim, Limelight, 2 July, 2015, https://limelight-arts.com.au/news/beethoven-and-verdi-lower-blood-pressure-new-study-claims/.
5 Kriyananda, *Art as a Hidden Message*, 120.
6 Philosophical Library, 1955; Citadel, 1994. https://www.barnesandnoble.com/w/talks-with-great-composers-arthur-m-abell/1101338887.
7 Kriyananda, *Art as a Hidden Message*, 85.

8 Kriyananda, "Music, Creativity, and Mystical Experience," from a talk by Swami Kriyananda at Ananda World Brotherhood Village, March 1996.
9 Kriyananda, *A Place Called Ananda*, 257.
10 Kriyananda, *Art as a Hidden Message*, 104.
11 Kriyananda, "Music, Creativity, and Mystical Experience."
12 Cooper, Lyz, "Your Healing Voice – The benefits of singing for health and well-being," British Academy of Sound Therapy, https://www.britishacademyofsoundtherapy.com/wp-content/uploads/2020/07/Your-Healing-Voice-Article-sing-for-health-research-3.pdf.
13 "Music as Medicine," John Hopkins Medicine, https://www.hopkinsmedicine.org/center-for-music-and-medicine/music-as-medicine.
14 "17 Surprising Health Benefits of Playing an Instrument," Music Notes, May 6, 2018, https://www.musicnotes.com/now/featured/17-surprising-health-benefits-of-playing-an-instrument/.
15 Galli-Curci, Amelita, "Sing! Oh, Sing!," *East-West*, September-October 1927.
16 Kriyananda, "Music, Creativity, and Mystical Experience."

Chapter Five

1 Yogananda, "Vibratory Healing," *Inner Culture*, September 1936.
2 Kriyananda, *Awaken to Superconsciousness*, 179.
3 Yogananda, "Vibratory Healing," *Inner Culture*, September 1936.
4 Yogananda, "Prelude," *Cosmic Chants*.
5 Kriyananda, *Awaken to Superconsciousness*, 183-184, 179.
6 Kriyananda, *The New Path*, 283.
7 Kriyananda, 279.
8 Yogananda, *Autobiography of a Yogi*, 159.
9 Kriyananda, *Art as a Hidden Message*, 146.
10 One example is a mantra to Lord Shiva often sung on Mahashivaratri: Shivaya Parameshwaraya Chandrashekaraya, Namah Om, Bhavaya Guna Sambhavaya Shiva Tandavaya Namah Om.
11 Kriyananda, Retirement Speech, Portland, Oregon, May 5, 1996.
12 Yogananda, *Autobiography of a Yogi*, 326.
13 Kriyananda, *Awaken to Superconsciousness*, 184.
14 Yogananda, *Autobiography of a Yogi*, 462-463.
15 Yogananda, "Prelude," *Cosmic Chants*, 11.
16 Yogananda, xii.
17 Yogananda. Yogananda recorded his Cosmic Chants on the album "Songs of My Heart," https://bookstore.yogananda-srf.org/product/songs-of-my-heart-2/. Swami Kriyananda spiritualized these chants and recorded some of them in the album "Kriyananda Sings Yogananda," https://www.crystalclarity.com/products/kriyananda-chants-yogananda.
18 Kriyananda, *The Art and Science of Raja Yoga*, 246-247.
19 Kriyananda, *Awaken to Superconsciousness*, 181.
20 Yogananda, "Prelude," *Cosmic Chants*, xi.
21 Yogananda, "Vibratory Healing," *Inner Culture*, September, 1936.
22 Kriyananda, "Whisper to God," unpublished article.
23 Kriyananda, *Awaken to Superconsciousness*, 180.
24 Yogananda, "Prelude," *Cosmic Chants*
25 Yogananda, 52.
26 Kriyananda, *Awaken to Superconsciousness*, 180.
27 Yogananda, *Advanced New Super Cosmic Science Course*, Lesson 1.

28 Yogananda, "Prelude," *Cosmic Chants*, xi.
29 Yogananda, xii.
30 Kriyananda, *Awaken to Superconsciousness*, 180-181.
31 Yogananda, "Vibratory Healing," *Inner Culture*, September 1936.
32 Recordings of many of these chants as well as songs by Kriyananda are available for purchase from Crystal Clarity Publishers, https://www.crystalclarity.com/collections/music; Ananda Sangha Publications, https://www.anandapublications.com; Yogananda Edizioni, https://www.anandaedizioni.it/categoria-prodotto/cd-e-dvd/cd/.
33 Yogananda, *Cosmic Chants*.
34 Yogananda, xii.
35 Kriyananda, *Awaken to Superconsciousness*, 188.
36 Yogananda, "Prelude," *Cosmic Chants*, xi.

Chapter Six

1 Cornell, Joseph Bharat, Crystal Clarity Publishers, *Deep Nature Play: A Guide to Wholeness, Aliveness, Creativity, and Inspired Learning*, https://www.crystalclarity.com/products/deep-nature-play.
2 Cornell, Joseph Bharat, *Flow Learning: Opening Heart and Spirit Through Nature*, Crystal Clarity Publishers, https://www.crystalclarity.com/en-eu/products/flow-learning
3 Witt, Elain, "The Waterfall Effect: Negative Ions Give Positive Results," *Alpenwild*, September 22, 2019, https://switzerlandtravel.swisshikingvacations.com/the-waterfall-effect/.
4 Burch, Kelly, "Thalassotherapy," Business Insider, July 31, 2023, https://www.businessinsider.com/doctors-explain-why-people-feel-better-near-the-ocean-2023-7
5 Hesse, Herman, *Siddhartha*, published in 1922 in German; English publication by New Directions, January 1, 1951.
6 Kriyananda, *The Promise of Immortality*, 336-337.
7 Kriyananda, *The Hindu Way of Awakening*, 69-70.
8 "Health Benefits of Houseplants (13 Plants With Benefits)," Garden for Indoor, https://gardenforindoor.com/health-benefits-of-houseplants.
9 Flower essences based on the spiritual qualities of plants are the subject of the book *The Essential Flower Essence Handbook*, by Lila Devi, https://www.crystalclarity.com/products/the-essential-flower-essence-handbook. Also see https://spirit-in-nature.com in the USA; https://yoganandafloweressences.com in India.
10 Hanson, Kelsey, "4 Surprising Health Benefits of Indoor Fountains," Sunnydaze Decor, https://sunnydazedecor.com/blogs/news/4-surprising-health-benefits-of-indoor-fountains.
11 "The Therapeutic Benefits of Running Water," *Universal Rocks*, February 9, 2019, https://www.universalrocks.com/blog/thetherapeutic-benefits-of-running-water.

Chapter Seven

1 Kriyananda, *Living Wisely, Living Well*, May 5, 65.
2 Mukamal, Reena, "How humans see colors," June 8, 2017, American Academy of Ophthalmology, https://www.aao.org/eye-health/tips-prevention/how-humans-see-in-color. "The visible spectrum for humans falls between ultraviolet light and red light. Scientists estimate that humans can distinguish up to 10 million colors."
3 Pope, Sarah, "The Fascinating Impact of Color on Health," *The Healthy Home Economist*, https://www.thehealthyhomeeconomist.com/the-fascinating-impact-of-color-on-health/.

4 The citations about the quality of colors are from Kriyananda's book, *Living Wisely, Living Well,* for the month of May; *Do It NOW!*; and *A Renunciate Order for the New Age,* Chapter Three.

Chapter Eight

1 Kriyananda, *A Place Called Ananda,* 313.
2 Kriyananda, *Art and Science of Raja Yoga,* Step Three—V. Healing.
3 Holland, Oscar, "Biophilic Skyscraper," October 14, 2022, CNN Style, https://edition.cnn.com/style/article/capitaspring-singapore-skyscraper-biophilic/index.html.
4 Silverman, Sherri, "Vastu," Hindupedia, https://hindupedia.com/en/Vastu.
5 Kriyananda, *A Place Called Ananda,* 312.
6 Kriyananda, *Space, Light, and Harmony: The Story of Crystal Hermitage,* 10.
7 Kriyananda, 46.
8 Kriyananda, *Cities of Light,* 56.
9 Kriyananda, 57.

Chapter Nine

1 Yogananda, "Second Coming of Christ," *Inner Culture,* October-December 1940.
2 Kriyananda, *The Promise of Immortality,* 322-323.
3 Kriyananda, 323.
4 Yogananda, *Autobiography of a Yogi,* 204, 205.
5 Kriyananda, *The Promise of Immortality,* 322.
6 Kriyananda, *Rays of the Same Light,* Week Six, 59.
7 Yogananda, *Autobiography of a Yogi,* 10.
8 Kriyananda, *The Promise of Immortality,* 322.
9 Kriyananda tells stories of saints he met in India in his book, *Visits to Saints of India.*
10 Yogananda, *The Essence of Self-Realization,* 13:2.

Chapter Ten

1 Yogananda, "The Meaning of Lent," *East-West,* January-February 1929.
2 Kriyananda, *The Hindu Way of Awakening,* 32, 38.
3 Yogananda, *Advanced Course on Practical Metaphysics,* Lesson 2.
4 Yogananda, "The Second Coming of Christ," *Inner Culture,* January 1935.
5 "Padre Pio's Celebration of Mass Was a Journey of Faith," Padre Pio da Pietrelcina, https://www.padrepiodapietrelcina.com/en/mass-padre-pio/.
6 Tessione, Paolo, "Padre Pio and the phenomenon of levitation," Io Amo Gesù, October 18, 2019, https://www.ioamogesu.com/padre-pio-e-il-fenomeno-della-levitazione-checose-alcuni-episodi/.
7 Yogananda, *Autobiography of a Yogi,* 336-337.
8 Yogananda, "The Second Coming of Christ," *Inner Culture,* September 1938.
9 Kriyananda, from an unpublished talk, "Pilgrimage to Joy," 1989.
10 Yogananda, "How to Keep the Church Steadfast," *East-West,* September 1933.
11 Detailed descriptions about Kriya can be found in Paramhansa Yogananda's *Autobiography of a Yogi*; in Swami Kriyananda's *The New Path* (references are in the Bibliography); and on these websites: www.ananda.org; www.anandaeurope.org; and www.anandaindia.org.
12 Yogananda, "Unique Methods of Spiritual Healing," New Super Cosmic Science Course, Lesson 2.
13 Yogananda, "Meditations and Affirmations," *Inner Culture,* October-December 1949.

Chapter Eleven

1 Kriyananda, *The Art and Science of Raja Yoga*, 298.
2 In 1939 Semyon and Valeria Kirlian developed a high-frequency, high-voltage instrument that captures the light produced by photons emitted by the coronal discharge of objects.
"Kirlian photography," Wikipedia https://en.wikipedia.org/wiki/Kirlian_photography.
3 Kriyananda, *Awaken to Superconsciousness*, 165-166.
4 Kriyananda, *The Art and Science of Raja Yoga*, 295.
5 Kriyananda, *Awaken to Superconsciousness*, 173-174.
6 Kriyananda, *The Art and Science of Raja Yoga*, 295.
7 Kriyananda, *Patanjali Demystified*, 1-29.
8 Kriyananda, *Awaken to Superconsciousness*, 174.
9 Kriyananda, 175.
10 A recording of this mantra is available from www.crystalclarity.com; www.anandapublications.com; and www.anandaedizioni.it/.
11 Yogananda, *Advanced New Super Cosmic Science Course*, Lesson 5.
12 Kriyananda, *Awaken to Superconsciousness*, 175.
13 Kriyananda, *Conversations with Yogananda* No. 421.
14 Kriyananda, *Awaken to Superconsciousness*, 175.
15 Kriyananda, *The Art and Science of Raja Yoga*, 295.
16 Yogananda, "Acquiring Magnetism," *Inner Culture*, July 1941.
17 Kriyananda, *Awaken to Superconsciousness*, 170-171, 175.
18 Kriyananda, *Awaken to Superconsciousness*, 175, 176.
19 Yogananda, "Spiritualizing Astrology," *Inner Culture*, April 1941.
20 Yogananda, *Autobiography of a Yogi*, 164-165.
21 Yogananda, *The Essence of Self-Realization*, 10:21.
22 Kriyananda, *The Art and Science of Raja Yoga*, 295-296.

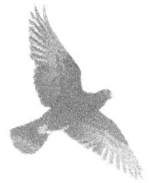

EPILOGUE
TRANSITION AND TRANSCENDENCE

I AM THY BIRD OF PARADISE WISHING TO FLY IN THY ASTRAL AIRPLANE
~ *Paramhansa Yogananda* ~

Thine astral airplane of earthly parting came to take my soul away. I wondered through what strange skies I was to soar, and to what lands I was to travel.

I asked the mystic Pilot of Cosmic Law whither I was going. The Silent One answered, soundlessly:

"I am the Pilot of Life, mistakenly called the terrible Death by ignorant earth-folk. I am thy brother, uplifter, redeemer, friend-unloader of thy gross burden of body-troubles. I come to fetch thee away from the valley of thy broken dreams to the highland of light, where poisonous vapors of sorrow can never climb.

"I have mercilessly broken thy cage of flesh-attachment, that thy soul-bird may be free. I have broken thy chains of disease and mental fears. Thy long imprisonment behind the bars of bones made thee unwillingly become used to the cage. Thou didst want thy freedom always. Now, why art thou fearfilled, when thou hast won thy long-craved freedom?

"O bird of paradise! Hop into My plane of omnipresence! Fold thy long-fluttering wings and restfully ride with me, anywhere, everywhere, in thine ethereal home!" [1]

EPILOGUE CHAPTER ONE

Overcoming the fear of death

> So when this corruptible shall have put on incorruption, and this mortal shall have put on immortality, then shall be brought to pass the saying that is written, Death is swallowed up in victory. O death, where is thy sting? O grave, where is thy victory?
> —Holy Bible: First Corinthians. 15:54-55[*]

> This Self is not born, nor does it perish. Self-existent, it continues its existence forever. It is birthless, eternal, changeless, and ever the same. The Self is not slain when the body dies.... Just as a person removes a worn-out garment and dons a new one, so the soul living in a physical body (removes and) discards it when it becomes outworn, and replaces it with a new one. Weapons cannot cut the soul; fire cannot burn it; water cannot drown it; wind cannot wither it away! The soul is never touched; it is immutable, all-pervading, calm, unshakable; its existence is eternal
> —The Bhagavad Gita 2:20, 22-24[†]

> Die happily and look forward to taking up a new and better form. Like the sun, only when you set in the west can you rise in the east.[1] —Rumi

---

[*] This and all Bible citations are from the King James Bible.
[†] This and all Bhagavad Gita citations are from Yogananda, *The Bhagavad Gita According to Paramhansa Yogananda*.

People formerly believed that the mystery of life after death would never be solved, because no one had ever returned from the grave to tell their story. But with the publication of Dr. Raymond Moody's book *Life After Life*,[2] the veil was finally lifted. Moody's interviews with patients who had survived clinical death reveal detailed descriptions of their experiences. Since then, millions have reported "near-death experiences (NDEs). Extensive research has identified some common characteristics of these experiences.[3]

1. Sudden peace and relief from pain.
2. Perception of a relaxing sound or other-worldly music.
3. The subjects' consciousness or spirit ascending above their body, sometimes viewing medical professionals' attempts at resuscitation.
4. The person's spirit leaving the earthly realm and ascending rapidly through a tunnel of light in a universe of darkness.
5. Arriving at a brilliant "heavenly place."
6. Being met by "people of the light," usually deceased friends and family, in a joyous reunion.
7. Meeting a deity, often in a form from their religious tradition, or as an angelic being that emitted pure love and light.
8. Undergoing an instantaneous life review, and understanding how all of the good and bad they had done had affected themselves and others.
9. Returning to their earthly body and life, either because they were told that it was not their time to die, or because they were given a choice and decided to return for the benefit of their family and loved ones.

Happy Winingham, whose story will be told in greater detail in the next chapter, was in a severe automobile accident in which she suffered a heart attack and died while she was being transported to the hospital. She later recalled her death experience.

I went through a tunnel of light and emerged into a big, open space where I was surrounded by a powerful presence. This presence consisted of many souls and emanated pure light, pure golden warmth, pure nurturing comfort, and an overwhelming feeling of love. It seemed that I had merged with all these souls. We were all one and yet individual, too. Nothing else existed; nothing else mattered. It felt like home.... I am no longer afraid.... death is merely a transition, an opportunity for joyous freedom.[4]

After-death experiences are reported not only by pious people, but also by those who have done things in their lives of which they were not proud. In Dr. Moody's study, similar experiences were reported by a professional assassin, a person who had attempted suicide, and many who had caused harm to others. As a result of their experiences, all of the subjects no longer feared death, having realized what the Bible and Bhagavad Gita describe as the immortality of the soul. Upon returning, they were able to understand the deeper meaning and purpose of their lives.

These studies confirm the experience of Paramhansa Yogananda and of the spiritual masters of many traditions.

> **Death gives new robes to the Soul actors,
> in which to play new dramas on the stage of Life.
> Death, above all else, is a transition to a better
> land, a change of residence. Let us see it as
> a door through which bravely-marching Souls
> of earthly Life can enter to find the all-alluring,
> all-charming region of our ever-luminous,
> ever-peaceful Common Cosmic Home.
> Mortal fears, heartaches, dreams, and illusions
> fade, and the darkness of death changes into
> another infinitely more beautiful universe.[5]**

Yogananda also refers to the sound that many people experience as they are propelled through a tunnel.

The slipping of the electrical body from the physical body gives birth to the hum of released vita-electrons. This Cosmic uplifting sound, every Soul, virtuous or sinful, of necessity must astrally hear after death, during the transition from the physical to the Astral world.[6]

The secret of immortality

We need not wait for the end of this earthly life to experience our immortality. These words by Swami Kriyananda are meant to help us embrace our identity as the deathless soul.

You are not your body. You are not your thoughts, your desires, your changing personality. Your body has a certain age, but you, yourself, have no age! Your body may tire or become unwell, but you yourself, the fatigueless soul, cannot tire, can never know disease!

Tell yourself always, "I am a child of eternity!" Don't be identified with your outward form, nor with change, but live in timelessness. It is our identity with change that creates the illusion of passing time. Feel that, through all outward changes, you, the immortal soul, remain the same. Death itself will be but one more change; be not identified with it. Then, when death comes, you shall rise in eternal freedom! [7]

The affirmation that accompanies this excerpt, when practiced on waking, before sleep, and after meditating, holds a power to replace the fear of death with the hope of life everlasting.*

* See Volume Two, Part VIII for details on how to practice affirmations effectively.

Affirmation

**I am a child of eternity! I am ageless.
I am deathless. I am the changeless Spirit
at the heart of all mutation!**

In addition to *affirming* our immortality, in deep meditation we can we realize it as an actual experience.

> Make a stronger effort to contact God through deep meditation, and get acquainted with the forgotten, deathless, indestructible real Soul which is hidden behind the false pleasure-infested, perishable, pretending-to-be-your-own, body.[8]

> For in deep meditation the soul merges into that light. The long tunnel, yogis explain, is the spine, through which the energy and consciousness must pass before one can leave the body by the doorway of the spiritual eye—whether temporarily, in ecstasy, or finally, in death. St. Paul described this experience also. "I assure you," he wrote, "by the certainty of Jesus Christ which we possess, I die daily."
> (I Corinthians, 15:31)
>
> Deep meditation resembles the actual death experience, *with this important exception: One can return from meditation at will.* In deep meditation, as also in death, the energy and consciousness rise through the tunnel of the spine, and become centered in the brain.[9]

Paramhansa Yogananda taught meditation techniques* that give us an experience of the freedom and bliss of the deathless state.

> The Bliss acquired by meditation becomes a permanent mansion of the soul, which not even the most-dreaded death can destroy.[10]

---

* For residential and online courses in meditation, visit: https://anandaindia.org/meditation/; https://www.ananda.org/meditation/; https://corsi.ananda.it/en/category/0000027-meditation/.

EPILOGUE CHAPTER TWO

Give Up or Fight

> We must never give up even though we are old, discouraged, and at death's door. We must try to improve every minute of our existence, for life continues after death into the better land of the Astral plane, and into new, encouraging surroundings on the physical plane.[1]
> —YOGANANDA

> The consciousness one brings to death determines his future existence—whether in this world, in a higher world, or in eternity.[2]
> —KRIYANANDA

Illness — especially serious long-term illness, chronic disease, or degenerative conditions — confronts us with a challenge: Will we passively accept our "fate" and allow the disease to run its course, or should we instead use our full willpower, faith, and intelligence at least to put up a good fight, if not to eliminate the condition?

During fleeting illnesses such as a cold, flu, headache, or gastric disturbance, we can generally apply our intelligence and energy to relieve the symptoms and accelerate a healing. But when we are faced with a chronic or potentially fatal disease, we will need to dig deep to discover our hidden powers.

Swami Kriyananda answered someone who asked this personal question: *"How much effort should I put forth to remain alive?"*

> Think of what a job it is to be reborn and
> come back again as a baby, then to grow up,
> and then take who knows how many years before
> you remember your spiritual aspiration once
> again, and decide to take that responsibility
> seriously. Think of the risks involved, also,
> of further detours and of consequent pain!
> I suggest that, as long as you feel able to make a
> spiritual effort, you do your best to stay alive now
> and keep working toward your salvation.[3]

Some people are able to fully recover from an incurable disease, as we see in the very first story of this trilogy, "Live or Die."* This story tells how Happy Winingham responded after she was diagnosed with an incurable and fatal disease.

❋ Happy again ❋

Her name suited her perfectly – Happy! Full of energy and creatively gifted, Happy delighted in her friends, who felt uplifted in her presence and were infected by her natural enthusiasm for life.

Happy was passionate about sharing and serving. She loved theater, music, and dance, and she wrote, directed, and performed in plays about spiritually inspiring historical figures.

Uncharacteristically, Happy began to feel her energy flagging. Where she had been enthusiastically engaged, she now felt tired and less interested. When mysterious aches and pains appeared while she trained to run a marathon, she sought medical help and was subjected to a broad range of tests. No one could have suspected the diagnosis: Happy had AIDS. The doctors suspected that the virus had entered her body years earlier. Long dormant, it had now become active.

---

* See page 5-6 in Volume One.

Life-saving medications were still in the experimental stages, and the doctors told Happy that she could expect to live perhaps eighteen months. She was uncertain how to respond – should she accept the diagnosis and prepare to leave this world, or should she fight hard to prolong her life? She asked her spiritual guide, Swami Kriyananda, for his counsel.

"If you die, you'll just have to start over in a new incarnation," he told her. "It may take you a long time to get to where you are now. If it were I, I would keep trying to live until I couldn't meditate anymore, or until I felt that the treatments or the body itself were an insurmountable obstacle to spiritual progress.

"You have a wealth of techniques in Yogananda's teachings that you already know. Use them: deepen your meditation, use the affirmations, do the Energy Recharging exercises more often and more conscientiously. Chant, pray, and find ways to share your journey with others."

His advice was a great comfort. By following his instructions, she became Happy again. During the ten remaining years of her life, Happy progressed remarkably in her meditations. She chanted, and she sang affirmations from Yogananda's poems and writings. Regular practice of the Energization Exercises built her body's immunity, revitalizing the cells. There were ups and downs, during which she was occasionally at death's door. But when she was strong, she shared her remarkable journey with others through her play, *The Ribbon Dance* which she performed for AIDS awareness and support groups around the country, bringing hope, comfort, and joy to thousands, and receiving numerous awards for her work with AIDS awareness in high schools.

To friends and strangers alike, Happy became an embodiment of a favorite affirmation she had composed: ***"God's power, vitality, good health and strength, flow through me, flow through me."*** [4]

✵ LIVING GRACEFULLY ✵
WITH AN ILLNESS

It was strange, unexpected, and humanly unpredictable: I have multiple sclerosis, a degenerative autoimmune disease that cannot currently be cured.

One afternoon, going up the stairs to meditate, I couldn't put my right foot down because I felt a sharp pain. I did my meditation, hoping that it was just a strained muscle. But afterward it was the same – I couldn't walk. I went to the emergency room, where an MRI showed plaque deposits in some parts of my brain and along my spine, a sure indication of MS.

At the time of the diagnosis, I had been engaged in spiritual practices for three years. I was meditating, energizing, participating in yoga classes, and creating space in my life for the search for God.

I was, and still am, a civil rights lawyer and lecturer in law and communication, as well as a coach with a transpersonal orientation. Freelancing gives me the opportunity to combine my work life, which is necessary for my livelihood, with my spiritual life, which is necessary to answer the existential question of my life: what did I come to this earth to do? I am finding the answer: to return to God.

You could say that I was prepared for this illness, and in many ways I was. I knew that I had serious inner work to do. I understood the nature of duality and the law of karma, and this kept me from being angry. During the Covid isolation period, I was able to spend time in silence and meditation, reading the lives of the saints and watching spiritual teachings on the internet. I was able to work remotely as a teacher and counselor, which opened channels that I continue to use.

At first I hoped that everything would go back to the way it had been, like a normal illness. But as the years have passed, I have come to understand how to accept the situation and teach myself to live with it. The pains are signals that I need to adapt the rhythm of my life. When I feel pain, I chant Aum and pray, and the pain lessens, or at least I am comforted in knowing that one day it will pass because I will have cleared the negative karma. I have learned to be flexible in my daily routine. I can concentrate for about an hour and a half, and then I need to rest a while before engaging in work or spiritual activities.

I can honestly say that I am grateful for my situation, which is teaching me what I need to learn: non-attachment to my role, to things, to habits, to people, to everything that is considered normal in life. Because I have to stay in a moderate climate, I change houses five times a year. I am able to move with few material things, and I am learning to adapt to the life of each place, to the people and their habits. I have few friends, because I am constantly leaving them to move to another suitable location. It is a great test of loneliness, but I have learned that soul friends are everywhere.

Every day is a divine gift for me. The greatest gift of all is my ability to smile and trust that even though my body may never be healed, I have faith in the divine plan, and my soul is moving closer and closer to God.
–**Federica**, *Italy*

EPILOGUE CHAPTER THREE

Letting Go

> Love not your body-prison...Why tie
> the infinite soul to a bony post of flesh?
> Let go, cut the cords of flesh-consciousness,
> body-attachment, hunger, pleasure,
> pain, and bodily and mental discomforts.
> Relax; loosen the soul from the grip of
> the body. Let not the heaving breath
> remind you of the bars of the body.
> Sit still in breathless silence, expecting
> every minute to make the dash for
> freedom into the Infinite.[1]
>
> —YOGANANDA
>
> As you are not likely to identify yourself
> with one breath, or with one day in your life,
> so, tell yourself, this identity you've
> accepted with this one body is illusory also.
> You, in your true essence, are eternal! [2]
>
> —KRIYANANDA
>
> Those who at death can fix their minds
> at the point between the eyebrows,
> calling deeply to God in their hearts,
> will go to Him.[3]
>
> —KRIYANANDA

When our life's mission is finished, or when it is no longer possible to make progress, it will be time to move on.

> Death comes to a dutiful Soul as its
> promotion to a higher state. It comes to
> an unsuccessful Soul to give it another
> chance in a different environment.
> The wise man experiences through death
> an infinitely better, safer haven.[4]

Death may arrive unexpectedly, even in the prime of life. In that moment, all of our activities, our friends and family, and our desires and aspirations will vanish, replaced by either a feeling of profound loss, or a sense of relief and freedom.

> Death is an ordeal everyone must face...
> The sudden realization that everything one has
> known, all the people to whom one has related,
> all the work one has set into motion,
> the many people who are—for good or for ill—
> dependent on one, all the things one may
> have left undone, and above all the sum total
> of one's bad and/or virtuous deeds: The loss
> of all these must be faced and accepted as a fact,
> then relinquished into eternity and turned
> to some fresh resolution for the future.[5]

Whether death calls us suddenly or at the end of a long illness, we will want to prepare for this important final appointment.

> The most important moment of life is, in a very
> true sense, its last moment. For death is when we
> take our final exam. The thought uppermost in
> the mind at that time will determine whether our
> future takes us upward, or sideways, or downward:

upward, toward greater spiritual clarity and freedom; sideways, toward further involvement in desires and worldly attachments; or (the least fortunate) downward, toward greater darkness, confusion, and ignorance. The Bhagavad Gita, India's best-loved scripture, says that if our last thought is of God, it is to Him we will go.[6]

A practice that Swami Kriyananda used, with the following variations, contributed to his complete sense of freedom at his passing. You might like to incorporate these practices in your nightly routine.

To make them as effective as possible, first make a mental or physical list of your attachments to people, places, projects, responsibilities, opinions, your hopes for the future, and your unfulfilled desires. You can keep the list in your meditation room and/or on your bedstand.

VISUALIZATION
Release Your Attachments

Nothing is ours. No one belongs to us. Mentally, we should make a bonfire of our love for God, and cast into it all attachments, all desires, all hopes and disappointments. It helps mentally to examine one's heart every evening, and liberate it anew of all desires. Pluck out from your heart any burrs of new attachments that you find clinging there. Cast them joyfully into the fire of devotion.

Pray to God energetically, "I destroy all my attachments. They are no longer mine, Lord. I am free in Thee!"[7]

✻

Every night think of all your desires, all
your attachments, all your involvements and
responsibilities. Mentally build a bonfire and
cast them into that fire, recognizing that you
could die this very night and you want to die free.
Give everything it back to God—it doesn't belong
to you. The more you live that way, the more
you will find (a) sense of inner freedom.[8]

※

Make it a point, every night before you
fall asleep, to check the feelings in your heart.
See whether any burrs of attachment still
cling there, affixed by desires you may have
developed during the day. If you find any such
'burr,' mentally build a fire and cast that burr
into it. Watch with a smile of relief as
each burr disintegrates to ashes.[9]

※

Every night when you go to sleep,
give everything back to God. It helps even
to build a fire mentally and cast into that
fire every attachment, every desire, every
self-definition. Say, "I belong to you, God.[10]

※

If you feel any attachments, visualize a cord
leading out to them from your heart.
With a sharp knife mentally sever that cord,
or, if it seems thick, hack at it with an axe.
Feel every attachment being cut off, leaving
you with the blessing of inner freedom.[11]

※

> Meditate sometimes on the freedom of the vast blue sky. Visualize a balloon. Think of it as symbolizing all your likes and dislikes, all your worldly desires and attachments. Release the string of ego by which you hold this balloon in your grasp. Watch the balloon soar upward, growing smaller and smaller with distance—until only the vast blue sky is left.
>
> Or see the balloon sailing for a time in the skies of divine freedom; consider how insignificant it seems, alone in infinity. Then mentally prick the balloon, and watch it vanish instantaneously into the infinite, blue void. You are that void! [12]

An early "Life Review"

Those who have had near-death experiences nearly always describe the "life review" as an important stage in the soul's passage to the next world. Swami Kriyananda suggests that we conduct such an evaluation *before* we die. Below are some items on his "final exam" checklist* that you might like to consider, to keep your life moving in a positive direction and to prepare yourself for the moment of transition.

- Go over your life up to the present moment. Concentrate on the happy times, rather than on the sad… Do not avoid reflecting on the mistakes you may have made. Try, instead, to view those mistakes positively.
- If you remember having ever hurt anybody, or perhaps having acted unjustly toward him, mentally send him blessings. Visualize him (or her) floating in the ocean of God's bliss.

---

* Kriyananda's article, "The Final Exam," is included in the online Appendices.

- If ever you've desecrated your own higher self-image, face that memory frankly, but calmly and dispassionately. Don't seek justification for your mistakes. And don't beat yourself mentally and emotionally for having done wrong. Rather, say to God, "It was You, Lord, acting through my ignorance. ... I won't cling to that folly any longer. I release it!"
- If ever you have spoken or acted inconsiderately toward another human being, even perhaps only in haste, recreate that scene in your mind, and then ask God to bless everyone whom you may ever have hurt. Project rays of love and bliss outward from your heart to all who have ever had to bear the brunt of your anger, impatience, unkindness, or cruelty.
- If ever you've held a negative thought toward anyone...raise your feelings to a level where you find yourself thinking of that person with kindness.
- If ever you've spoken critically of, or mocked anyone, even mentally, offer him now your heartfelt kindness and good wishes for his eventual wisdom and inner freedom.
- Pray for all beings. Bless them in God's light. Send them His love. Reflect that everyone on earth, no matter how deeply deluded he may be, is, in his own way, seeking eternal bliss. Reflect also that it is *everyone's destiny* to find that bliss, no matter how long a journey it is. [13]

When death approaches

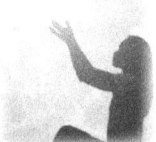

We cannot always know when death is approaching. Those who are suffering from a debilitating illness or a terminal disease will have the opportunity to complete their life's work consciously and constructively. Doctors will sometimes advise terminal patients to "get their affairs in order." It's good advice for settling not only our practical accounts but also, and even more importantly, our spiritual ones.

In the "Live or Die" story, we saw how a patient who had received a "death sentence" decided to put his life in order by doing the things he had always dreamed of doing – he would check off the items on his "bucket list." Paula's story tells how she spent her last days in a manner that continues to inspire those who knew her, or who hear her story.

✻ Paula's Farewell Party* ✻

The doctors said that Paula had three days to live, and so it turned out. The operation to excise the tumor was abandoned – the tumor had surrounded her heart and now was inoperable. Her many years on the spiritual path, and a previous close call with death, had prepared her. But how many of us are truly ready to hear that final news?

Paula called her close friends to join her. Many stayed in the hospital all day, while some slept overnight on the floor. Her brother arrived from Italy, and they relived their life together, growing up as close friends. Paula had followed her brother to the spiritual path, eventually becoming the leader of an Ananda community. As they touched on their shared memories, it was clear that Paula was letting go of each experience, and each person.

She called many friends, some in other countries, to tell them how much she appreciated their friendship and the things they had done together. There was never a note of regret in her voice, not even for the relationships that had not been harmonious. She touched them and let them go, like balloons set free to soar in the sky until they disappeared in the sunlight.

The atmosphere in her room was permeated with a serene joy, even a sanctity. She had a kind word or a message of love for each visitor. Paula would not let anyone be sad. Food was arranged for everyone. Paula had always enjoyed a cup of good coffee, and she smiled and laughed as she sipped and shared her gift of friendship with everyone. The doctors brought her flowers, the nurses were sad when their shift ended, and everyone loved being in her room. Hour after hour the layers of desires and attachments fell away, until all that remained was who Paula had always been: a person who loved and cared about everyone, the personification of sweetness.

As the end neared, Paula asked those present for their help. "This is hard. I don't know how to do this. Chant

---

* Paula's story is told in Nalini Graeber's *Transition with Grace*, 262-273.

with me. You have to help me." When she was assured that everyone was present, she started to tear off the petals of flowers and hand them out so that there would be a ceremony at the end. Her brother observed that from that point she saw him no longer as her older brother but as a soul. She removed the oxygen tubes from her nose and consciously left her body while her friends chanted Aum to send her soul into the light.

With joyful tears they sang Ananda's farewell song:

> Go with love, may joyful blessings
> Speed you safely on your way.
> May God's light expand within you.
> May we be one in that light someday.

There are many lessons we can glean from the grace with which Paula completed her life. She reviewed her life in her own breathtakingly sweet way, bringing light and freedom to each experience and 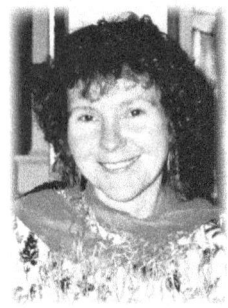 freeing herself from emotional attachments. She thanked those who had helped her, and asked forgiveness for any conscious or unintended harm she might have done. She kept her friends close and asked them in all simplicity and humility for their help. It was Paula herself who created an atmosphere of joy so that others would not experience sadness at her passing.

At her memorial service, Swami Kriyananda said: "There have been very few experiences in my life that can be compared with the inspiration of Paula's passing. It was beautiful. It was filled with joy. It was filled with humor. It was filled with happiness. She went in a spirit of great freedom."

Closure

We want to prepare to experience those final days and hours, to the extent we are able, in an uplifted state of consciousness, and in self-offering to God.

The thoughts with which one leaves his body
have a great influence on his future state...
Feelings of guilt will hinder you from making
further progress, acting as affirmations of failure.
Cast guilt, therefore, from your heart...
say to God, simply, "Take me as I am, Lord.
I know, now, that I want you alone...."

Mostly, dwell on happy thoughts. Tell yourself,
and tell God, "This life has been a dance in
Your bliss. Even the hard tests You've sent me have
helped me. I've learned so much from them;
I'm grateful for all of them; they have given me
priceless insights. But now, Lord, I offer everything
up to You. It was Your life I lived, not mine.
Let me rest eternally, from now on, in Your love...."

Dwell on thoughts of God's eternal love for you,
and for all creatures. Dwell more on His
forgiveness: on His utter *acceptance* of you as,
through all eternity, His very own.[14]

Affirmation

Nothing on earth can hold me! My soul,
like a weightless balloon, soars upward
through skies of eternal freedom![15]

EPILOGUE CHAPTER FOUR

Helping a Dying Friend

> Angels visit hospitals to give strength and comfort to those who suffer physically. Sometimes, they heal those for whom the doctors have abandoned all hope. Often, they help to ease the dying in their struggles to win release from their physical bodies.[1]
>
> —KRIYANANDA

If we are called to help someone in the final stages of their life, we may discover that it can be an occasion for deepening the relationship, for playing an important role in the person's life, or for fulfilling a karmic debt, as well as for facing our own fears and limitations.

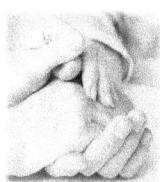

If the situation stretches over months or years, our involvement may become unbearably stressful, and even injurious to our health. How can we know the best course, in the innumerable moments when we will have to make decisions large or small? What is the extent of our responsibility? How can we keep ourselves from becoming mentally and emotionally depleted?

By approaching these situations from a superconscious perspective, we can be sure that if the universe places us in such a situation, it is because we have something to offer, and also something to gain. Even doctors do not have the ultimate responsibility for the lives of others: the karma of each person is supreme. It is enacted through the instruments of health care providers, and the friends and loved ones who have been divinely chosen to play a role, giving and gaining. To play our role well, we need to be centered in the present moment, in a calm and intuitive frame of mind, our bodies charged with vital energy and our minds clear and alert.

Whether or not to inform those dying of their condition, and to what extent, will be the doctors' responsibility. It will also depend on their wishes. If you are a primary caregiver or close friend, you may have to ask with urgency and intensity for inner, divine guidance regarding whether or not to encourage them to keep trying to heal, or to help them prepare for the soul's transition from the physical body. Something to keep in mind is that their soul will be aware of what is needed, and that it is trying to communicate it to them, and possibly to you as well. Remaining in a calm and energized state when you are with them will help you read the signs and receive the messages.

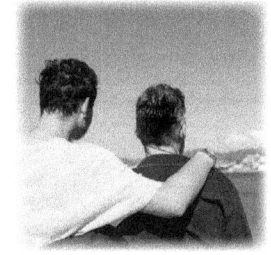

Much can be learned during the final stages of life, even if physical healing is no longer possible. If the dying person is spiritually prepared, we can help them use whatever spiritual practices they may know to help them meet the situation with inner spiritual strength. We can also help them avoid negative thoughts, regrets, and recriminations by helping them stay focused on the happy moments of their lives, and encouraging them to express gratitude to the people who have loved and supported them.

The doctors' prognosis may not be infallible, as we saw in the story "Live or Die." Our circumstances also can change through the application of divine laws, such as prayer, affirmation, Life Force Recharging, and meditation. If they are receptive, you can help them stimulate their willpower to magnetize divine grace. Swami Sri Yukteswar said: **"Everything in future will improve if you are making a spiritual effort now."** [2]

Here is a true story about helping a dying friend recover.

❈ Deathbed reprieve ❈

Sarah is a magnetic soul, bursting with energy and vitality. At the supermarket one day she met her friend Cristina, who was stricken with cancer. Sarah offered to show Cristina the benefits of the Life Force Recharging Exercises and how they help us tap into a higher source of healing energy. But Cristina wasn't attracted, and Sarah didn't insist.

Over the ensuing years they lost sight of each other. Then Sarah received a call from Cristina's husband, who told her that Cristina was dying and was asking for her.

Sarah rushed be by her longtime friend's side. Although Cristina was confined to her bed, Sarah guided her slowly and patiently through the process of opening the doorway of the medulla oblongata and using her imagination to send the healing life force from that point to twenty parts of her body. Though Cristina's willpower was weakened by her illness, Sarah's powerful positive magnetism was able to stimulate her friend's will bit by bit, more and more.

Cristina was no longer able to tense her muscles, but she did her best to place her attention on the part to be recharged. Often, she would fall asleep, while Sarah stayed by her side, praying for her. When Cristina awoke they would start where they had left off: "Tense the left foot, now the right one..."

Sarah continued to help her friend in this way for seven hours, and when she felt that the Lord had accomplished what He wanted through her, she said goodbye, leaving Cristina feeling deeply at peace.

Late that night, Cristina's husband called, and in a state of euphoria announced that his wife had gotten out of bed! Shortly after, she recovered completely.

Cristina had been given another chance. She deliberately and consciously recalled when and why she had come to the point of dying, and her feelings of regret for not having paid attention to the important things in her life. She had given too much time to her work, to worries, and to material things, and there had been a sense of emptiness.

She now began to devote quality time to her husband and two children, giving them her full attention and love. She improved her relationships with her colleagues at work, and generally began to give greater consideration to others.

She lived three more years, cancer-free, then she died of a heart attack. We must all die; what matters is how we have lived. When Cristina left her body, she was content, knowing that she had accomplished something of real value. —**Told by Premi**, *Ananda Assisi.* (*The story is true, but the women's names have been changed.*)

※ ※ ※

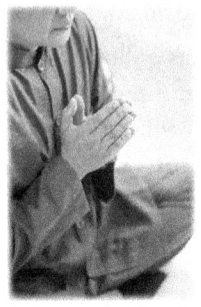

How can prayer help them?

Spiritual masters possess a power to intercede and change the course of our destiny. Yogananda repeatedly saved the life of his advanced disciple, Sister Gyanamata. Although it is unlikely that our prayers would have such power, are they therefore useless? Whatever the condition of the physical body, the soul is ever awake and aware, and it will be comforted and encouraged by our prayers that the person be infused with the wisdom and courage either to fight on or to go into the Light.

Create a calm, uplifting environment

Whatever a person's faith or doubts, a comforting environment will ease their transition. It will be easier to arrange the environment for them in a private home or hospice, but it may even be possible to an extent in a hospital. In addition to ensuring that they are physically comfortable, there are many things we can do to support them.

- Make sure there is adequate and appropriate lighting, avoiding dark and depressing atmospheres.
- Keep them engaged for as long as possible in whatever activities they can manage.
- Provide soothing music, appropriate to their tastes. If they are sharing the room with others, arrange for them to have comfortable headphones. If they have a religious or spiritual background, choose chants, affirmations, prayers (for example, inspiring recitations of the *Hail Mary* if they are Catholic) or mantras from their spiritual tradition. A continuously playing recording of the chanting of the cosmic

vibration of Aum, even if barely audible, can charge the environment with refined vibrations and serve as a bridge between the physical and astral worlds.

- If they are able to watch videos, make sure they have a good screen, and help them choose uplifting programs. The film *Life After Life**, that includes interviews with people who have experienced dying, could help them face their own transition with serenity.

- Read aloud from uplifting materials, and provide positive or entertaining audiobooks.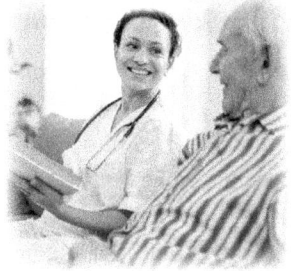

- Arrange for them to have regular massage treatments from loving hands, especially on their feet, hands, and head.

- Keep your conversation with them positive, by helping them remember happy times and encouraging them to express their gratitude for the good things and people in their life. If it's appropriate for them and yourself, talk to them of the beauty of the life that awaits them.

- Invite friends to visit; and if the dying person follows a spiritual tradition, arrange for small groups of their friends to sing, chant, pray, and meditate with them.

Stay fit

To be of the greatest possible help, you should be calm and energized. Fatigue, burnout, and depression are always a risk without a deliberate effort to prevent them. *As guidelines:*

- Eat regular, nutritious meals.
- Have daily exercise, outdoors in the fresh air.
- Do the Life Force Full Body Recharge† whenever your energy begins to flag.

* Available for view at https://www.youtube.com/watch?v=z56u4wMxNlg.
† See Volume One, Part IV.

- Take breaks while they are sleeping or when others are with them, so you can detach emotionally. Taking a full day or a weekend off when possible will help you keep going.
- Be sure to have all of the medical, mental health, and social service resources required, and be in touch with trusted friends for your own support.

During sleep or unconsciousness

We should be careful with our spoken words in the presence of a dying person, even if they are sleeping or in a coma. The physical senses close down as the body approaches death, but the sense of hearing is the last to go. The soul's awareness isn't limited to the physical senses, and they can sense our thoughts. Praying for people in this state can make a profound psychological and emotional difference.

As long as the soul inhabits the body, there may be a possibility that the person's willpower can be awakened to help reverse the process. Yogananda tells this story.

> **The sense of hearing is the last to leave the consciousness.... That is why it is extremely unwise to even whisper within the hearing of a dying person: "All is over; he is about to die."**
>
> **Once two students, a brother and sister, had a singular experience. The sister lay dying in a room, with her brother and doctors in attendance. When the brother left the room for a moment to get some water, the doctors exclaimed: "All is over; her pulse has failed." There was a spasm and she lay apparently dead. As soon as the brother came back, he ordered everybody out of the room. He then shook his sister vigorously, crying: "Sister, your teacher told you to make the effort and you will live."**

In a few moments her pulse came back; she breathed, sat up, and told of the following experience: "My entire body was paralyzed, but I could hear the footsteps of my brother leaving the room. I was making an effort to stir the life force in my inert body by will, but as soon as I heard the doctors say: 'All is over,' I gave up the will to live and I witnessed a complete inertia in my outer muscles and internal organs, and a blinding flash of light in the head, followed by intense darkness, which I could see. But again, in this state I heard my brother coming toward me, and as soon as he urged me to use my will power and wake up, I revived my will to live, and here I am. My consciousness was able to resuscitate itself into the inner organs, muscles, and the senses, which had become inert before." [3]

Swami Kriyananda suggests yet another way to help a dying person.

Q. *If someone sinks into a coma, or seems perhaps dead already, might it help him to chant AUM in his presence?*

A. Yes, definitely. Chant softly, especially in the right ear. Yogananda said the sense of hearing is the last to go. A person may appear dead, but may not yet have withdrawn completely from the body. By chanting AUM, or by calling to him in the right ear, you may actually bring him back to life.[4]

If you are certain that the situation is irreversible, you may be able to help them overcome the fear of dying by gently guiding them to release their soul from the prison of the body.

> Place your finger on his forehead at a point midway between the eyebrows. This is the seat of will power, concentration, and ecstasy in the body. Direct energy through your finger to that point, and try to draw that person's energy up in focus there.[5]

> Anyone dear to the person who is dying, will do well...to place his forefinger on the person's forehead, at the point midway between the eyebrows, and, sending energy there, encourage him (or her) to focus the body's energy completely at that point.[6]

We can gain immeasurably by caring for a dying friend, by finding our inner strength, facing our fears, and taking full advantage of the opportunity to give our unconditional love.

If you happen upon an accident where someone is unconscious and may be dying, or is already dead, you can, if you feel so inspired, place your index finger at their spiritual eye and pray for their soul. We may never know, and can only imagine, the solace that this gesture of selfless love may give them.

Reciprocity

We can become so absorbed in our role as a caregiver that we fail to see how much the situation and the person for whom we are caring have to offer. Every relationship involves give and take, and the delicacy of this situation can bring rewards not otherwise available. Victoria's story is a touching conclusion to this Epilogue and to the entire *Healing with Life Force* trilogy.

❈ BEING HELPED BY A DYING FRIEND ❈

She was ninety-nine, with dementia, but for much of the time Nancy's mind was crystal clear, her humor was delightful, and her wisdom was deep.

I was her companion and caregiver during the months before her passing. Our time together enriched my life immeasurably.

In the afternoon, I would do the Energization Exercises while she watched me. She was enthusiastic about the exercises – she would wait expectantly, with beaming eyes, for me to begin.

I taught her several of the exercises, and she loved to practice them. She was able to feel energy entering through the medulla oblongata and flowing down to her hand as she tensed and relaxed it. She marveled as she watched the muscles vibrate, as if she were observing a masterpiece.

Watching her practice was energizing for me as well – to witness the devout concentration and joy with which she felt the energy, and her childlike wonder in the process.

It was clear that she preferred feeling the energy over taking a snooze in the sun. I believe her practice helped her stay vibrantly alive until the end.

When I told her about Paramhansa Yogananda, she took to him right away. She kept his photograph in her bedroom, and she often told me how she had spoken to Yogananda the previous night. She described their relationship: "He embraces your life – it's a good feeling. It doesn't mean you're told what to do; with a Guru, you just go into the right sphere of being, and somehow he can enter your life in a real spiritual way, without it being a 'religious' way."

Age may not always bring us wisdom, but in Nancy's case it was so. These are some of the pearls she shared with me in her last days:

"Be open in life to see things not as you expect but in a different way, and accept that. Not that you're wrong, but just be open to seeing things in a different way. It's important to be flexible. That's why children need to be brought up to meet different people of all age groups, countries, and cultures, so that they can cope with life as an adult, where you need to be flexible."

"Giving to others makes your soul grow, doesn't it? Happiness is all there is — if you're happy, you give to life, and if you're not, you take from life."

"Don't talk about one friend to the other. Value their privacy, and respect it."

"We're all equal. All human beings are equal inside, so I never put myself above or below anyone."

"In order to progress in life, you need self-discipline and belief in yourself. You don't always know the right things about yourself – what you're about, who you are, where you are, and how you can touch others with the same feeling you find in yourself. It's self-knowledge, and that's a happiness, really – to find that part of yourself and be able to connect with it."

"I'm not afraid of death. It comes to us all, but if we are calm, then we can transition."

In the beginning, I thought that I would be helping this soul with her transition, but in the end it was she who helped me understand life. –**Victoria**, *UK*

NOTES | EPILOGUE

Title Page
1 Yogananda, *Whispers from Eternity*, No. 44.

Chapter One
1 AZ Quotes, https://www.azquotes.com/quote/569160.
2 Moody, Raymond, *Life After Life*, https://www.goodreads.com/book/show/28790866-life-after-life; and https://near-death.com/raymond-moody/, available to view on YouTube at https://www.youtube.com/watch?v=z56u4wMxNlg.
3 "Near-death experience," Wikipedia, https://en.wikipedia.org/wiki/Near-death_experience.
4 Graeber, Nalini, *Transitioning in Grace*, 37.
5 Yogananda, "Life After Death," *East-West*, November 1933.
6 Yogananda, "Mystic Meaning of Resurrection," *Inner Culture*, April 1934.
7 Kriyananda, "Immortality," *Affirmations for Self-Healing*, 116.
8 Yogananda, "Interpretation of the Bhagavad Gita," *Inner Culture*, June 1934.
9 Kriyananda, *Rays of the Same Light*, Week 23, 73.
10 Yogananda, "Second Coming of Christ," *Inner Culture*, November 1936

Chapter Two
1 Yogananda, "Mystic Meaning of Resurrection," *Inner Culture*, April 1934.
2 Kriyananda, *The Essence of the Bhagavad Gita*, Verse 7:30, 339.
3 Kriyananda, "The Final Exam," *Religion in the New Age*, 113-114. The full text of this article is in the online Appendices.

Chapter Three
1 Yogananda, "To Free the Soul from the Body," *Metaphysical Meditations*, 88.
2 Kriyananda, "How Old Are You?"
3 Kriyananda, *The Essence of the Bhagavad Gita*, Verse 7:30, 340.
4 Yogananda, "Life After Death," *East-West*, November 1933.
5 Kriyananda, *The Essence of the Bhagavad Gita*, Verse 7:30, 338-339.
6 Kriyananda, "The Final Exam," *Religion in the New Age*, 99.
7 Kriyananda, "Non-attachment," *Affirmations for Self-Healing*, 70.
8 Kriyananda, from a talk Ananda World Brotherhood Village on September 30, 1995.
9 Kriyananda, "The Final Exam," *Religion in the New Age*, 101.
10 Kriyananda, from the Memorial service for Paula Lucki.
11 Kriyananda, "The Final Exam," *Religion in the New Age*, 111.
12 Kriyananda, *The Art and Science of Raja Yoga*, 214.
13 Kriyananda, "The Final Exam," *Religion in the New Age*, 105-111.
14 Kriyananda, 118, 124.
15 Kriyananda, "Non-attachment," *Affirmations for Self-Healing*, 71.

Chapter Four
1 Kriyananda, *How To Be a True Channel*, 60.
2 Yogananda, *Autobiography of a Yogi*, 119.
3 Yogananda, *Advanced New Super Cosmic Science Course*, Lesson 5.
4 Kriyananda, "The Final Exam," *Religion in the New Age*, 112.
5 Kriyananda, 126.
6 Kriyananda, *The Essence of the Bhagavad Gita*, Verse 7:30, 340.

Poem "I will be Thine always"
Yogananda, *Whispers from Eternity*, No. 195.

I will be Thine always

I may go far, farther than the farthest star,
but I will be Thine always!
Devotees may come, devotees may go,
but I will be Thine always.

I may bound over the billows of many lives,
forlorn beneath the skies of loneliness,
but I will be Thine always.

The world may leave Thee,
while engrossed with Thy playthings,
but I will be Thine always.
Thou mayest take everything away
that Thou gavest me,
but I will be Thine always.

Death, disease, and trials may
riddle and rend me, and yet, while the
embers of memory shall flicker, look into
my dying eyes and they will mutely say,
"I will be Thine always."

My voice may become feeble,
fail and forsake me, and yet,
with the silent, bursting voice of my soul,
I will whisper to Thee,
"I am Thine always."

GLOSSARY

Ahankara. The ego, from the Sanskrit, meaning "I act."

Aum. The all-pervading sound emanating from Cosmic Vibration, also known as the Pranava, the Amen, and the Amin.

Babaji. Called "Mahavatar" ("Great Avatar") by Yogananda, Babaji reintroduced the ancient science of Kriya Yoga in the modern age. In *Autobiography of a Yogi*, Yogananda writes: "Babaji's mission in India has been to assist prophets in carrying out their special dispensation."

Bhagavad Gita. The major scripture of Hinduism, the teachings of Lord Krishna to his disciple Arjuna, delivered on the battlefield of Kurukshetra, as told in the epic story, Mahabharata.

Chakras. Plexuses or centers in the spine, from which energy flows out into the nervous system, and through that system into the body, sustaining and activating the various body parts.

Chitta. The feeling aspect of consciousness.

Christ Consciousness. Consciousness of Spirit as immanent in every unit of vibratory creation.

Cosmic Consciousness. Consciousness of Spirit transcending finite creation.

Day of Brahma. The aeons-long period of cosmic manifestation. At the dawn of a Day of Brahma, all creation, remanifested, emerges from a state of unmanifestation – the Night of Brahma.

Dharana. One-pointed concentration.

Dharma. Virtue, righteousness, right action.

Dhyana. Absorption in deep meditation.

Ego. The soul identified with and attached to the material body and the material creation.

Gunas. The three basic qualities that comprise the universe: *sattwa guna*, the elevating quality, that which most clearly suggests divinity; *rajas*, the activating element in nature; *tamas*, the darkening quality, that which obscures the underlying unity of Life.

Guru. The spiritual preceptor who introduces the disciple to God and guides his inner journey from the darkness of ignorance to the light of Self-realization.

Ida. One of the two parallel nerve channels in the astral spine, *ida* begins and ends on the left side of the spine. The energy passes upward through it and causes inhalation.

Karma. Action that is motivated by the ego, and which at some time, in one form or another, returns to the one who initiated it.

Krishna. One of the incarnations of Lord Vishnu, Krishna was a king at the time of the war of Kurukshetra, as told in the epic, Mahabharata. He is the guru of the warrior Arjuna, and his instructions to his disciple at the beginning of the war form the Bhagavad Gita, India's principle scripture.

Kriya Yoga. An ancient science developed in India for the use of all God-seekers. Its technique is referred to and praised by Krishna in the *Bhagavad Gita*, and by Patanjali in the *Yoga Sutras*. It consists of the careful, conscious circulation of energy around the spine in order to magnetize it and redirect the mental tendencies toward the brain.

Kundalini. Life Force which lies dormant at the base of the sushumna in the astral body. Spiritual enlightenment requires that this force be awakened and through specific practices caused to rise upward and reunite with Spirit at the *sahasrara chakra*, the thousand-petalled lotus.

Kutashta Chaitanya. The state of Christ Consciousness, or the awareness of the presence of Spirit in every atom of creation. Located at the Spiritual Eye, the Kutastha, is a reflection of the medulla oblongata: a field of dark blue light surrounded by a golden halo, in the center of which is a five-pointed star. The golden aureole represents the astral world; the blue field inside it, the causal world and the omnipresent Christ consciousness; the star in the center, the Spirit beyond creation.

Lahiri Mahasaya. Yogananda's "param guru," Lahiri Mahasaya was the guru of Swami Sri Yukteswar. He initiated thousands into the practice of Kriya Yoga.

Mahabharata. One of the two major Sanskrit epics of ancient India, the Mahabharata is both historical and allegorical. It contains an account of the war of Kurukshetra and also the Bhagavad Gita.

Maya. The instrument with which material manifestation was created, separating the creation from the Creator. It is a conscious force that perpetuates creation and keeps its inhabitants in ignorance of their true identity. Often referred to as Maha Shakti.

Medulla oblongata. The approximate physical location of the negative pole of the sixth chakra. It is the point at which cosmic energy enters the physical body.

Nadis. Subtle channels of life force in the astral body, comparable to the nervous system in the physical body.

Patanjali. An enlightened sage who described the science of Raja Yoga in his *Yoga Sutras*. He lived approximately in the second century BCE and is reputed to have written numerous spiritual treatises. Yogananda refers to him as an ancient Indian avatar, "the greatest of Hindu Yogis."

Pingala. One of the parallel nerve channels in the astral spine, pingala begins and ends on the right side of the spine. Energy passing downward through it causes exhalation.

Prana. Life force as it manifests in the human body and in all living creatures.

Pranayama. Control of the senses through withdrawal of energy.

Sanatan Dharma. The "Eternal Religion." The immutable truths that form the basis of religious and spiritual theologies, and moral and ethical codes.

Satchidananda. The description of the state preceding and beyond manifestation by India's great philosopher-saint, Swami Adi Shankaracharya: *Ever-existing, ever-conscious, ever-new Bliss.*

Swami Sri Yukteswar. Yogananda's guru, and a direct disciple of Lahiri Mahasaya, often mentioned in *Autobiography of a Yogi.*

Samadhi. Divine ecstasy. Union of the individual soul with the infinite Spirit.

Samskaras. Past tendencies. The traces of past karmas, both positive and negative, that carry over from life to life.

Spiritual Eye. The point midway between the eyebrows, within the frontal lobe of the brain, is described as the seat of the intellect, of willpower, and—in superconsciousness—of ecstasy and spiritual vision.

Sushumna. The astral spine, through which kundalini, having been magnetized to flow upward, begins its slow ascent toward enlightenment.

Vasana. A tendency or talent from past incarnations that influences current behavior.

Vedas. The four ancient scriptural texts of *Sanatan Dharma*: Rigveda, Samaveda, Yajurveda, and Atharvaveda.

Vritti. Eddies or whirlpools of energy that accompany ego-motivated thoughts and actions.

Yugas. Ages or cycles of time. The four ages are Kali Yuga (the age dark with ignorance), Dwapara Yuga (an age of energy), Treta Yuga (an age of awareness of the power of mind), and Satya Yuga, also called Krita (an age of high spiritual awareness).

Yamas and Niyamas. Described by Patanjali in his Yoga Sutras, the first two branches of the soul's journey to enlightenment, which consist of guidelines for conserving vital energy and directing it into constructive attitudes and actions.

BIBLIOGRAPHY

Becker, Robert. *The Body Electric: Electromagnetism and The Foundation of Life*. New York: William Morrow Paperbacks, 1998.

Clarity Magazine. Ananda Church of Self-Realization, Nevada City, California. Winter 2011.

Cornell, Joseph Bharat. *Deep Nature Play: A Guide to Wholeness, Aliveness, Creativity, and Inspired Learning*. Nevada City, CA, Crystal Clarity Publishers, 2018.

Cornell, Joseph Bharat. *Flow Learning: Opening Heart and Spirit Through Nature*, Nevada City, CA, Crystal Clarity Publishers, 2022

East-West. Self-Realization Fellowship. Monthly and bimonthly issues, November/December 1925–March 1934.

Graeber, Nalini. *Transitioning in Grace: A Yogi's Approach to Death and Dying*. Nevada City, CA: Crystal Clarity Publishers, 2019.

Inner Culture. Self-Realization Fellowship. Monthly issues, April 1934–December 1941.

Kriyananda, Swami. See also Walters, J. Donald.

Affirmations for Self-Healing. Nevada City, CA: Crystal Clarity Publishers, 2005.

Ananda Yoga for Higher Awareness. Nevada City, CA: Crystal Clarity Publishers, 2004.

Art as a Hidden Message. Nevada City, CA: Crystal Clarity Publishers, 1997.

"Astral Ascension Ceremony." Online Appendix.

Awaken to Superconsciousness. Nevada City, CA: Crystal Clarity Publishers, 2000.

"Baptism Ceremony." Online Appendix.

Cities of Light: A New Vision for the Future. Gurgaon, India: Ananda Sangha Publications, 2009.

Conversations with Yogananda. Nevada City, CA: Crystal Clarity Publishers, 2003.

Eastern Thoughts, Western Thoughts. Nevada City, CA: Crystal Clarity Publishers, 1975.

Education for Life. Gurgaon, India: Ananda Sangha Publications, 2006.

"A Festival of Light." Online Appendix.

God Is for Everyone. Nevada City, CA: Crystal Clarity Publishers, 2003.

"Grace vs. Self-Effort." Speaking Tree, *Hindustan Times*, January 29, 2004. https://www.hindustantimes.com/india/grace-vs-self-effort/story-CiQ5zfaJykdwz8uOKUeprN.html

Guidelines for Conduct of Members of the Ananda Sevaka Order. Nocera Umbra, Italy: Ananda Sangha Publications, 2020.

A Handbook on Discipleship. Nevada City, CA: Crystal Clarity Publishers, 2010.

The Hindu Way of Awakening: Its Revelation, Its Symbols. Nevada City, CA: Crystal Clarity Publishers, 1998.

Hope for a Better World! Nevada City, CA: Crystal Clarity Publishers, 2002.

"How Old Are You?" Speaking Tree, *Times of India*, date unknown.

"How Well Do You Get Along with Others?" *Clarity Magazine*, Ananda Church of Self-Realization, Winter 2011.

In Divine Friendship: Letters of Counsel and Reflection. Nevada City, CA: Crystal Clarity Publishers, 2008.

Intuition for Starters. Edited by Devi Novak. Nevada City, CA: Crystal Clarity Publishers, 2002.

Keys to the Bhagavad Gita. Nevada City, CA: Crystal Clarity Publishers, 1979.

"Lahiri Mahasaya's Birthday." Talk at Ananda Village, California, September 30, 1995.

Letters to Truth Seekers. Nevada City, CA: Crystal Clarity Publishers, 1973.

The Light of Superconsciousness. Edited by Devi Novak. Nevada City, CA: Crystal Clarity Publishers, 1999.

Living Wisely, Living Well. Nevada City, CA: Crystal Clarity Publishers, 2010.

Material Success Through Yoga Principles. Nevada City, CA: Crystal Clarity Publishers, 2005.

Meditation for Starters. Nevada City, CA: Crystal Clarity Publishers, 1996.

Money Magnetism: How to Attract What You Need, When You Need It. Nevada City, CA: Crystal Clarity Publishers, 1992.

The New Path: My Life with Paramhansa Yogananda. Nevada City, CA: Crystal Clarity Publishers, 2009.

Out of the Labyrinth. Nevada City, CA: Crystal Clarity Publishers, 2001.

A Place Called Ananda. Nevada City, CA: Crystal Clarity Publishers, 1996.

The Promise of Immortality. Nevada City, CA: Crystal Clarity Publishers, 2001.

"Radiant Health and Well-Being." YouTube video, Ananda Sangha Worldwide. https://www.youtube.com/watch?v=jRx_U2JS8HE

Rays of the One Light. Nevada City, CA: Crystal Clarity Publishers, 2007.

Rays of the Same Light. Nevada City, CA: Crystal Clarity Publishers, 1988.

Religion in the New Age. Gurgaon, India: Ananda Sangha Publications, 2010.

A Renunciate Order for the New Age. Nevada City, CA: Crystal Clarity Publishers, 2010.

The Road Ahead. Nevada City, California: Ananda Publications, 1973.

The Road Ahead. Nevada City, CA: Crystal Clarity Publishers, 1974.

Sadhu, Beware! A New Approach to Renunciation. Gurgaon, India: Ananda Sangha Publications, 2005.

"The Science of the Future." Talk at Unity in Yoga Conference, May 27, 1995.

Self-Expansion Through Marriage. Nevada City, CA: Crystal Clarity Publishers, 2012.

Space, Light, and Harmony: The Story of Crystal Hermitage. Nevada City, CA: Crystal Clarity Publishers, 2005.

Twenty-Six Keys to Living with Greater Awareness. Nevada City, CA: Crystal Clarity Publishers, 1989.

Visits to Saints of India, Nevada City, CA: Crystal Clarity Publishers, February 2019.

"Wedding Ceremony." Online Appendix.

"Whisper to God." Speaking Tree, *Times of India*, date unknown.

"You Don't Have to Be Sick." YouTube video, Ananda Sangha Worldwide. https://www.youtube.com/watch?v=V9ApjBHI29U&abchannel=AnandaSanghaWorldwide

Your Sun Sign as a Spiritual Guide. Nevada City, CA: Crystal Clarity Publishers, 2013.

Yours—the Universe! Nevada City, CA: Hansa Publications, 1967.

Laubach, Frank. *Letters by a Modern Mystic.* London, United Kingdom: SPCK Publishing, 1937.

Sivananda, Swami. *Japa Yoga.* Rishikesh: The Sivananda Publication League, 1942.

Walters, J. Donald (a.k.a. Swami Kriyananda). *How to Be a Channel.* Nevada City, CA: Crystal Clarity Publishers, 1987.

Secrets of Friendship. Nevada City, CA: Crystal Clarity Publishers, 1992.

Secrets of Health and Healing. Nevada City, CA: Crystal Clarity Publishers, 2018.

Secrets of Success and Leadership. Nevada City, CA: Crystal Clarity Publishers, 2017.

Yogananda, Paramhansa. *The Attributes of Success.* Los Angeles, CA: Self-Realization Fellowship, 1944.

Autobiography of a Yogi. Gurgaon, India: Ananda Sangha Publications, 2004. Reprint of the 1946 first printing, published by The Philosophical Library, Inc., New York, New York.

The Bhagavad Gita According to Paramhansa Yogananda. Edited by Swami Kriyananda. Nevada City, CA: Crystal Clarity Publishers, 2008.

The Essence of the Bhagavad Gita, Explained by Paramhansa Yogananda, As Remembered by His Disciple Swami Kriyananda. Nevada City, CA: Crystal Clarity Publishers, 2006.

The Essence of Self-Realization: The Wisdom of Paramhansa Yogananda, Recorded, compiled, and edited by his disciple Swami Kriyananda. Nevada City, CA: Crystal Clarity Publishers, 1990.

How to Love and Be Loved. Nevada City, CA: Crystal Clarity Publishers, 2007.

The Rubaiyat of Omar Khayyam Explained. Edited, with occasional comments, by J. Donald Walters. Nevada City, CA: Crystal Clarity Publishers, 1994.

"Spiritual Interpretation of the Bhagavad Gita." *Inner Culture,* August 1938–December 1941.

Whispers from Eternity. Edited by Swami Kriyananda. Nevada City, CA: Crystal Clarity Publishers, 2008.

Yogananda, Swami. "Advanced Course on Practical Metaphysics, 1926." Lessons 1-12. Los Angeles, CA: Self-Realization Fellowship, 1926.

"Advanced Super Cosmic Science Course, 1934." Lessons 1-6. Los Angeles, CA: Self-Realization Fellowship, 1934.

Cosmic Chants. Los Angeles, CA: Self-Realization Fellowship, 1938.

"Interpretation of the Bhagavad Gita." *East-West,* April 1932–March 1934.

"Interpretation of the Bhagavad Gita." *Inner Culture,* April 1934–February 1936.

Metaphysical Meditations. Los Angeles, CA: Self-Realization Fellowship, 1932.

"New Super Cosmic Science Course, 1934." Lessons 1-6. Los Angeles, CA: Self-Realization Fellowship, 1934.

Praecepta Lessons, Volumes 1-5. Los Angeles, CA: Self-Realization Fellowship, 1934–1938.

Psychological Chart. Los Angeles, CA: Self-Realization Fellowship, 1925.

Scientific Healing Affirmations. Los Angeles, CA: Self-Realization Fellowship, 1924.

Songs of the Soul. Los Angeles, CA: Self-Realization Fellowship, 1923.

"Spiritual Interpretation of the Bhagavad Gita." *Inner Culture,* May 1937–July 1938.

"Super Advanced Course No. 1, 1930." Lessons 1-12. Los Angeles, CA: Self-Realization Fellowship, 1930.

"Yogoda Course, 1925." Lessons 1-12. Los Angeles, CA: Self-Realization Fellowship, 1925.

Yogoda, Tissue-Will System of Body and Mind Perfection. Boston, MA: Sat-Sanga, 1923.

Yogoda, Tissue-Will System of Body and Mind Perfection. Boston, MA: Sat-Sanga, 1925.

PHOTO & ILLUSTRATIONS

Cover Background: KingKahn-Internet2011, Freepik
p. 10: Ananda Image Bank
p. 11 : Ananda Image Bank
p. 12: Storyset, Freepik
p. 14: Ananda Image Bank
p. 17: Timo Stern, Unsplash
p. 20 : Freepik
p. 23: Tejindra Tully
p. 26: RAStudio, Freepik
p. 31: Ruby Stoppe
p. 32: Ananda Image Bank
p. 39 : JyotishArt.com
p. 42: Ananda Image Bank
p. 44: Freepik
p. 48: V.Ivash, Freepik
p. 53: User17938247, Freepik
p. 55: BiZkettE1, Freepik
p. 59: Aryavan Bryan McSweeney
p. 60: Freepik
p. 65: Swami Kriyananda
p. 70: jcomp, Freepik
p. 77: elena_kalinicheva, Freepik
p. 89: bluext72, Freepik
p. 106: GarryKillian, Freepik
p. 111: Freepik
p. 113: Sirilakshmi.com
p. 116: IconicBestiary, Freepik
p. 124: Santima.Studio, Freepik
p. 131: ann_isme, Freepik
p. 132: Mamboh, Freepik
p. 139: rawpixel.com, Freepik
p. 142: WayHomeStudio, Freepik
p. 146: macrovector, Freepik
p. 151: Ananda Image Bank
p. 152: Photoangel, Freepik
p. 154: Pookpiik, Freepik
p. 160: Ananda Image Bank
p. 163: catalyststuff, Freepik
p. 168: Freepik
p. 169: Ananda Image Bank
p. 173: Shantidev, meditationart.eu
p. 176: Vector Stock
p. 178: Freepik
p. 179: IrynaShek, Freepik
p. 182: madaniaart, Freepik
p. 186: TanyaBosyk Freepik
p. 187: pikisuperstar, Freepik
p. 189: dooder, Freepik
p. 192: Freepik
p. 195: Ananda Image Bank
p. 198: syarifahbrit, Freepik
p. 201: Freepik
p. 203: Volha, Freepik
p. 206: Freepik
p. 209: Vecstock, Freepik
p. 210: Public Domain
p. 213: Gpointstudio, Freepik
p. 215: Ananda Image Bank
p. 219: Freepik
p. 225: IsometricWorld, Freepik
p. 226: onetime, Freepik
p. 227: Midjourney 5.1, Freepik

p. 228: Ananda Image Bank
p. 229: Public Domain, ClipArt
p. 230: Helen Stratton, Public Domain
p. 232: Ananda Image Bank
p. 237: Andrea Roach
p. 238: Ananda Image Bank
p. 243: Ananda Image Bank
p. 246: Public Domain
p. 250: Wirestock, Freepik
p. 253: Public Domain
p. 254: Swami Kriyananda
p. 255: Ananda Image Bank
p. 257: Ananda Edizioni
p. 258: katemangostar, Freepik
p. 262: Storyset, Freepik
p. 263: kjpargeter, Freepik
p. 265: Kuldeep Gangwani
p. 268: Public Domain
p. 270: Swami Kriyananda
p. 271: Freepik
p. 273: Swami Kriyananda
p. 275: Public Domain
p. 276: Nikkized, 123rf.com
p. 277: valeria_aksakova, Freepik
p. 278: Racool_Studio, Freepik
p. 279: Freepik
p. 280: Swami Kriyananda
p. 281: Swami Kriyananda
p. 282: Freepik
p. 284: Ananda Image Bank
p. 285: Tejindra Tully
p. 287: Freepik
p. 289: ozgurdonmaz, iStock Photo
p. 291: Ekrem Osmanoglu, Unsplash
p. 293: Philip Fruytiers, Public Domain
p. 296: Vinish K Sahini, Flikr
p. 300: Fly20061, Creative Commons
p. 302: embracingtheworld.org
p. 305: Sonika Agarwal, Unsplash
p. 306: Ananda Image Bank
p. 309: Pixabay
p. 310: Prabhu Ravichandran, Unsplash
p. 314: Tejindra Tully
p. 315: Mateus Campos Felipe, Unsplash
p. 317: Aryavan Bryan McSweeney
p. 318: Jonathan Borba, Unsplash
p. 321: Eileen Lee, Aura Aura
p. 324: Nainizul, Freepik
p. 325: allahfoto, Freepik
p. 328: Federcap, Freepik
p. 333: Tejindra Tully
p. 336: Public Domain
p. 343: Ananda Image Bank
p. 352: Savvas Kalimeris, Unsplash
p. 356: Gustave Doré, Public Domain
p. 361: Freepik
p. 372: jcomp, Freepik
p. 374: Ananda Image Bank
p. 377, 378, 380, 381: Freepik
p. 384: Yanalya, Freepik
p. 398, 399: Ananda Image Bank
p. 400: Andrea Roach
p. 401: photopheeasia, Freepik

PARAMHANSA YOGANANDA

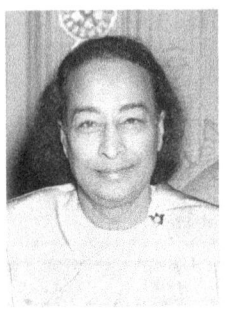

Known worldwide as the author of *Autobiography of a Yogi*, and revered as India's "spiritual ambassador to the West," Paramhansa Yogananda brought the ancient teachings of *Sanatan Dharma* into the modern age as the "Science of Self-realization."

He lived in the United States from 1920 until his passing in 1952. From his original center in Boston, he travelled widely across the country, giving lectures in most of the major cities. So popular were his lectures that as many as 5000 people attended them in some of America's largest auditoriums.

Unique among spiritual masters who possess the gift of healing, Yogananda rarely displayed his spiritual powers, preferring instead to help others learn to become their own healers.

During his early years in America, he often focused his lectures on healing-related topics, such as "Scientific Spiritual Healing," and "Magnetic Healing." His written lessons gave practical advice on such topics as "The Divine Magnetic Diet," "How to Convert the Hands into Healing Batteries of Life Force," and "Amazing Health Recipes for Healing and Prolonging Life." As a regular feature of his monthly magazines, he wrote "Health, Intellectual and Spiritual Recipes," practical advice for creating harmony between body, mind, and soul.

One of his earliest and most popular books, *Scientific Healing Affirmations*, remains a pillar of his teachings.

Through his writings and the exemplary lives of those who live and teach his methods, Yogananda continues to influence and uplift people all over the world, by showing them the way to a happier, healthier, and more deeply fulfilling life.

> *"As a bright light shining in the midst of darkness, so was Yogananda's presence in this world. Such a great soul comes on earth only rarely, when there is a real need among men."*
>
> – HIS HOLINESS THE SHANKARACHARYA *of* KANCHIPURAM –

SWAMI KRIYANANDA

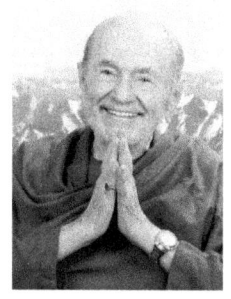

Directly after reading *Autobiography of a Yogi*, young Donald Walters (soon to become Swami Kriyananda) traveled from New York City to Los Angeles to meet the author, Paramhansa Yogananda. Yogananda accepted him as a disciple at their first meeting. For the next three and a half years Kriyananda was trained by Yogananda in the two missions the master gave him: to write and to lecture.

To prepare him for these responsibilities, Yogananda had Kriyananda study all of his writings, including his books, correspondence lessons, and his commentaries on the Bhagavad Gita and the Christian Bible. Yogananda appointed him as head of the monks, as a main speaker at his churches, and conferred on him the authority to give initiation into Kriya Yoga.

Kriyananda was present when Yogananda spoke passionately about the importance of establishing "world brotherhood colonies," based on principles of "simple living and high thinking." He silently vowed to make Yogananda's vision a reality, and in 1969 he founded the first such community, the Ananda World Brotherhood Village in northern California, to be followed years later by sister communities in America, Italy, and India.

Faithful to his Guru's wishes, Kriyananda gave thousands of lectures, and published more than 140 books teaching people everywhere how they can integrate their daily lives with spiritual ideals.

From 2003 until his passing in 2013, Kriyananda lived and taught in India. His daily talks on Indian television were viewed by millions. They include "A Way to Awakening" based on his book *Conversations with Yogananda*, and a second series of talks based on Yogananda's commentaries on the Bhagavad Gita.

> "Not only did Kriyananda walk in the footsteps of an enlightened master, it [is] obvious that he himself became an embodiment of Yogananda's teachings."
> – MICHAEL BERNARD BECKWITH, author, *Spiritual Liberation* –

ABOUT THE AUTHOR

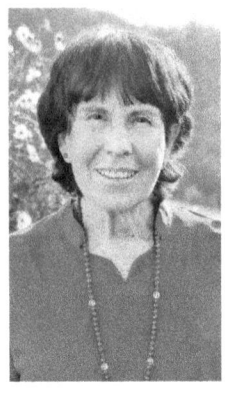

SHIVANI LUCKI left her legal studies and a promising career in Washington, D.C. when she realized her quest for truth and justice would not be fulfilled in the classroom or courtroom. Her gypsy journey across the United States eventually led to California where she began a serious practice of yoga and meditation with Swami Kriyananda, who introduced her to the idea of intentional communities through his book, *Cooperative Communities — How to Start Them and Why*.

With a small backpack, a sleeping bag, and a heart full of hope, she arrived on June 22, 1969, at the fledgling Ananda community. She was twenty-four years old. Recognition was instantaneous: This was the way of life she had long been seeking. She resolved to dedicate her life to Yogananda's ideal of "World Brotherhood Colonies," for "plain living and high thinking."

Her special passion has always been the self-healing techniques of Yogananda, taking as her unique mission to find and share these mostly out of print or never published teachings. One day she hoped to found an institute for healing based on Yogananda's methods.

Shivani has earned a worldwide reputation as one of the foremost teachers of meditation, specifically Kriya Yoga, an ancient method Yogananda re-introduced to the world in modern times. She helped establish two Ananda communities—one in California, and one near Assisi, Italy—and the Yogananda Academy of Europe. Fulfilling her dream, she founded the Life Therapy School for Self-Healing. Since 1985 she and her husband have lived in the Ananda Assisi community.

"Shivani possesses a luminosity that disperses all self-doubt and fear. To know her is to exchange endless ego traps for clarity, joy, and inner security."

—*Jagadish*, *Thailand*

⁓ *In Appreciation* ⁓

*E*very creative endeavor is a journey. We may believe we know where we are headed and how to get there – but it doesn't always work out that way. Inspiration is never static, and the creative process, like life itself, develops through many stages.

While my goal was crystal clear for me at the outset – to present the full scope, depth, and practical healing power of Paramhansa Yogananda's techniques for achieving physical vitality, mental peace, and spiritual realization – the path to the goal became a profound process or personal discovery. Discoveries came, of course, through meditating on the principles and practicing the techniques, and through the many people who kindly commented on the text, and shared their personal stories of healing. As the book grew from infancy to adulthood, it gradually discovered its destiny as a trilogy instead of a single encyclopedic tome.

I have acknowledged the true authors of these books in the Dedication. Here, I add my deep appreciation to **Nandini Cerri**, director of Yogananda Edizioni in Italy, who for years encouraged me to write, and supported me at every step of the way.

Many friends, teachers, and healthcare practitioners read parts of the book, offering their thoughtful insights and suggestions. My thanks to them all, especially to: **Jagadish Photikie, Jennifer Hansa Black, Hana Mukti Božanin, Dr. Donatella Caramia, Dr. Abhilash Kumar, Latha Gupta, Nayaswami Lakshman, David Sanjaya Connolly**, and **Prisha Kirby**.

Of exceptional note, I offer my deepest appreciation to my Aquarian brothers: **Rambhakta Beinhorn**, who sensitively and expertly edited the books; and **Tejindra Scott Tully**, whose inspired design for the covers and text makes the book a pleasure to read and a brilliant examplar of graphic artistry.

Let me not forget my husband, **Arjuna Lucki**, who endured long absences while I was sequestered in my writing hideaway; and my many friends and colleagues who, during my absence from usual duties, took the helm and taught my classes with masterful skill.

May I presume to thank you as well, **dear reader**, for sharing the inspiration you garner from these pages with those in need of healing?

Together may we bring Light and Healing to the world!

HEALTHY LIVING with CRYSTAL CLARITY

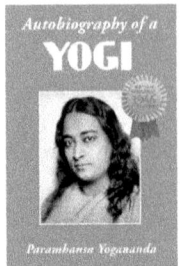

Autobiography of a Yogi
Paramhansa Yogananda

Autobiography of a Yogi is one of the world's most acclaimed spiritual classics, with millions of copies sold. Named one of the Best 100 Spiritual Books of the twentieth century, this book helped launch and continues to inspire a spiritual awakening throughout the Western world.

Yogananda was the first yoga master of India whose mission brought him to settle and teach in the West. His firsthand account of his life experiences in India includes childhood revelations, stories of his visits to saints and masters, and long-secret teachings of yoga and Self-realization that he first made available to the Western reader.

This reprint of the original 1946 edition is free from textual changes made after Yogananda's passing in 1952. This updated edition includes bonus materials: the last chapter that Yogananda wrote in 1951, also without posthumous changes, the eulogy Yogananda wrote for Gandhi, and a new foreword and afterword by Swami Kriyananda, one of Yogananda's close, direct disciples.

Also available in Spanish and Hindi from Crystal Clarity Publishers.

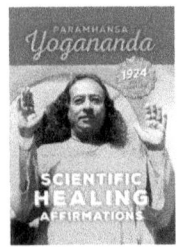

Scientific Healing Affirmations
Paramhansa Yogananda

Yogananda's 1924 classic, reprinted here, is a pioneering work in the fields of self-healing and self-transformation. He explains that words are crystallized thoughts and have life-changing power when spoken with conviction, concentration, willpower, and feeling. Yogananda offers far more than mere suggestions for achieving positive attitudes. He shows how to impregnate words with spiritual force to shift habitual thought patterns of the mind and create a new personal reality.

Added to this text are over fifty of Yogananda's well-loved "Short Affirmations," taken from issues of East-West and Inner Culture magazines from 1932 to 1942. This little book will be a treasured companion on the road to realizing your highest, divine potential.

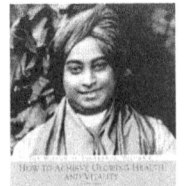

How to Achieve Glowing Health and Vitality
THE WISDOM OF YOGANANDA SERIES, VOLUME 6
Paramhansa Yogananda

Yogananda explains principles that promote physical health and overall well-being, mental clarity, and inspiration in one's spiritual life. He offers practical, wide-ranging, and fascinating suggestions on having more energy and living a radiantly healthy life. Readers will discover the priceless Energization Exercises for rejuvenating the body and mind, the fine art of conscious relaxation, and helpful diet tips for health and beauty.

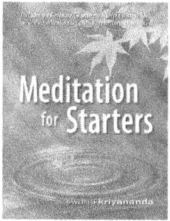

Meditation for Starters
Swami Kriyananda

Have you wanted to learn to meditate, but just never got around to it? Or tried "sitting in the silence" only to find your mind wandering? Do you wish you had a meditation guidebook that explained clearly what to do, step-by-step? If so, *Meditation for Starters* is for you.

Learn meditation from a true expert, with more than 60 years of experience. Swami Kriyananda has helped tens of thousands of people successfully start a regular meditation routine.

This award-winning book provides everything you need to begin a meditation practice. Easy-to-follow instructions teach you how to relax the body, focus your attention, and interiorize your mind. With only a little practice you will experience the enhanced awareness and joyful calmness that was missing in your life.

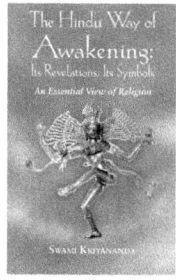

The Hindu Way of Awakening
ITS REVELATION, ITS SYMBOLS:
AN ESSENTIAL VIEW OF RELIGION
Swami Kriyananda

Hinduism, as it comes across in this book, is a robust, joyful religion, amazingly in step with the most advanced thinking of modern times, in love with life, deeply human as well as humane, delightfully aware of your personal life's needs, for the teaching in this book is no abstraction: It is down-to-earth and pressingly immediate.

This book brings order to the seeming chaos of the symbols and imagery in Hinduism and clearly communicates the underlying teachings from which these symbols arise - truths inherent in all religions, and their essential purpose - the direct inner experience of God.

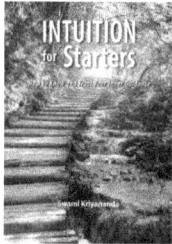

Intuition for Starters
HOW TO KNOW & TRUST YOUR INNER GUIDANCE
Swami Kriyananda

Is there a way to know how to make the best choice? Yes! through developing our faculty of intuition.

Often thought of as something vague and undefinable, intuition is the ability to perceive truth directly not by reason, logic, or analysis, but by simply knowing from within.

This book explains how within each of us lies the ability to perceive the answers we need and shows how to access the powerful stream of creative energy which lies beneath the surface of our conscious mind: the superconscious.

Step-by-step exercises, advice, and guidance reveal intuition to be an ally and an accessible fountain of wisdom to be found within each of us.

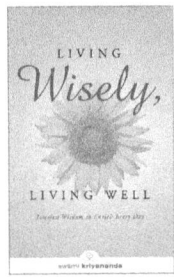

Living Wisely, Living Well
Swami Kriyananda
Winner of the 2011 International Book Award for Self-Help: Motivational Book of the Year.

Want to transform yourself? This book contains 366 practical ways to improve your life—a thought for each day of the year. Each saying is warm with wisdom, alive with positive expectation, and provides simple actions that bring profound results.

See life with new eyes. Discover hundreds of techniques for self-improvement. This distillation of a lifetime of wisdom will wake you up to dynamic inner growth. So take time off from the "same old you." Read this book, put into practice what it teaches, and in a year's time you won't recognize yourself.

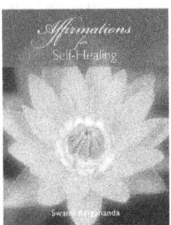

Affirmtions for Self-Healing
Swami Kriyananda

This inspirational book is the ultimate self-help manual, a powerful tool for personal transformation. These 52 affirmations and prayers—one for each week of the year—will help you strengthen positive qualities in yourself such as good health, willpower, forgiveness, security, happiness, and many others. Affirmation is a proven method of influencing the subconscious mind and replacing those negative thoughts with positive statements of well-being. Each of the affirmations in this book reaches the subconscious in a language it can hear and understand. Where other methods fail, these affirmations are sure to succeed.

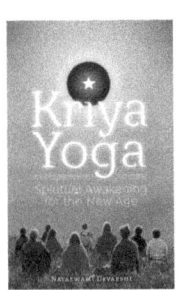

Kriya Yoga
SPIRITUAL AWAKENING FOR THE NEW AGE
Nayaswami Devarshi

Both instructive and inspiring, this book shows the aspiring devotee both how and why to take up the lifelong practice of Kriya Yoga. Learn the pitfalls to look out for along the way, and how to reach ultimate success on your journey to Self-realization.

Simultaneously, this book is a roadmap for those already practicing Kriya Yogi. Through real-life stories from longtime Kriyabans, learn the attitudes and practices that help or hinder your progress on the spiritual path.

"I wasn't sent to the West by Christ and the great masters of India to dogmatize you with a new theology," Yogananda often told his audiences. "I want to help you toward the attainment of actual experience of Him, through your daily practice of Kriya Yoga."

He added, "The time for knowing God has come!"

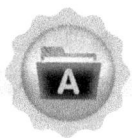

APPENDICES
A treasure trove of inspiration awaits you!

The online Appendices for this volume are reserved just for you. Scan the QR code or enter the internet address below, and discover many additional resources to help deepen your understanding on your path to self-healing and Self-realization.

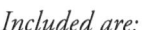
Included are:

- *Four original lessons by Paramhansa Yogananda*
- *A Wedding Ceremony*
- *Articles by Yogananda and Kriyananda on material and spiritual success*
- *Guidelines for helping those who are gravely ill, and preparing for our own transition*
- *Twenty musical compositions by Swami Kriyananda*

www.healinglifeforces.com/volume-3/

HEALING LIFE FORCE COMMUNITY
Sign up today and you will receive:

- *Healing Tips videos by the author*
- *Live sessions with the author*
- *Blogs on healing techniques in daily life*
- *Insights, invitations and much more.*

Scan the QR code or enter this internet address to join!
www.healinglifeforces.com

Your HEALING JOURNEY with PARAMHANSA YOGANANDA continues!

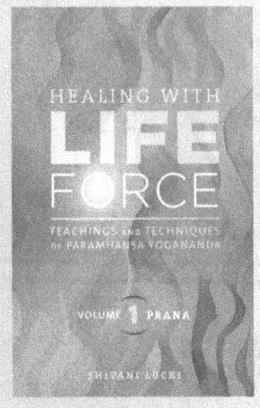

HEALING WITH LIFE FORCE
VOLUME ONE

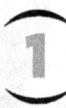

PRANA

Volume One, *Prana*, takes us back to the very beginning, when Life Force becomes the power that fashions creation. Yogananda shows us how to harness that power and use it to infuse our bodies with vitality. That force also gives rise to the eternal struggle between the soul and the ego, the root cause of all disease. Through the pages and practices of this book, you will learn how to reconcile these two protagonists through techniques of meditation; how to regenerate the cells and organs of your body with **Yogananda's Energization Exercises**; and how to nourish yourself and keep your body free from impurities with his dietary and detox recipes. A fascinating section in this volume presents Yogananda's techniques for utilizing the sun's power for self-healing.

"All methods of healing are really indirect ways of rousing the life energy, which is the real and direct healer of all diseases."
—YOGANANDA

"The greater the will, the greater the flow of energy."

"Remember it. Emblazon it in your mind. Repeat it to yourself several times a day. This single truth can revolutionize your life."
—KRIYANANDA

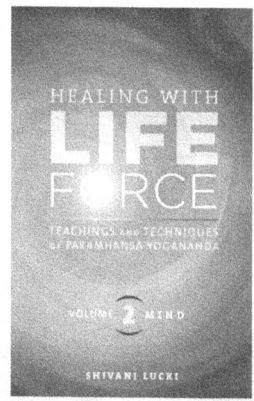

Healing with Life Force
Volume Two

2
Mind

Our mind is the most important self-healing instrument that we possess – once we learn to be its master. In Volume Two you will be introduced to its multi-dimensional capacities that can be developed and used to prevent illness and reverse symptoms of disease.

Superpowers of the Conscious Mind:
Concentration, willpower, visualization

Superpowers of the Subconscious Mind:
Memory and Habit development

Superpowers of the Superconscious Mind:
Intuition

Using these superpowers, you will learn to:

Eradicate unhealthy habit grooves and establish good ones

Create a positive mental outlook with the use of scientific healing affirmations

Attract divine grace and receive inner guidance for aspects of your life.

Channel healing life force to others

> "All disease has its roots in the mind.
> If the mind can produce ill health,
> it can also produce good health."
> —Yogananda

Available at CrystalClarity.com in October, 2024

nce